Prehospital Medicine
The Art of On-Line Medical Command

Prehospital

Medicine

The Art of On-Line Medical Command

Editors

Paul M. Paris, MD, FACEP

Ronald N. Roth, MD, FACEP

Vincent P. Verdile, MD, FACEP

A JEMS BOOK

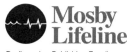

Mosby
Lifeline

Dedicated to Publishing Excellence

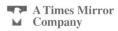

A Times Mirror
Company

A JEMS BOOK

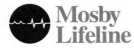
Mosby
Lifeline

Dedicated to Publishing Excellence

A Times Mirror
Company

Vice President and Publisher:	David Dusthimer
Editor-In-Chief:	Claire Merrick
Acquisitions Editor:	Rina Steinhauer
Developmental Editor:	Melissa Blair
Project Manager:	Chris Baumle
Project Supervisor:	Shannon Canty
Design Manager:	Nancy McDonald
Designer:	Ellen C. Dawson
Cover Photography:	Tony Stone Images, Inc.
Manufacturing Supervisor:	Andrew Christensen

Printed in the United States of America
Composition by Accu-Color, Inc.
Printing/binding by R.R. Donnelley

Mosby-Year Book, Inc.
11830 Westline Industrial Drive
St. Louis, Missouri 63146

ISBN 0-8151-6849-7

96 97 98 99 00 / 9 8 7 6 5 4 3 2 1

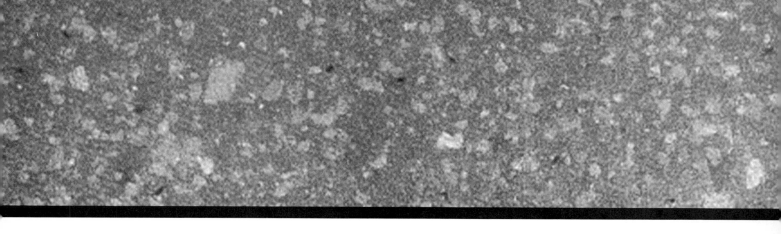

Dedication

Paul M. Paris

To the City of Pittsburgh Paramedics, who have provided 20 years of exemplary care to the citizens of Pittsburgh and 15 years of field education to the residents and faculty of the University of Pittsburgh Affiliated Residency in Emergency Medicine.

Vincent P. Verdile

Without the support and understanding of my wife Lou-Ann, the work ethic given me by my parents, and the education garnered from Paul M Paris, M.D. and the men and women of Pittsburgh EMS this book could never have been accomplished.

Ronald N. Roth

This book is dedicated to my family, Sheila and Michael, for their love and support during this and the many other "projects" over the years. A special thanks to the professional paramedics of Pittsburgh EMS, my friends and colleagues since 1978.

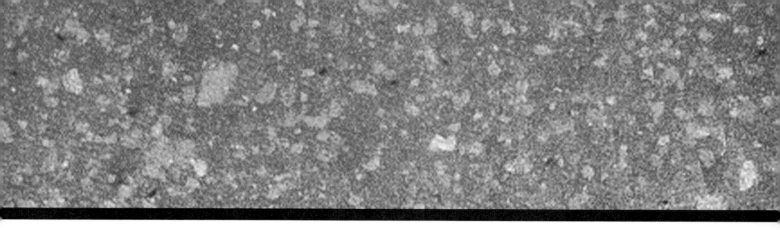

Contributing Authors

James G. Adams, MD, FACEP
Director of Clinical Operations
Department of Emergency Medicine
Brigham & Womens Hospital
Harvard Medical School
Boston, MA

Hector M. Alonso-Serra, MD
EMS Fellow
Department of Emergency Medicine
University of Pittsburgh School of Medicine
Pittsburgh, PA

William J. Angelos, MD, FACEP
Director, Emergency Department
Presbyterian University Hospital
Assistant Professor of Emergency Medicine
University of Pittsburgh School of Medicine
Pittsburgh, PA

Daniel J. Cobaugh, PHARM D
Director, Finger Lakes Poison Control Center
University of Rochester
Rochester, NY

Adrian D'Amico, MD, FACEP
Director of Emergency Medicine
Citizens General Hospital
Pittsburgh, PA

Eric Davis, MD, FACEP
Regional EMS Medical Director
Monroe-Livingston County
Associate Professor of Emergency Medicine
Department of Emergency Medicine
University of Rochester
Rochester, NY

Theodore R. Delbridge, MD, MPH, FACEP
Assistant Professor of Emergency Medicine
EMS Fellowship Director
Department of Emergency Medicine
University of Pittsburgh School of Medicine
Associate Medical Director
City of Pittsburgh, Bureau of EMS
Pittsburgh, PA

Susan M. Dunmire, MD, FACEP
Assistant Professor of Emergency Medicine
Department of Emergency Medicine
University of Pittsburgh School of Medicine
Pittsburgh, PA

Thomas D. Fowlkes, MD
Emergency Physician
Chief Medical Director
Priority EMS
Memphis, TN

Susan M. Fuchs, MD, FAAP
Associate Professor of Emergency Medicine
Department of Emergency Medicine
University of Pittsburgh School of Medicine
Pittsburgh, PA

Carl W. Gossett, MD, FACEP
Vice Chairman
Residency Director
Assistant Professor
Department of Emergency Medicine
Scott & White
Temple, TX

A.J. Heightman, MPA, EMT-P
Director, JEMS Communications
Conference Division and Emergency Care Information
    Center (ECIC)
Carlsbad, CA

Michael J. Leicht, MD
Associate Professor
Department of Emergency Medicine
Director of Lifeflight
Geisinger Medical Center
Danville, PA

Vince N. Mosesso, Jr. MD, FACEP
Assistant Professor of Emergency Medicine
Department of Emergency Medicine
University of Pittsburgh School of Medicine
Associate Medical Director
City of Pittsburgh Bureau of EMS
Pittsburgh, PA

Robert E. O'Connor, MD, FACEP
Medical Director, Office of Paramedic Administration
State of Delaware
Clinical Associate Professor
Department of Emergency Medicine
Medical Center of Delaware
Newark, DE

Paul M. Paris, MD, FACEP
Chairman and Professor
Department of Emergency Medicine
University of Pittsburgh School of Medicine
Medical Director
City of Pittsburgh
Department of Public Safety
Medical Director
Center for Emergency Medicine of Western Pennsylvania
Pittsburgh, PA

Ronald N. Roth, MD, FACEP
Assistant Professor of Emergency Medicine
Department of Emergency Medicine
University of Pittsburgh School of Medicine
Associate Medical Director
City of Pittsburgh, Bureau of EMS
Pittsburgh, PA

Sandra M. Schneider, MD
Professor and Chairman
Department of Emergency Medicine
University of Rochester
Rochester, NY

Ronald D. Stewart, MD
Minister of Health
Office of the Minister
Halifax, Nova Scotia

Michael P. Sullivan, MD, FACEP
Attending Physician
St. Joseph's Hospital
Department of Emergency Medicine
Bellingham, WA

David Thompson, MS, MD, FACEP
Assistant Professor of Emergency Medicine
Department of Emergency Medicine
East Carolina University School of Medicine
Medical Director, East Care
Greenville, NC

Vincent P. Verdile, MD, FACEP
Associate Professor of Emergency Medicine
and Vice Chairman
Department of Emergency Medicine
Albany Medical College
Medical Director
City of Albany Department of Fire and Emergency
    Services
Albany, NY

Donald M. Yealy, MD, FACEP
Associate Professor and Vice Chairman
Department of Emergency Medicine
University of Pittsburgh School of Medicine
Pittsburgh, PA

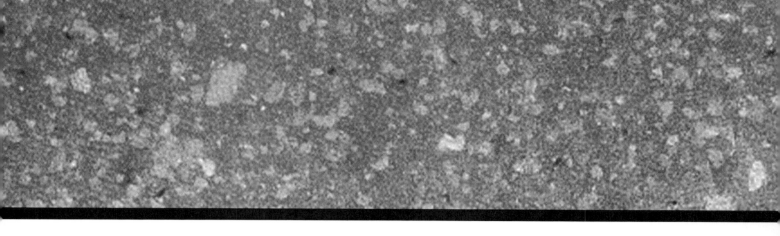

Publisher's Acknowledgments

The editors wish to recognize and thank the following individuals who shared their insights and expertise throughout the review process.

Barbara Aehlert, RN
Director EMS Education
Samaritan Health Systems
Phoenix, Arizona

R. Jack Ayres
Clinical Associate Professor of Hospital Administration
The University of Texas Southwestern Medical Center
Clinical Associate Professor of Emergency Medicine
    Education
Department of Health Care Sciences, Dallas, Texas
Director, Emergency Legal Assistance Program
Parkland Memorial Hospital
Dallas, Texas

Marilyn K. Bourn, RN, MSN, NREMT-P
EMS Educator, Division of Emergency Medicine
Senior Instructor, Department of Surgery
University of Colorado Health Sciences Center
Denver, Colorado

Jeff Clawson, MD
Medical Director, Medical Priority Consultants
Medical Director, Gold Cross Ambulance
Chairman, Board of Certification
National Academy of Emergency Medical Dispatch

James N. Eastham, Jr., ScD
Associate Professor, Emergency Health Services
    Department
University of Maryland Baltimore County
Catonsville, Maryland

Robert A. Felter, MD, FAAP
Chairman, Department of Pediatrics and Adolescent
    Medicine
Tod Childrens Hospital, Youngstown, Ohio
Professor of Pediatrics
Northeast Ohio Universities College of Medicine

Mark A. Kirk, MD
Director, Medical Toxicology Fellowship
Associate Medical Director, Indiana Poison Center
Department of Emergency Medicine
Methodist Hospital of Indiana
Indianapolis, Indiana

William Koenig, MD, FACEP
Medical Director, LA County EMS
Pasadena, California

A.J. Macnab, MD (London), FRCPC
Director, Pediatric Transport Program
Division of Critical Care
British Columbia's Childrens Hospital
Vancouver, British Columbia

William Raynovich, MPH, NREMT-P
Senior Program Director
EMS Academy
University of New Mexico
Albuquerque, New Mexico

Mick J. Sanders, EMT-P, MSA
St. Charles, Missouri

C.J. Shanaberger, JD
Lakewood, Colorado

James F. Veronesi, RN, MSN, CEN, HP
President and Senior Instructor, Armstrong County EMS
    Council
Staff Nurse, Emergency Department, Allegheny General
    Hospital
Pittsburgh, Pennsylvania

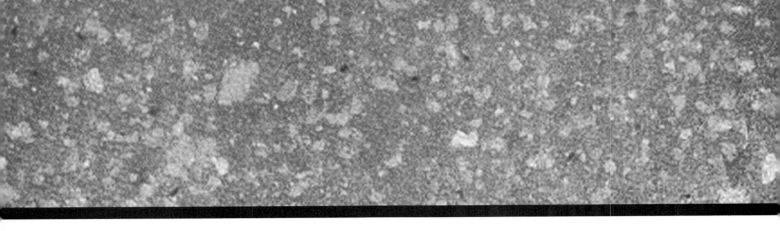

Authors

James G. Adams, MD, FACEP

Hector M. Alonso-Serra, MD

William J, Angelos, MD, FACEP

Daniel J, Cobaugh, PHARM D

Adrian D'Amico, MD, FACEP

Eric Davis, MD, FACEP

Theodore R. Delbridge, MD, MPH, FACEP

Susan M. Dunmire, MD, FACEP

Thomas D. Fowlkes, MD

Susan M. Fuchs, MD, FAAP

Carl W. Gossett, MD, FACEP

A.J. Heightman, MPA, EMT-P

Michael J. Leicht, MD

Vince N. Mosesso, Jr. MD, FACEP

Robert E. O'Connor, MD, FACEP

Paul M. Paris, MD, FACEP

Ronald N. Roth, MD, FACEP

Sandra M. Schneider, MD

Ronald D. Stewart, OC, MD, FACEP, FRCPC, DSc (honorary)

Michael P. Sullivan, MD, FACEP

David Thompson, MS, MD, FACEP

Vincent P. Verdile, MD, FACEP

Donald M. Yealy, MD, FACEP

Foreword

The evolution of specialties in the field of medicine has often depended upon the unfolding of knowledge and the development of technology pertaining to a particular organ or system malfunction. Over the last two decades a demanding speciality of prehospital medical practice has arisen, in part because of technology, but more as a result of patient need and the influence of the environment in which that need must be met. "Prehospital medical command", the practice of "remote patient care" via prehospital teams and radio, is an important part of the developing subspecialty of Emergency Medical Services (EMS). Its origins are rooted firmly in the "team" concept in emergency medicine, a concept in which members of that team have a defined role and remain clearly interdependent. In no other specialty is the team approach to care so crucial or defining of the specialty, as it is in emergency medicine. In the case of prehospital medical command, this is more than a concept, it is essential to its practice.

The epitome of a true team in action is the interchange between a physician and a field team, in which that field team acts as the eyes, ears, and hands of the remote-care physician. True interdependence is seen in the exchange, and a true continuity of care is provided for those cared for in the early stages of their illness or injury.

In the earlier days of EMS, it was felt that in-hospital care providers had to be present on-scene before field teams could safely provide "advanced" life support. Nurses and physicians ran with rescue teams, some of which were located within hospitals and fire departments. It was soon demonstrated that safe and adequate care could be delivered by well-trained technicians without supervisors being present. Hospital-based personnel soon happily retreated to the rather cloistered confines of the coronary care unit or emergency department. However, telemetry—the transmission of electrocardiographic tracings via radio or telephone—remained as the umbilical cord nourishing the security of both field and hospital personnel.

Little thought, and less research, was given to the question of whether any of this made any real difference to patient outcome. The removal of supervising physicians and nurses occurred largely as the techology of telemetry improved and the economic realities of the system took hold. At first glance there appeared to be little difference in outcome when on-scene supervision by nurses ended and telemetry and field teams took over.

The pendulum then swung gradually in the other direction. If on-scene supervision appeared not to influence outcome, could not remote supervision via radio also be dispensed with? The era of protocol-EMS was upon us. It is not difficult, glancing back over the past 20 years, to see why this trend took hold. Although the natural desire of paramedics for more independence of action played a part, more important was the feeling of many field teams that the remote supervision provided by some physicians and nurses was inadequate, inexperienced, inappropriate to field conditions, and often fell short of meeting patients' needs. The reason most commonly cited for such deficits was a lack of appreciation of the prehospital environment by in-hospital personnel. But perhaps the greater impact on the quality of advice provided was the lack of formal training required of nurses or physicians to provide medical command, often an add-on task to those faced with the demands of a busy emergency department.

Between the two extremes—on-scene supervision and prehospital care by protocol only—lay various combinations of interchange between in-hospital and prehospital teams. Modern EMS systems in most urban areas have no on-scene physician supervision. In those systems in which physicians do respond to field emergencies, the purpose of the response is more for physician training than for physician intervention. And although in American EMS systems the emergency physician is seldom part of the field team, most would agree that there is no substitute for field experience in the training of "street-wise" EMS physicians.

Whether the role of the physician in the system be on-scene supervision, medical command via radio, quality improvement, or training and education—or all of these—the EMS physician must be well-schooled in the essentials of prehospital care. This philosophy forms the solid foundation of this text, the unique nature of which can be seen from the approach taken by the authors. Conspicuously, and wonderfully, absent from this work is the assumption, often implied, that the practice of prehospital medicine is not much different than treating patients in the emergency department. Indeed, the special nature of field medicine is recognized at every turn, and the peculiar nature of directing care via radio permeates every chapter and verse.

That this text adopts this approach is less surprising when one peruses the list of authors and considers their experience in the field of EMS systems. This is no "ivory tower" effort. These physicians frequently vacate the ivory tower, go into the streets, and learn from those doing the job in the field. Their approach is fresh, practical, and represents their daily contact with other members of the EMS team.

"Prehospital Medicine: The Art of On-Line Medical Command" represents a milestone along the EMS roadway. It provides, perhaps for the first time, guidelines for the management of patients in the prehospital setting. These guidelines are specific and practical to the field environment and composed by a new generation of EMS physicians trained in this subspecialty. They will do much to elevate the standards expected of EMS systems. They may well improve care in the field. They may even save lives.

Ronald D. Stewart, OC, MD, FACEP, FRCPC, DSc(hon)
Minister of Health, Province of Nova Scotia   Halifax, NS

Contents

PART III Special Concerns

PART 1

Basic Elements of Advanced Life Support Systems

The first section of this text, Basic Elements of Advanced Life Support Systems, highlights the four elements that distinguish Advanced Life Support (ALS) from Basic Life Support (BLS) systems. The essence of providing state-of-the-art Advanced Life Support revolves around physicians who are EMS knowledgeable and intimately involved in all elements of the system, communication systems that allow physicians to be in direct contact with field providers, a set of invasive procedures that each of the providers is trained to do, and availability and knowledge of drugs that can be used in a variety of medical conditions. Most importantly, they should be capable, motivated field clinicians. In designing continuous quality improvement programs for any ALS system, each of these specific four elements needs to be addressed individually. If one were to use the chain analogy, a case can be made that an ALS system is only going to be as strong as the weakest of these four links. Each of these elements has made great advances over the past two decades. The foundation of this text will be providing comprehensive support to each of these crucial system components.

Contemporary Medical Direction

Contemporary medical direction of emergency medical services (EMS) systems entails broad oversight to ensure that the prehospital medical care being delivered is effective. Medical directors must have a working familiarity with the history of their EMS systems, the capabilities of their systems and personnel, the political landscape of the EMS and layperson community, and the current relevant biomedical science impacting prehospital medical care. One tool available to physicians for providing optimal EMS system oversight and for translating EMS science to field practice is direct medical control. This chapter provides an overview of the recent history of EMS in the United States and the obligations of medical oversight, followed by a discussion of the issues pertaining to direct medical control. The intent is to establish a framework by which the principles and practices of on-line medical command can be realized by any physician who finds himself or herself with the need to begin medical care outside of the hospital.

History

The complexion of modern EMS is the result of an explosive evolution that began just 30 years ago. In 1966 the National Academy of Science–National Research Council reported that accidents were the leading cause of death for persons between the ages of 1 and 37 years and the fourth leading cause of death overall.[1] The report, "Accidental Death and Disability: The Neglected Disease of Modern Society," pointed out that the health-care system in the United States was ill-prepared to deal with the injury epidemic.[1] It became the impetus for a series of efforts directed toward improving EMS systems.

The National Highway Safety Act of 1966 placed an emphasis on developing highway safety programs and included guidelines for programs to improve emergency medical care.[2] Federal funds subsequently helped to finance EMS system equipment, personnel, and administrative costs. The Emergency Medical Services Systems Act of 1973 (PL93-154)[3] focused specifically on EMS systems development and provided the federal funding that made the rapid growth of EMS systems possible. By then, EMS sys-

THEODORE R. DELBRIDGE, MD, MPH, FACEP   VINCENT P. VERDILE, MD, FACEP   MICHAEL P. SULLIVAN, MD, FACEP

tems were expanding based on models that had demonstrated increased survival when advanced treatment started at the scene of cardiac patients.

The lay public, through media exposure, became aware of exceptional advances in a few urban areas and sought the same standard of prehospital care for their communities. Subsequently, the scope of prehospital emergency care extended well beyond cardiac patients and traffic accident victims, to include every age group and nearly every conceivable malady. In less than 30 years, the term EMS has changed from one connoting well-intentioned advanced first aiders to systems that use sophisticated communications, technical gadgetry, and an ever-expanding list of pharmacological agents provided by well-trained paramedics to treat patients in the field.

Growth and development of all EMS systems have not been uniform, with economics, demographics, and governance all influencing the shape and size of an EMS system. Consequently, the manner in which these systems are managed or medically directed is also quite variable. Administrative and medical oversight management components, working in concert, are required to ensure efficient operations and delivery of quality state-of-the-art care. The initial EMS growth spurt found many public safety officials flung into the realm of street medicine, often catching them off guard and without consistent medical input.

Since early EMS system development, physicians have participated in direct medical control, providing EMS field personnel with the orders they require to care for patients. It was not until the 1980s, however, that medical direction, more recently termed medical oversight, was viewed as a requisite component of EMS systems. Physicians affiliated with EMS systems have served to a varying extent from full-time salaried system administrators or medical directors to informal, unpaid medical advisors or consultants.

Emergency Medical Services Physicians

EMS physicians have a special interest in EMS issues and medical oversight and surface from many different medical specialties. Paralleling the growth of EMS, emergency medicine has evolved into a recognized medical specialty. The first residency program to train new physicians exclusively for the practice of emergency medicine was not established until 1972. Currently, however, there are more than 110 emergency medicine residency pro-

grams, graduating more than 800 emergency medicine specialists each year.[4] Emergency medicine achieved recognition as a primary board specialty by the American Board of Medical Specialties in 1989.

Emergency physicians in training are exposed to the principles and practice of medical oversight of EMS systems but unfortunately not to the same extent at all residency programs.[5] A model curriculum for EMS education within emergency medicine residency programs has been published by the Society for Academic Emergency Medicine and serves as a guide for requiste EMS learning.[6] In Pittsburgh, emergency medicine residents acquire EMS-related knowledge and skills by providing direct medical control for the city's EMS system, which frequently entails responding directly to the scene of certain emergency situations.[7] Other residency programs require emergency medicine residents to spend time observing or providing care on ambulances.[5,8,9] As the number of emergency medicine residency programs continues to expand, so does the number of physicians entering practice with some knowledge of the principles of EMS system medical oversight.

Emergency physicians often serve as a natural manpower pool to fill medical oversight responsibilities. In many states, emergency physicians provide the majority of on-line medical direction.[10] The nature of their practice requires emergency physicians to have routine interactions with EMS personnel and to continue care that was initiated in the field.

Physicians with an active interest in EMS now effect the business of national organizations, including the American College of Emergency Physicians (ACEP), which currently supports an EMS committee and an EMS section. An EMS committee is also a part of the organizational structure of the Society of Academic Emergency Medicine (SAEM). The National Association of EMS Physicians (NAEMSP), with more than 1000 members, provides a forum for EMS physicians to exchange information and effect leadership for national EMS issues. Approximately 76% of the physician members of NAEMSP consider their specialty to be emergency medicine, but other represented disciplines include family medicine, internal medicine, surgery, and pediatrics.[11] Additionally, the availability of educational programs for physicians in areas such as EMS quality improvement, provider training, and base station operations has expanded. In Pennsylvania, for example, physicians who provide orders to EMS personnel from a radio base station must complete a 1-day base station physician course. Token EMS medical directors and advisors are changing or being replaced by EMS physicians with enthusiasm, commitment, and a greater knowledge of EMS system workings.

Medical Oversight

The traditional paradigm of medical care practiced throughout the United States, including the prehospital setting, is that it is carried out directly or supervised by licensed physicians. Field EMS personnel who function as advanced life support (ALS) providers perform their duties under the authorization of their systems' medical directors, who assume some degree of vicarious liability by providing such authorization. In most states, medical direction of paramedic systems is mandated by law.[12] In large urban areas, EMS medical direction may be a full-time job, while it remains a part-time and often volunteer job in most areas of the country.

Authorities in some regions have also recognized the value of physician oversight of prehospital basic life support (BLS) care, as well.[12] As a result, a growing number of BLS EMS systems are being required to establish formal relationships with responsible physician medical directors.[10] Unfortunately, most prehospital medical care today is provided by BLS personnel without medical oversight. Ideally, BLS medical care should come under the purview of EMS knowledgeable physicians, to ensure quality, enhance education, and improve outcomes for our patients.

Medical oversight is a complex task that involves the direction of the EMS system and providers in the overall clinical management of patients.[12] It can be divided into two broad activities: indirect medical control and direct medical control.[12] Indirect medical control refers to all the "behind the scenes" activities that help ensure a system is competent, efficient, and optimally caring for its patients (Box 1-1). It is a time-consuming and energy-expending endeavor that requires physicians to be knowledgeable about operational, financial, and political issues.[12] Indirect medical control is ultimately responsible for the quality of patient care delivered by the EMS system. The developmental history of the system, its administration, the political climate, and available resources all affect how the goals of indirect medical control are met.

Direct (on-line) medical control refers to the moment-to-moment contemporaneous medical direction of EMS personnel in the field. Direct medical control provides the best example of EMS providers functioning as the eyes and

Box 1-1	Components of Indirect Medical Control

- Personnel Selection and Retention
- Total Quality Management Program
- Training and Education Program
- Development of Treatment and Transport Protocols
- Development of a Medical Control Plan
- Disaster/Hazardous Materials Management Plan
- Equipment and Medication Standards
- Budget, Billing, and Purchasing Negotiations

ears of the physician. It acknowledges the concept of EMS personnel serving as physician extenders. Interestingly, just as the growth and development of EMS systems has not been uniform, the manner and degree to which direct medical control is applied has not been standardized. In current practice, direct medical control varies greatly among EMS systems, in terms of both who provides it and the expectations of how frequently it must be used in patient care. One might intuit that as the acuity of the patient rises, so should the involvement of the on-line medical control physician. Also, keeping in mind the limits of the educational experience of most ALS providers, it becomes apparent that medical or surgical conditions that fall outside of traditional ALS teachings would necessitate more physician input. Between these points are a vast number of diverse clinical conditions that would undoubtedly benefit from a tincture of medical input.

Protocols and Standing Orders

Similar to all medical care, the care delivered by EMS personnel in the prehospital setting generally follows a set of guidelines or standards called *protocols.* As part of indirect medical control activities, the EMS system medical director, or in some cases a medical oversight committee or equivalent, is responsible for developing and implementing patient care protocols. They are frequently developed with input from the regional medical community and field personnel to ensure that they are state-of-the-art, widely accepted, and feasible to implement.

Protocols must have a clear objective or raison d'etre. Each must have explicit criteria for its application and take into account possible field conditions. Application criteria should be objective and readily assessable/measurable by field personnel to avoid erroneous misuse or nonuse.

Protocol content should be clear and precise, contain indications and contraindications to proceeding, and include expected outcomes of interventions. At what point in the delivery of patient care EMS field personnel should be required to contact the individual(s) providing direct medical control is system dependent and is often the topic of research inquiries and controversy.

Standing orders, when used by EMS systems, exist as components of protocols. Unlike guidelines, standing orders are directives for care that have been pre-authorized by the medical director in cases when certain indications and lack of contraindications exist. Use of the term standing orders implies that no contact with the medical control physician is necessary before initiating the specific treatment(s). The classic example of the use and importance of standing orders is in the treatment of patients in ventricular fibrillation. It would not be prudent for an ALS provider to take the time to contact direct medical control for directives to defibrillate a patient. Since time to defibrillation is such a crucial issue, it must be allowed under a standing order portion of the cardiac arrest treatment protocol.

Besides the issue of timely administration of medical therapies, standing orders also have a role in EMS systems for other reasons. For example, in rural EMS systems, topography or distance may prevent contemporaneous on-line medical direction and therefore reliance on standing orders to deliver patient care is a necessity. Another instance might be air medical EMS systems (see Chapter 17), which also can face situations where direct medical control is not feasible. Implicit in the implementation of an all standing order system is the need for rigorous quality assurance measures to monitor patient care activities. Overall, the willingness of EMS systems to adopt standing orders for invasive and pharmacologic interventions is multifactorial and varies greatly among EMS systems.

Compliance by field personnel, acceptance by the medical community, and basis in current EMS biomedical research all require continuous monitoring if protocols are to remain effective. Protocols and standing orders, once developed, require that an investment be made in the education of field personnel, who must be intimately familiar with them if they are to be appropriately and successfully used. Quality improvement activities should detect misuse of protocols and standing orders and ensure that their appropriate application yields the desired results. For example, realization that a new trauma protocol is extending on-scene times or that field personnel

cannot reliably identify correct patients for a specific standing order might indicate the need for education or protocol revision.

Direct Medical Control

Direct (on-line) medical control allows a medical director to influence the clinical care being delivered by an EMS system on a minute-to-minute basis. Because it must be provided on a 24 hour-per-day basis, direct medical control is a medical oversight activity likely to be delegated by the EMS medical director to other EMS knowledgable physicians. Availability of direct medical control, via radio, telephone, or on the scene has many distinct advantages, particularly when compared to standing orders alone (Box 1-2). First, direct medical control enables authorization for paramedics to deviate from routine system protocols when indicated by infrequently occurring circumstances. As long as the deviation remains within the scope of their capabilities, it allows the ALS providers an opportunity to adjust the delivery of health care to the patient's needs. An example of this might be the administration of sublingual nitroglycerin beyond the protocol limits of 0.4 mg every 5 minutes for chest pain to 0.8 mg or more every 2 minutes for the patient with chest pain, accelerated hypertension, and severe pulmonary edema.

Additional benefits of direct medical control include contemporaneous quality improvement, education of EMS personnel, and enhanced communications between field and medical oversight providers. The opportunity to discuss the patient's clinical presentation, alternatives to treatment, and expected outcome is extremely valuable for the paramedic, the physician receiving the patient, and ultimately the patient. A 35-year-old, morbidly obese female patient, on birth control pills, with a 20 year smoking history and in a long leg cast who develops chest

Box 1-2	**Advantages of On-line Medical Command**

- Protocol selection
- Protocol deviation
- Directed patient assessement
- Contemporaneous quality improvement
- EMS provider education
- Patient status awareness
- Patient ETA

pain and shortness of breath probably does not warrant treatment for ischemic heart disease. In an EMS system of standing orders only however, it is conceivable that this patient's complaint of chest pain might be the impetus for using nitroglycerin, which would offer her nothing and potentially cause some harm. In a direct medical control EMS system, this is far less likely to occur.

Radio communication with physicians was the early standard for providing direct medical control. Among EMS systems, several different configurations for creating this communications link have been developed.[13] Emergency medical services systems may use either single or multiple base stations to receive direct medical control. In most cases, direct medical control originates from base stations located in hospital emergency departments. In systems with several base station hospitals, determining which hospital to contact may be a function of either the geographic region in which the EMS unit is operating or the facility that will be receiving the patient. New York City provides direct medical control for its EMS personnel via physicians located at a central communications center. In Pittsburgh, radio traffic from EMS units requiring direct medical control is routed through a single communications center, but the physicians who speak with the field personnel are mobile and communicate via portable UHF radios. Clearly, many different configurations can be made to work satisfactorily. The medical control plan must consider all factors that will facilitate the delivery of timely medical input.

For some EMS systems, direct medical control is provided by physician surrogates, such as specially trained mobile intensive care nurses (MICN). San Diego and parts of Chicago are examples of cities with systems using MICNs who work from protocols to provide direct medical control for the majority of radio consultations from the field.[13] Physician backup is available for complex situations or clinical conditions that require deviation from existing protocols. There are, of course, advantages and disadvantages to every system. One might argue that having physician surrogates operate from protocols may seem no better than increasing the number of the system's standing orders. However, when MICNs or paramedic communicators receive calls from the field, they are removed from the often emotionally charged environment in which EMS personnel are operating, can refer to written protocols, and may provide calm prompting for the consulting provider. Because these medical control providers are typically dedicated to EMS communications,

they are in a good position to obtain often sought patient follow-up information and relay it to field personnel. Medical oversight physicians, however, may become further removed from the delivery of prehospital emergency care. Greater attention is required to avoid potential loss of system familiarity and to communicate with field personnel who value interactions with medical oversight physicians. Nevertheless, it appears that many different approaches to providing direct medical control can be made to work effectively for EMS systems.

In the early development of ALS EMS systems, the ability to transmit ECG data from the field to the medical control facility was deemed to be necessary to provide medical orders for patients with cardiac related complaints. Subsequently, it was demonstrated that when telemetry was used, paramedics had extended on-scene times and that its use did not affect the outcome of patients with life-threatening dysrhythmias.[14] Furthermore, physicians receiving the telemetry had unacceptable rates of rhythm misinterpretation.[15] Although misinterpretation may have simply been the result of poor signal quality, in the final analysis it is more important for field EMS personnel to recognize which patients require cardiac monitoring and to sharpen their own ECG rhythm interpretation skills.

The ability of hospitals to receive transmitted ECG data from the field may again become important as communications technology improves and EMS personnel are able to perform 12 lead ECGs. Technological and therapeutic evolution might require medical control physicians to interpret 12 lead ECGs for evidence of ischemia. Interpretation of reliable data from the field will allow either prehospital or expedited emergency department administration of thrombolytic therapy for appropriate patients.[16]

The Effectiveness of Direct Medical Control

One of the greatest difficulties in EMS has been defining outcome measures that effectively assess our performance as a system providing medical care. The same might be said of the process of providing direct medical control. Some EMS physicians have questioned the value of mandating direct medical control for every patient encounter. One concern that is often raised is that a requirement to establish radio contact with a medical control facility prolongs EMS unit on-scene times. Evaluations of on-scene times relative to a need to seek medical control, however, have not been consistent. Furthermore, other than for seriously injured patients, no study to date has analyzed the effect of the length of scene time with patient outcome in a meaningful way. We do not know for instance if the medical needs of acutely ill asthmatic patients, congestive heart failure patients, or status epilepticus patients are jeopardized or helped by a few minutes longer on scene because of on-line medical direction. One might infer, however, that physician input into the care of these seriously ill patients might have some measurable effect on their morbidity and mortality. Unfortunately, it would require a clinical trial of enormous magnitude to show a statistically and clinically significant difference in patient outcome with and without on-line medical direction.

Erder found that paramedics spend an average of 8 minutes longer on the scene when they call for medical control.[17] The study, however, conducted in Philadelphia, was not controlled, and other confounding factors in patients' conditions may well have accounted for differences in on-scene and total prehospital times. Pointer noted that when a California EMS system changed from requiring medical control to completely operating with standing orders, a statistically significant decrease of approximately 4 minutes in total prehospital time occurred.[18] Patient outcomes were not assessed, however, making the implication of a 4-minute-longer scene time undeterminable. When Gratton evaluated the overall duration of prehospital care, after a system's change from requiring radio contact to no radio contact before treating unstable trauma patients, no significant difference could be appreciated.[19] Similarly, no difference was detected in on-scene times after a comparison of prehospital cardiac arrest resuscitations conducted with and without direct medical control via radio.[20]

Only recently has the importance of evaluating prehospital time intervals in a standardized fashion been fully appreciated.[21] One must consider the consequences of events that are or are not able to be occurring simultaneously. With trauma for example, it is universally acceptable to reduce prehospital time to an absolute minimum, since restorative care can never be accomplished by the EMS system. For other types of patients however, there is a less tangible trade-off between potential benefits derived from a more thorough assessment or initiation of treatment and additional time spent at the scene. Confounding factors, such as time to access the patient, barriers to patient removal from the scene (physical and

otherwise), bystander interference, and others, must also be considered. In addition, the fact that EMS systems do not routinely provide ongoing or follow-up care, are not well integrated into the hospital quality improvement program, and often care for patients whose outcome reflects the natural progression of the disease process rather than the results of a procedure or intervention, makes the evaluation of prehospital time intervals as a piece of the overall health-care delivery system extremely difficult.

In one study, when direct medical control via radio was provided to paramedics, physicians in urban EMS systems directed deviations from protocol in 2%-5% of cases.[17,22] Physicians provided unanticipated orders beyond standard therapies, such as intravenous fluids, $D_{50}W$, and oxygen, when patients had respiratory distress, abnormal vital signs, or some other significant sign/symptom.[22] In a rural Pennsylvania study, direct medical control resulted in physician orders in 19% of cases.[23] Approximately one-half of the orders were for interventions already included in protocols but that had not yet been initiated. Although orders resulting from direct medical control are often not for care beyond that which is included in protocols, physicians and paramedics continue to feel that radio communication is medically helpful or critical in 17.4% and 12.9% of cases, respectively.[24] Furthermore, when considering the number of patients that are cared for by EMS providers annually, these seemingly small percentages translate into significant numbers of patients who benefit from on-line medical control.

Patient outcome differences with and without the benefit of direct medical control have been difficult for EMS systems to objectively evaluate. However, EMS personnel achieved return of spontaneous circulation in 24% and 19% of cardiac arrest patients treated with and without the benefit of direct medical control, respectively.[20] The study required greater numbers of patients for the found differences to reach statistical significance. Additionally, in the Philadelphia EMS system, 5.5% of patients experienced an overall clinical improvement when direct medical control was obtained by field personnel, as opposed to 3.2% who improved when there was no direct medical control.[17]

A distinct advantage of direct medical control is the ability to affect paramedics' patient assessments, either by prompting performance of a technique or modifying conclusions based on the information provided. In Arizona, when skilled observers accompanied paramedics on ambulances throughout the state, they found that the

EMS providers did not obtain a heart rate or blood pressure for 37% of 227 patients who they evaluated.[25] This was in complete disregard of statewide protocols indicating the need for obtaining complete vital signs for all patients. Of those transported to a hospital, 19.4% had no blood pressure taken. Of even greater concern was that, for those who were not transported, 49.1% had no blood pressure taken.[25] Clearly the benefit to the patient of on-line medical command would be the moral authority to gather all the necessary and available patient related data before selecting and implementing a treatment protocol.

Some reports have identified a concern for the accuracy with which EMS personnel are able to differentiate specific patient problems. In a Los Angeles study, 23% of the patients who paramedics had assessed and treated as having pulmonary edema were actually found in the emergency department to be suffering from chronic obstructive pulmonary disease (COPD), pneumonia, or another pulmonary disease.[26] Other investigations have confirmed 10%-30% misassessment rates, compared to emergency department diagnoses by advanced EMS personnel.[27,28] Misassessment may have significant consequences. Patients who were suffering from COPD exacerbations, but were erroneously treated as if they were had congestive heart failure, experienced higher mortality rates than those COPD patients who received no prehospital treatment.[28] An on-line medical control physician will be able to influence the direction and quality of ALS provider assessement and reassesment in the care of patients with respiratory and other medical conditions necessitating therapy.

The added value of on-line physician input is exemplified by a report from Pittsburgh. Paramedics, with the benefit of direct medical control, correctly differentiated congestive heart failure and bronchospasm in 86% and 92% of cases, respectively. Treatment administered, whether prehospital impression is correct, is appropriate, as determined by the ED diagnosis, for 98% of bronchospasm and 92% of congestive heart failure cases.[29]

There may be other less tangible benefits of routinely providing direct medical control. For example, the field radio report may be a hidden pearl in the educational development of less experienced EMS providers. The report, by its nature, must be succinct and accurate. A standard format fosters clear and concise problem oriented thinking that may translate into less frequent omission of critical patient information and better patient care. Direct medical control also serves as one mechanism for achieving continuous quality improvement. With regard to patients who are evaluated by EMS personnel but not transported, direct medical control appears to be one factor that improves the EMS system's documentation for these events.[30] Direct medical control is often responsible for ensuring that patients are appropriately transported to the hospital when they had initially refused.[31]

Direct Medical Control Paradigms

To date, no system has been able to perform a controlled, randomized study of patient outcomes when direct medical control was or was not available to demonstrate the most effective model. Retrospective controls for prospective and descriptive studies do not account for other system changes or advancements that may have occurred concurrently. More importantly, which objective patient outcomes to evaluate remains unclear. One cannot definitively demonstrate the value of a specific model for delivering direct medical control, whether it is for selected or for all ALS EMS responses, without a well-controlled study using discreet outcome measures that are relevant and specific to the prehospital phase of care.

In some EMS systems, direct medical control is provided by PGY II and PGY III emergency medicine residents who are supervised by a faculty physician.[5,7,8] Under certain situations, the resident physicians respond directly to the scene, providing on-scene direct medical control. This field experience often serves to enhance the level of care provided, offers contemporaneous quality improvement, and offers an expanded educational opportunity for the residents. In fact, physicians have a legacy of responding to field emergencies prior to their relative absence over the past 30 years. The residents in one program find that most field responses are educationally valuable and that they benefit from the increased physician-paramedic interactions.[32]

The most traditional configuration for direct medical control is the emergency department base station command facility with the on-duty physician providing directives over a radio system.[13,33] Permutations of this model with different types of on-line commanders and communication equipment are workable alternatives and are described elsewhere in this chapter. Each EMS jurisdiction must determine what configuration of on-line medical control is most effective for their system, given the resources available, the number of patient encounters requiring physician input, the acuity of the patients treated, and the incidence of misdiagnosis or incorrect therapy discovered in the quality management program. Cellular and digital telephone technology will undoubtedly expand the type of direct medical control systems.

Some EMS physicians have proposed that direct medical control is not necessary for all ALS-level EMS responses.[17,22] Some EMS systems may use standing orders as a means to avoid the need for direct medical control.[13] Nevertheless, the ability to provide direct medical control, at least for certain subsets of patients, remains crucial for the operation of most EMS systems. Physicians should be available for consultation from field personnel when any of the following conditions arise: 1) a non-protocol intervention is being contemplated, 2) a clinical situation deviates from a protocol, 3) field personnel feel that physician input would be helpful, 4) a patient is refusing treatment or transport, 5) field personnel and a physician surrogate medical control provider disagree, or 6) a physician surrogate requests physician input. There may certainly be other situations in which physician-provided medical control may prove helpful. These might include prolonged resuscitation calls, termination of resuscitative efforts, patients in shock, the presence of a physician wishing to assume control at the scene, and multiple casualty incidents with triage considerations. Implementation of direct medical control tends to be a function of the level of training of the field personnel, the resources available to them, and the operating philosophy of the medical control physicians and EMS system medical director.

One final paradigm for direct medical control is still evolving. As health-care delivery systems are being redefined, EMS systems and providers are being considered for new roles. Expanding the scope of practice of EMS providers under direct medical control ensures physician participation at a level that might not be possible with other physician extenders or allied health professionals. The advantages of on-line medical control for expanded health care practices by EMS personnel will undoubtedly be important as these systems develop.

Summary

Until the proper investigations occur demonstrating the effectiveness or ineffectiveness of direct (on-line) medical control, it can be safely assumed that in nearly every community, EMS providers will require some medical

direction. Past practices indicate that the local emergency department will more likely than not be looked upon as the resource for direct medical control. It is imperative therefore, for each of us who interact with EMS professionals who are acting on our behalf in the care of patients, to strive to be the very best on-line medical commanders as possible. This textbook attempts to improve our ability in this regard by offering insights into the principles and practices of on-line medical direction that heretofore were not available.

Physicians continue to have a heightened interest in EMS. Contemporary medical direction consists of a system of medical oversight that efficiently incorporates both direct and indirect medical control. It connotes renewed vitality and enthusiasm of EMS physicians to improve the scientific evaluation both of the prehospital care provided to the community and of the systems that deliver that care and to incorporate new knowledge into advanced, efficient systems of care that improve patient outcomes. Direct medical control allows EMS physicians to immediately impact the delivery and quality of prehospital emergency medical care using a rapidly evolving fund of knowledge. It enhances communication between medical oversight and EMS field personnel and positively effects system-wide education and quality improvement activities.

REFERENCES

1. National Academy of Science, National Research Council: *Accidental death and disability: the neglected disease of modern society,* Washington, DC, 1966, National Academy Press.

2. National Highway Safety Act of 1966: Public Law 89-564, Washington, DC, 1966.

3. Emergency Medical Services Systems Act of 1973: Public Law 93-154, Title XII of the Public Health Service Act, Washington, DC, 1973.

4. *Graduate Medical Education Directory 1995-1996,* Chicago, American Medical Association, 1995, pp 362-379.

5. Paris PM, Benson NH: Education about prehospital care during emergency education residency training: the results of a survey, *Prehosp Disaster Med* 5:209-215, 1990.

6. Swor RA, Chisolm C, Krohmer J: Model curriculum in emergency medical services for emergency medicine residencies, *Ann Emerg Med* 18:418-421, 1989.

7. Stewart RD, Paris PM, Heller MB: Design of a resident in-field experience for an emergency medicine residency curriculum, *Ann Emerg Med* 16:175-179, 1987.

8. Dinerman N, Pons PT, Markovchick V: The emergency medicine resident as paramedic: a prehospital in-field rotation, *J Emerg Med* 8:507-511, 1990.

9. Boyle MF, Eilers MA, Hunt RL, et al.: Objectives to direct the training of emergency medicine residents on off-service rotations: emergency medical services, *J Emerg Med* 8:791-795, 1990.

10. Snyder JA, Braen JM, Ryan SD, et al.: Emergency medical service system development: results of the statewide emergency medical service technical assessment program, *Ann Emerg Med* 25:768-775, 1995.

11. National Association of EMS Physicians: Personal communication, July 1995.

12. Racht EM, Reines HD: Medical oversight. In Kheul AE, editor: *Prehospital systems and medical oversight,* ed 2, St Louis, 1994, Mosby, pp 181-185.

13. Braun O: Direct medical control. In Kheul AE editor: *Prehospital systems and medical oversight,* ed 2, St Louis, 1994, Mosby, pp 196-216.

14. Cayten C, Oler J, Walker K, et al.: The effect of telemetry on urban prehospital cardiac care, *Ann Emerg Med* 14:976-981, 1985.

15. Pozen MW, De'Agostino RB, Sytkowski PA, et al.: Effectiveness of a prehospital medical control system: an analysis of the interaction between emergency room physician and paramedic, *Circulation* 63:442-447, 1981.

16. Auferheide T, Hendley GE: The diagnostic impact of prehospital 12 lead electrocardiography, *Ann Emerg Med* 19:1287-1380, 1990.

17. Erder MH, Davidson SJ, Chaney RA: On-line medical command in theory and practice, *Ann Emerg Med* 18:261-288, 1989.

18. Pointer JE, Osur MA: Effect of standing orders on field times, *Ann Emerg Med* 18:1119-1121, 1989.

19. Gratton MC, Bethke RA, Watson WA, et al.: Effect of standing orders on paramedic scene time for trauma patients, *Ann Emerg Med* 20:52-55, 1991.

20. Hunt RC, Bass RR, Graham RG, et al.: Standing orders versus voice control, *JEMS* 7:26-31, 1982.

21. Spaite DW, Valenzuela TD, Meislin HW, et al.: Prospective validation of a new model for evaluating emergency medical services systems by in-field observation of specific time intervals in prehospital care, *Ann Emerg Med* 22:638-645, 1993.

22. Hoffman JR, Luo J, Schriger DL, et al.: Does paramedic-based hospital contact result in beneficial deviations from standard prehospital protocols?, *West J Med* 153:283-287, 1989.

23. Wuerz RC, Swope GE, Holliman CJ, et al.: On-line medical direction: a prospective study, *Prehosp Disaster Med* 10:174-177, 1995.

24. Thompson SJ, Schriver JA: A survey of prehospital care paramedic/physician communication for Multnomah County (Portland), Oregon, *J Emerg Med* 1:421-428, 1984.

25. Spaite DW, Criss EA, Valenzuela TD, et al.: A prospective evaluation of prehospital patient assessment by direct in-field observation: failure of ALS personnel to measure vital signs, *Prehosp Disaster Med* 5:325-333, 1990.

26. Hoffman JR, Reynolds S: Comparison of nitroglycerin, morphine and furosemide in treatment of presumed prehospital pulmonary edema, *Chest* 92:586-593, 1987.

27. Tresch DD, Dabrowski RC, Firetti GP, et al.: Out-of-hospital pulmonary edema: diagnosis and treatment, *Ann Emerg Med* 12:533-537, 1983.

28. Wuerz RC, Meador SA: Effects of prehospital medications on mortality and length of stay in congestive heart failure, *Ann Emerg Med* 21:669-674, 1992.

29. Macleod BA, Lorei J, Wolfson AB: The accuracy of prehospital diagnosis in patients with dyspnea (abstract), *Ann Emerg Med* 19:459, 1990.

30. Cone DC, Kim DT, Davidson SJ: Patient-initiated refusals of prehospital care: ambulance call report documentation, patient outcome, and on-line medical command, *Prehosp Disaster Med* 10:3-9, 1995.

31. Stark G, Hedges J: Patients who initially refuse prehospital evaluation and/or therapy, *Am J Emerg Med* 8:509-511, 1990.

32. Hutton KC, LaCovey MA: Prospective evaluation of in-the-field medical command with emergency response duties as part of an emergency medicine residency curriculum (abstract), *Prehosp Disaster Med* 5:303, 1990.

33. Roush WR: Medical accountablity. In Roush WR, editor: *Principles of EMS systems,* ed 2, Dallas, 1994, ACEP.

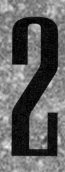

Communications
PART 1: EMERGENCY MEDICAL SERVICES COMMUNICATIONS FOR THE BASE STATION PHYSICIAN

At the heart of every EMS is a unique communications system. A basic need of EMS personnel is to communicate with others. On a daily basis, prehospital care providers must communicate with their dispatch center, other prehospital care providers, police, fire services, and receiving hospitals. Prehospital care providers are the physician's eyes and ears in the field. They communicate their findings to the physician, and in return physicians communicate their orders back to the provider. With today's technology, there are many different modes of communications, each with individual advantages and disadvantages. It is essential that the base station physician have a basic understanding of the communications system related to his or her local EMS.

Communications Equipment

The two-way radio and the telephone are essential components of most communications systems.

Telephones

In general, the telephone "landline" provides excellent quality and reliability. The conversation between the physician and the field team is confidential, although the conversation should be recorded for quality assurance purposes. Unfortunately, the availability of a telephone at the scene of a prehospital care response cannot be guaranteed. In addition, during a disaster, telephone lines may become inoperable. Telephone communications allow simultaneous transmission of speech in two directions (Duplex communication). This allows one party to interrupt another party in mid-conversation. With the new cellular telephone technology, access and availability problems of the standard telephone have been overcome and many services now rely on cellular telephones for communications with medical command facilities. Unfortunately, the cost

RONALD N. ROTH, MD, FACEP   A.J. HEIGHTMAN, MPA, EMT-P

of cellular telephones and air time associated with them limits their use by some services. Although the standard telephone conversation is private, cellular telephone conversations are transmitted over frequencies that can be monitored by individuals with the correct equipment. Therefore, some discretion should be used when conversing via cellular telephone. The availability of cellular technology depends on the availability of cells (radio telephone receiver transmitters). Although the geographic areas covered by cells continue to expand, cells may not be present in some areas, especially in rural areas.

Radios

Despite cellular telephone technology, two-way radios remain an essential component of most EMS systems. It is imperative that the base station physician understand some basic principles associated with two-way radio communications. EMS radio communications may be transmitted over any of four radio frequency bands, low band VHF, high band VHF, UHF (ultra high frequency), and the 800 and 900 band. Each of these frequency bands has advantages and disadvantages for use by EMS (Table 2-1). The frequency allocations within the individual bands are assigned by the Federal Communications Commission (FCC). The FCC licenses the use of EMS frequencies and has developed rules for their use.

VHF Low Band

VHF low band operates on frequencies between 32-50 megahertz (MHz). The VHF low band transmissions have the longest range when compared to other EMS frequencies. VHF low band transmissions follow the curve of the Earth and can travel great distances. However, despite their long range, low band transmissions suffer from poor quality and are easily interfered with by buildings, electrical equipment, and land masses. VHF low band poorly penetrates structures, making it a poor choice for inner city communications. However, the properties of the VHF low band may prove advantageous to communications in wide open rural areas. Due to the susceptibility of interference, the VHF low band is limited to voice communications. VHF low band radios operate on a simplex mode, that is, the same frequency is used for both transmitting and receiving communications. Transmissions can only occur in one direction at a time (Simplex communications). Therefore, one party cannot interrupt a second transmitting party during a transmission. Therefore, proper communications procedures are essential. Transmission should be kept brief and adequate time for the receiving party to reply to a transmission should be given.

VHF High Band

VHF high band operates over a frequency range of 150-174 MHz. Unlike low band transmissions, VHF high band signals travel in a straight line and do not follow the curvature of the Earth. Therefore, the range of high band is considerably less than the range of low band transmissions. VHF high band provides better quality transmissions and is less susceptible to disturbances than

Table 2-1	Comparison of Radio Frequencies			
Frequency	**Operating MHz**	**Mode of Transmission**	**Advantages**	**Disadvantages**
VHF low	32-50	simplex	■ travels great distances	■ interference ■ voice comm. only ■ over-crowded
VHF high	150-174	simplex	■ better quality	■ low range ■ interference ■ over-crowded
UHF	450-470	simplex or duplex	■ excellent structure penetration	■ shorter range (can be overcome with repeater system)
800-900 MHz	800-900	simplex or duplex	■ excellent quality ■ structure penetration ■ flexible ■ private	■ shortest range ■ requires repeater systems ■ expensive equipment and technology

low band transmissions. Unfortunately, solid structures such as buildings interfere with VHF signals. Therefore, transmission from within buildings may be difficult. Like low band transmissions, VHF high band transmissions are Simplex communication. Unfortunately, both the VHF low and high bands suffer from extreme overcrowding. It is not uncommon to have several services sharing individual frequencies, making communications at busy times extremely difficult, if not impossible. The VHF frequency 155.340 MHz has been reserved for ambulance use throughout the country.

UHF Band

UHF band operates between 450-470 MHz. Like VHF, UHF signals follow in a straight line, although their range is shorter than VHF. The UHF frequency has excellent structure penetration and provides for a better signal quality, allowing for telemetry data to be transmitted over these frequencies. The FCC has designated specific frequencies (medical channels) for EMS use. Two of these channels are reserved for dispatch, with the remaining channels used for EMS communications and telemetry. These channels are used only by EMS personnel for medical communications and therefore suffer less congestion than VHF or UHF frequencies. Unlike the VHF frequencies, the UHF band can with the proper equipment use simplex or duplex communications. UHF systems are frequently used with repeater systems. Repeater equipment receives transmissions from a relatively low wattage transmitter, such as a hand-held portable, then relays them to the receiving facility, thereby increasing the effective range of the transmission.

800-900 MHz Frequency

As would be expected, the 800-900 MHz system has the shortest range of the available frequencies but provides excellent quality and structure penetration. Many frequencies are available within the 800-900 MHz range. Due to their short range, all 800 MHz frequencies require repeater systems. The 800-900 MHz frequency bands use trunking systems that coordinate the use of repeaters by computers, increasing efficiency, flexibility, and privacy. An 800-900 MHz frequency system requires expensive equipment and technology.

Satellite Technology

New technology and the increased use of satellite communications have created the potential for using satellites to link physicians with field providers in very remote locations. Relatively small antenna sizes, lightweight suitcase sized equipment, and decreasing costs make satellite communications feasible for select EMS providers.

The frequency ranges used for satellite communications include the L band (1.5-1.6 gigahertz [GHz]), S band (2.5-2.7 GHz), and the Ka band (20-30 GHz). Satellites in orbit above the Earth could potentially link physicians with field teams almost anywhere on the planet.

Other Equipment
Repeaters

Repeater equipment picks up signals from low power units, such as portable radios, and relays them to the receiving facility via another frequency, telephone line, or microwave. Repeaters extend the range of radios. Repeaters may be located in the responding vehicle or can be strategically located on towers in the response area.

REPEATER SYSTEM

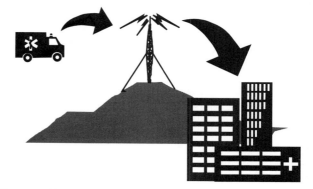

Base Station Remote

A transmitter and receiver at a fixed location (such as a dispatch center) is called a base station. Equipment that can control the base station at the site removed from the base station is called a remote site. Often the remote and base station are connected together by landline. Therefore, the remote station has all the advantages and power of the base station without the expense or space requirements of a base station. A medical command hospital may serve as a remote to a site at a distance from the EMS main base station.

Squelch

Squelch is a method to suppress unwanted noise or communications from being received. A circuit in the radio shuts off the speaker until a signal is received. This can be set to a noise level or a particular tone transmitted along with the voice or telemetry communication. Codes can be programmed into radio to allow only reception of transmissions with the proper squelch code. This convenience, sometimes called a private line, allows you to hear only private transmissions.

Types of Communication

Simplex

In simplex communication, all units receive and transmit on the same frequency, therefore you cannot talk and listen simultaneously. Proper communication etiquette is required to prevent missed transmissions. You may recall the terms "roger" or "over and out" popularized many years ago to signal a change in transmission direction.

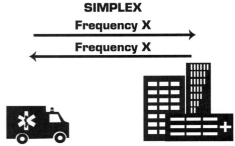

SIMPLEX

Frequency X

Frequency X

The field unit and the hospital alternately transmit and receive on the same frequency.

Duplex

Duplex communication separates transmission and reception to allow simultaneous talking and listening.

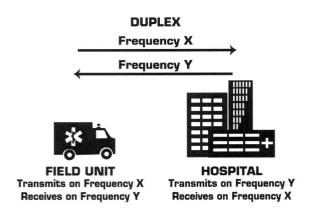

DUPLEX

Frequency X

Frequency Y

FIELD UNIT
Transmits on Frequency X
Receives on Frequency Y

HOSPITAL
Transmits on Frequency Y
Receives on Frequency X

Radio Etiquette

Although protocols for radio use vary from system to system, a few guidelines are offered to improve radio efficiency and professionalism. See Part 2 of this chapter

for an in-depth discussion of the interpersonal aspects of medical command communications.

1. Press the TRANSMIT key for approximately 1 second before you begin talking. This prevents your first few words from being cut off as the system activates. For example:

   "Do not defibrillate the patient" might sound like "defibrillate the patient" if the first few words of the transmission are lost.

2. Give the name of the unit being called first, then give your identification. Example:

   "Medic One, this is MD-36."

3. Keep transmissions brief and commands simple. Ask for additional information when needed. If the added information will not alter your treatment plan, do not ask for it. It is desirable to have a brief discussion with the medics on difficult or confusing cases. Do not be afraid to ask the medics for their suggestions and observations.

4. Be professional and use discretion. There are potentially thousands of people listening to your conversation with scanners, and in addition many systems record their radio transmissions.

5. When you given an order, make sure that it is repeated back to you by the field team.

6. Always say something when the medics call. Silence is deadly and makes the field team very uneasy. If you need time, tell the medics to (Stand By) while you put together your thoughts.

7. When you stand a new call, identify yourself to the medics by name.

   "Medic 5, this is Dr. Roth, MD-9, go ahead."

8. When ordering drugs, be specific. Do not say,

   "Give an amp of Narcan."

   Narcan comes in a variety of sizes and may be given IV, IM, SQ, sublingual, and endotracheal.

   Be very careful when ordering epinephrine.

   Example:

   "Give 0.3 cc of 1:1000 epinephrine SQ."

9. The medics are your eyes, ears, and hands in the field. Respect them. We are all on the same team, with patient care as our ultimate goal.

Summary

Communications systems are a vital component of all EMS systems. Rapidly expanding communications technology allows for a wide variety of communications options. Each system option has distinct advantages, disadvantages, and unique features that the command physician must understand. Just as important as the technical aspects of a communications system is the command physician–field provider interaction. Clearly, the overall success of an EMS communications system relies heavily on the mutual trust and respect between the physician and the field provider.

Suggested Readings

Augustine JJ: Communications. In Kuehl AE, editor: *Prehospital systems in medical oversight,* ed 2, St Louis, 1994, Mosby, pp. 118-124.

Feh H: A primer on radio communications, *JEMS* 1980; 5:22-34.

Forrest RT: Two way communicating systems, repeaters boost range, but require special system design and equipment, *APCO Bulletin* 1990;58:57-60.

Johnson MS, Van Cott CC: The FCC may be listening, update on EMS communications, *JEMS* 1992;17:19-27.

Van Cott CC: EMS communications: the trends and technologies of emergency medical services, *APCO Bulletin* 1994;60:18-21.

SAMPLE CASES

CASE #1

MEDIC: Command this is medic 57 on Med channel 4. We are seeing a 67-year-old man with a history of heart problems and CHF who presents now with severe shortness of breath, typical of his CHF attacks.

His vital signs are a pulse of 110, respirations of 40 and a BP of 80/palpation. We have started an IV of D_5W at KVO and we have administered a sublingual nitroglycerin tablet and my partner is pushing 100 mg of furosemide IV...

BASE MD: (attempting to interrupt) Medic 57, why don't you hold off on that furosemide and I wouldn't give any more nitroglycerin.

MEDIC: ...after the furosemide we plan on giving morphine 2 mg IV. How do you copy?

DISCUSSION

As much as this physician would like to abort the medics' treatment scheme, in a simplex radio system, only one party can speak at a time. Unlike a telephone, where both parties can talk and listen at the same time, with a simplex radio system, transmissions can only occur in one direction. Unfortunately, the Base MD must wait until the field medic completes his or her transmission.

CASE #2

MEDIC: Command this is medic 19, we are seeing a 77-year-old female with a history of heart problems and COPD who called us today because of severe shortness of breath. Her vitals are a BP of 200/110, pulse 95, respirations 28. She has peripheral edema and wheezing in all lung fields. What would you like us to do?

BASE MD: That's copied medic 19, why don't you give 40 mg of furosemide IV, administer an albuterol treatment, and start an IV of D_5W to run at 100 cc per hour. Also, why don't you give two nitroglycerin sprays now, then retake her BP and if her systolic BP is greater than 180, give two additional nitroglycerin sprays. However, if her systolic BP is less than 180 but greater than 120, just give one nitroglycerin spray. If she is still short of breath after four nitros, go ahead with a second albuterol. How did you copy?

MEDIC: Doc, you lost me after the 40 mg of furosemide.

DISCUSSION

Avoid overwhelming the field medic with a long series of orders. Remember, the medic may not be in the best of situations, (in the dark, outside in the cold, etc.) and may not be able to write down your orders. The Base MD should issue only a few orders at one time and group orders in a logical order. Ask for the results of the initial interventions before issuing additional orders (i.e., Start an IV of D_5W and then administer 40 mg of furosemide, then give me an update on the patient's condition.)

CASE #3

MEDIC: Medic command, this is medic 5109, we are 10-17 to your location with 2 victims of a 10-71 with a 10-26 of 15-20 minutes. 10-4?

(continued)

(continued)

BASE MD: Medic 5109, please repeat your message in English.

MEDIC: 10-9?

DISCUSSION

In an effort to make radio communications more "efficient," many services use codes to help relay information. A commonly used code system is the 10-code. (example, 10-4 means OK!) Unfortunately, a universal 10-code system does not exist. The term 10-71 may mean a shooting in one jurisdiction, while in a neighboring community 10-71 may be the code for "medic on lunch break." Codes are often unique to one service, therefore a physician communicating with medics from more than one service could potentially be required to learn several sets of codes.

Upon re-evaluating the efficiency of radio codes, many experts believe that codes do little to shorten transmission time and may increase confusion. As a result, many systems have abandoned codes for "plain English".

CASE #4

MEDIC: Command, this is medic 5105, we are on scene with a rather large 35-year-old male with a history of psychiatric problems who states he took 100 extra-strength Tylenol® tablets to help him sleep. The patient took these pills about 1 hour ago. He says he feels fine and does not want to go to the hospital with us. My partner and I think he should be transported. Do you have any suggestions?

BASE MD: That's copied. This guy took enough Tylenol® to kill his liver. You tell this guy, that if he will not cooperate, we will tie him down onto the stretcher, intubate, and paralyze him.

(At this point, the patient, who overheard the physician's comments, became extremely violent.)

DISCUSSION

The physician must remember that the patient and family members can often hear the communications between the physician and field team. Occasionally, this can be an advantage when attempting to convince patients to comply with the field team's treatment plan. In this scenario however, the physician's conversation actually put the field team at risk for serious injury. Communications with the field providers must be held in a professional manner, keeping in mind that others may be listening.

PART 2: INTERPERSONAL ASPECTS OF MEDICAL COMMAND COMMUNICATIONS

References to physician medical command communications often involve only the equipment or technical aspects of radio communications. However, in the high-pressure environment of prehospital EMS, a physician must be well-versed in the personal aspects of medical communications. This will ensure that the patient, physician, and field provider all receive appropriate consideration and support throughout the prehospital call.

Understanding the Prehospital Environment

The medical command physician must understand the prehospital care environment to fully understand and appreciate all associated communications and emotional aspects involved in the execution of each call.

It is very difficult for a base station physician to supervise an individual unless he or she is aware of the working environment. The plant manager of a large manufacturing plant would be hard pressed to evaluate the performance of an assembly line employee if he or she was never in that person's work area of the plant. Likewise, it is difficult for a physician to appreciate the work environment of prehospital personnel if he or she has never been there. The physician must know the prehospital environment to understand that there are often very legitimate reasons why the crew "is taking so long in the field."

Having to render ALS care in the middle of a noisy wedding reception, with three physicians from "out-of-town" in attendance, and trying to receive orders from a medical command physician over a portable radio, are challenges that should be experienced first hand by a base station physician. Physicians who provide medical command to prehospital personnel should spend at least one tour of duty with the most active ALS unit in their system to experience the focus areas and issues discussed throughout this chapter.

Environmental Factors

The Patient

The patient seen in the prehospital environment will often present challenges to the field provider that are seldom experienced by an emergency department physician. The patient with chest pain who is pale and diaphoretic but "denying" his symptoms takes on a new slant in the upper seats of bleachers at a professional football game, during midnight mass in St. Peter's Cathedral, or in the middle of the main dining room at an exclusive restaurant.

Field personnel frequently must attempt to convince the patient that he or she presents indications that a medical problem exists and should be evaluated at a hospital. If a crew exhausts their ability to convince that patient that he or she should be seen in a hospital, they will often call the Command Physician for "advice".

As referenced earlier, the base station physician must remember that the patient can often hear the physician's voice over the on-scene radio system. A paramedic will frequently say,

> "Doctor, I am with a 67-year-old male who is within close range of my radio system..."

to hint to the physician that some carefully worded radio statements would be helpful to him or her.

This potential for the patient to overhear the physician therefore becomes a powerful tool that can be used to assist the crew in convincing the patient to go to an emergency department. Helpful radio statements include—

> "I would like you to inform this patient that his symptoms indicate potential cardiac problems that should be seen immediately in an emergency department. If he refuses to go, be sure that he and his family fully understand the serious consequences of his decision."

> "I believe this gentleman should be seen in an emergency department. It is unlikely that he is experiencing "indigestion" at 6:00 in the morning after a full night's sleep."

Patient Location and Weather Conditions

Patient location, inclement weather, or rush hour traffic may delay treatment or transport of the patient to a hospital. These external factors must be understood by the base station physician to appreciate transportation delays that must not modify the treatment regimen for a particular patient. Ingenious command physicians avoid analgesic agents in critically injured multiple trauma patients in the field.

However, a crew working on a severely injured patient under a tractor-trailer at the bottom of a 50-foot embankment may request patient analgesia to assist with extrication. Normally the command physician may not want to have one administered to a prehospital trauma patient.

If a crew presents the base station physician with a patient whose hand is trapped in a piece of farm machinery and they appear to not know how to extract the hand from the machinery, the physician may be called upon to serve as an "air traffic controller" for the incident. In this capacity, the physician might offer suggestions to the crew about analgesia and sedation.

In cold winter environments, the base station physician must understand that there will be delays experienced while crews cut away clothing and obtain vital signs on patients that are hypothermic and riding in ambulance vehicles that are bouncing on heavy tire chains.

Family and Bystanders

A base station physician must realize that his or her voice is being transmitted over radio waves that will often be overheard clearly by bystanders, friends, and relatives. Therefore, words must be chosen carefully for general etiquette and medicolegal reasons. Imagine the impression that is imprinted in the minds of the patient's wife or son if they hear the base station physician order the ALS crew to "ZAP HIM AGAIN" or "DUMP IN AS MUCH EPI AS YOU CAN."

Even though the base station physician is frequently confronted with patients who have been "down in excess of 30 minutes" or have been "worked for over an hour," it is inappropriate and unprofessional to tell a crew over the radio:

> "I think you're wasting your time"
> or
> "I think this guy's heart has had it."

Families will remember and have more respect for the physician if professional statements are made to the crew like,

> "I believe we have done everything we can for this patient in the field, it's time to begin transport to the emergency department."

"Oh - By the Way" Communications

Base station physicians occasionally receive last minute "jewels" of information from field personnel that would have been nice to have known earlier into the call to better prepare the emergency department. In the heat of the moment, field personnel often forget to tell the physician that the patient is a United States Senator, is submerged in 3 inches of beer under a beer truck, or has been laying in cow manure under a farm tractor for 45 minutes.

After things have settled down in the emergency department, the physician should take the crew aside or have them call him or her later if they transported the patient to another facility and remind them that those "little details" are often important to prepare a busy emergency department or the public relations department of the hospital.

Presentation of a Living Will

One of the most difficult radio command calls handled by base station physicians is "living will" or "do not resuscitate" cases. The paramedic on the scene often gets caught between the wishes of the patient, family members, and his or her gut instinct to treat the patient's condition. The base station physician is once again called upon to filter all information and present a professionally worded position on what should be done for the patient.

The base station physician must consider all medical, legal, and emotional aspects of the case. The patient's legal and first-hand wishes must be considered, along with the emotional feelings of the crew trapped in the middle. (see Chapters 19 and 20).

Crime Scenes and Cases Involving Weapons

Whenever weapons are involved or the EMS crew is working at a crime scene, the base station physician must understand that the crew may have to alter normal procedures to administer care on the patients involved.

Police officers at the scene of a victim with a gunshot wound to the head may be confused as to whether the individual was shot by an intruder or shot himself in an attempt to commit suicide. The police might innocently tell the EMS crew to leave the patient alone because it is a crime scene and the patient is "beyond help." However, the crew may report to the base station physician that the

patient presents them with rapid pulses, a diminishing blood pressure, and irregular respirations.

The base station physician can be most helpful in these situations by supporting the EMS crew's efforts at resuscitation.

Other Physicians On-Scene

It is not uncommon for physicians to intervene at the scene of cardiac arrests that occur at wedding receptions, auto accidents involving entrapments, and mass casualty scenes. It is the nature of their business to intervene in life-threatening cases.

While orders emotionally barked at field personnel at a scene are usually appropriate or well-intended, these Good Samaritan physicians are not always aware of the crew's prehospital treatment protocols, the state laws that govern prehospital personnel, or the ambulance service's operating procedures. Nor are many physicians willing to accompany the patient to the hospital after they have given on-scene orders. The base station physician must also be aware that ALS personnel are also frequently confronted at the scene by psychiatrists, veterinarians, and dentists who announce themselves only as Doctors.

The base station physician will usually be told by the field crew that,

> "there is a Doctor (...XYZ) on the scene requesting that we follow his (or her) orders..."

The crew will be seeking the base station physician's advice on how to proceed. Usually, the base station physician will recommend one of the following courses of action:

- If the physician is known to the crew or the base station physician, the crew may be permitted to accept the on-scene orders, as long as they are in line with the field provider's treatment protocols. (Many states or regions also require the on-scene physician to accompany the patient to the hospital.)
- If the physician is unknown to the crew or base station physician, the base station physician will have the crew tell the physician that they are "sorry but they are required to follow the orders of their base station physician."
- If the on-scene physician becomes uncooperative or persists in disrupting the scene, the base station physician should ask to speak directly to the physician via radio or telephone.

Protocol Requirements vs Command Physician Demands

Field personnel will sometimes question or "challenge" a base station physician's orders because they feel the orders are not in compliance with their prehospital ALS protocols. Field providers may forget that prehospital protocols are meant to serve as guidelines to be followed by field providers in the event of radio failure or under other adverse situations, but the base station physician is allowed to augment or modify the protocols when it is in the best interest of patient care.

This issue can usually be resolved by the base station physician simply telling the field provider that he or she realizes his or her orders differ from their protocols but feels "XYZ" is indicated for proper treatment of the patient under these circumstances.

The Tape Recorder Can be Your Friend

Whenever possible, conduct base station activities over a tape recorded means of communications. Most communications centers have the ability to patch radio, telephone, and cellular communications through a tape or digital recorder. This ensures that physician orders and conversations with field personnel are maintained for later recovery and backup.

In addition, these cases can be retrieved and reviewed for quality improvement or continuing education purposes. Using a tape from a "good call" at a continuing education session not only reinforces proper procedures but also gives proper credit and praise to the EMS crew that managed the incident.

Most communications centers maintain tapes for at least 30 days, at which time they are reused throughout the next 30-day cycle. Therefore, if a physician desires to have a call or conversation retrieved or saved for later review, the appropriate communications supervisor or EMS system manager must be contacted as soon as possible after that call. Physicians should specify the date and time of the incident whenever requesting a tape excerpt.

Using Indirect Means to Recontact ALS Crews

If a base station physician is unable to reach an EMS crew with whom he or she has already been in contact, the physician can call that service's communications center and request that the ALS unit be alerted to recontact him or her. The physician should provide the unit number or paramedic's name to the communications center for reference when attempting to contact a unit in this manner.

A physician can often find out more specific information about a serious situation or major incident by contacting the ALS unit's communications center during the early stages of a serious call. Keep in mind that a crew may be too busy to chat with the base station physician during a hostage situation where gunfire is being exchanged or a bus accident where triage is underway.

It is very important that base station physicians realize that communications centers become inundated with telephone and radio traffic during major incidents and may also have other high-pressure calls underway at the same time the physician is calling. The physician may be asked to hold on the line or call back at a later time.

Physicians should not start their conversation saying,

"This is Doctor ....., what the hell is going on out at the scene?"
or
"Hey, this is Doctor....., I'm waiting for an update from..."

Physicians should understand and appreciate the high-pressure environment in which the communications center staff operate and approach them in a professional manner:

"Hi, this is Doctor....., I realize you are busy, but I need to speak to paramedic.... to give him further orders, could you get in contact with him for me and have him re-contact me?"

"Hi, this is Doctor....., I realize you are busy, but I need to hear an update on what's happening at the scene of that accident on the Interstate. Can you fill me in on what's going on out at the scene on Interstate 80?"

Communications center personnel are often the unrecognized heroes during a major incident. They will react positively if the base station physician recognizes them as key players in the incident and expresses an interest in tapping their brains about the particulars of the incident. However, physicians must remember and respect that the communications center staff may not have the staffing or time available to speak to them at the moment they call, and the communications center may have to call the emergency department back later when they get a free minute.

Controversies and Pitfalls

Field providers having problems carrying out care in the field, or exhibiting skill deficiencies, may use statements to rationalize care provided (or withheld). Examples include—

> "Doctor, the patient has no veins..."
>
> "Doctor, I'm having trouble reading you over the radio..."
>
> "Doctor, I don't think the patient will tolerate endotracheal intubation at this time..."
>
> "The patient is in symptomatic SVT but does not want to have ALS rendered to him through cardioversion"

The base station physician must try to determine the underlying reason for treatment difficulties and take appropriate action. If real radio equipment problems are presented, the physician should have the field unit or their communications center attempt to arrange for an alternate means of command linkage.

If the base station physician believes the field provider is nervous or concerned about a particular procedure, encouraging and coaching the provider can be helpful in getting him or her to relax and complete the necessary skills or treatment.

Some suggestions to counter the statements presented are—

> "I would like you to take your time and evaluate both arms for an acceptable IV site..."
>
> "If your radio is not functioning and you are still at the patient's home, contact me via telephone..."
>
> "Try an oropharyngeal airway. If your patient is breathing and can tolerate an oropharyngeal airway, you can attempt oral or nasal intubation."
>
> "If your patient is that unstable and in need of cardioversion, you must proceed with the procedure as ordered. Administer 5 mg of valium and prepare the patient for cardioversion."

If the reasons for difficulty in treating the patient in the field are unclear, the physician should evaluate the patient's actual condition upon arrival in the emergency department and take the time then, or at a later time, to discuss the situation with the field provider. If the physician feels additional evaluation or retraining is necessary, he or she should follow appropriate channels to ensure it is carried out so that the problem does not continue or accelerate. The physician may need to contact an ambulance service supervisor or medical director if the problem is not resolved to his or her satisfaction or is deemed serious in nature.

"Reading" the Crew's Emotional Status

A base station physician can often sense problems that are occurring in the prehospital arena by reading the emotional tone of the field provider's voice over the radio system. Occasionally, a paramedic will start out the radio conversation screaming or out of breath. This should alert the physician that this call needs priority attention.

Additionally, the physician may need to calm the paramedic and talk him or her through a difficult situation. Physicians should not talk down to the paramedic like a child who is in trouble, but rather like a teacher trying to guide a student. Physicians can gain control of a situation and put a paramedic back onto the right track by presenting medical orders in a firm but understanding manner similar to the following statements:

> "I want you to check both antecubital areas..."
>
> "Prepare for needle decompression. Select the midclavicular line, between the second and third intercostal space. Then make sure you insert your 16 gauge catheter on top of the third rib."

Remember that the emotions do not end with the crew's arrival at the hospital. Look at the crew's eyes, facial expressions, clothing, and demeanor when they arrive in the emergency department to get a sense of how emotionally involved they were in the call and how much they were operating on overdrive.

It may be necessary to take the crew aside after the storm has settled in the emergency department and afford them the opportunity to release their emotions, frustrations, or concerns. This helps relieve built-up stress and gives the physician the opportunity to make a few refinement points about treatment issues or techniques.

A physician should not miss this important opportunity to show the EMS crew that he or she cares about their work and realizes the pressures under which they work.

Receiving the Bedside Report from the Crew

The bedside patient report provided by field providers is an important part of the EMS system chain of events for every call.

Field providers are taught that they should not leave the emergency department until they "give report" to a physician or nurse relative to the patient's past and present medical history, as well as the care they rendered to the patient. When an EMS crew is ignored upon their arrival in an emergency department, they often feel as though their dedication and sincere efforts to positively impact patient care were not appreciated.

Base station command physicians should take the time to receive this important information or ensure that another staff member listens to the report with genuine interest.

It is also important that emergency department personnel understand why certain prehospital equipment and devices like automatic ventilators or vacuum splints were placed on the patient in the field. Physicians should not allow hospital personnel to remove equipment without understanding the crew's rationale for its use and being aware of the proper way to disengage or remove the item.

After the bedside report is given and the patient is being managed by the emergency department staff, the base station physician should take the ALS personnel aside, out of hearing range of the patient and other personnel not involved in the case, to discuss the case. The physician should also present any compliments or concerns he or she has relative to the care of the patient, radio report provided during the case, or information provided during the bedside report.

This is a great time for the physician to explain to the crew why he or she was so short with them over the radio (14 patients were backed up in the department), or why he or she did not order Lidocaine when the crew reported frequent PVCs with a bradycardic patient. The base station physician should also take this prime opportunity to briefly educate the crew about their patient's condition and what he for she feels could or should have been done differently.

SUMMARY

This chapter attempts to point out the complexity and importance of the interpersonal aspects of ALS communications, in addition to the technical and equipment aspects.

Being a good base station physician takes more than just being a good clinician. A good base station physician has to be able to simultaneously juggle the roles of a physician, air traffic controller, parent, and counselor to see each out of hospital mission through to a successful conclusion.

SAMPLE CASES

CASE #1

Paramedics have contacted command requesting orders for a 68-year-old male at a shopping mall complaining of palpitations. Medics note that this gentleman has a history of cardiac disease and was recently discharged from the hospital with an MI. He has been complaining of palpitations for the last 15 minutes along with moderate shortness of breath and chest discomfort. He is described as a diaphoretic male in mild-to-moderate distress with vital signs, pulse 160, respirations 18, BP 70/palp. His lungs have rales at the bases, and JVD is present. The monitor shows a regular rhythm, wide complex tachycardia.

The medics state that they realize their treatment protocols state this patient should be cardioverted, however, he "looks too good." They are requesting to just initiate a KVO line of D_5W and transport to the hospital. The patient is on their stretcher, they are moving to their truck and have a rolling time of 25 minutes to the hospital.

How would you proceed?

This patient is in a symptomatic wide complex tachycardia, most likely ventricular in nature. The paramedics are obviously reluctant to cardiovert this patient. Clearly, this patient would benefit from immediate cardioversion and it is up to the command physician to identify why the paramedics are reluctant. It is not uncommon for paramedics to be reluctant to perform invasive procedures on an awake patient. The field providers may be unclear on how to perform synchronized cardioversion since it is a relatively rare prehospital care procedure.

The command physician should emphasize to the paramedics that this symptomatic patient is most likely in ventricular tachycardia and requires cardioversion. Since the patient is already on the medic's stretcher, it would not be unreasonable to allow the medics to delay cardioversion briefly until the patient was moved to a semi-private area or to their truck if it was in close proximity. Once in a suitable location, the command physician could walk the field providers through the steps of cardioversion (i.e., adjusting the defibrillators' energy setting, pushing the synchronize button, holding the paddles in place, until the unit fired, etc.).

CASE #2

Paramedics call and state they are on the scene with a 22-year-old printing press operator who has become entangled in a piece of machinery. They note that the patient's right hand, wrist, and forearm have become entrapped in the printing press. The medics believe they will be able to disassemble the press and extricate the patient. However, this process may take 30 minutes. They note that the patient screams and thrashes about any time they try to loosen the machinery. They are calling medical command for advice. The patient has no significant past medical history, relates no allergies, is awake, alert, and oriented.

How would you proceed?

With adequate monitoring, this patient would benefit from analgesia and sedation. Unfortunately the prehospital care armamentaria is limited, however, most ALS field providers carry a narcotic and a benzodiazepine derivative. For this patient, the field providers could be instructed to initiate a large bore line in the unaffected arm and could be given orders to titrate appropriate doses of morphine and valium to provide adequate analgesia and sedation while maintaining the patient's level of consciousness and vital signs within defined parameters.

CASE #3

Paramedics are called to the office of a 64-year-old lawyer who has suffered several witnessed syncopal episodes during the day. The lawyer's secretary notes that he has passed out three times today and during the last event, which lasted approximately 15 minutes, the secretary was not sure if he was breathing. The paramedics state that although their physical exam was unremarkable and the patient's vital signs are stable, they have requested that the patient be transported to the hospital, however, he refuses. Paramedics called command requesting your advice.

How would you proceed?

Clearly, this is a difficult situation that would be very difficult to handle via the radio. Since the paramedics are in the lawyer's office, a conversation via telephone might be more appropriate. Ideally, this conversation could occur over a recorded phone line. The command physician could request that the field providers call the base station to discuss the case over the phone. In addition, the command physician could talk directly to the patient over the telephone to clearly identify the potential risk of not going to the hospital.

3

State of the Art ALS Procedures

Among the most controversial issues in EMS are those related to which procedures an EMT or paramedic (EMT-P) should be authorized to perform and the situations in which those procedures are indicated. Although many municipalities provide an ALS response for their community, several authors have questioned the value of the procedures that are performed.[1-7] However, other authors have shown that ALS procedures have definite advantages.[8-15] One of the major problems in trying to define appropriate procedures to be done in the field is that there are over two dozen levels of prehospital providers defined by the different state laws in this country. The new DOT EMT-Basic curriculum authorizes basic EMTs (EMT-B) to perform some advanced skills, such as endotracheal intubation and assisting patients in the administration of epinephrine for allergic reactions or with inhalation treatments for bronchospasm.[16] In addition, although states may allow a wide range of procedures in the prehospital arena, most medical directors significantly limit the procedures available to the providers in their system. Some medical directors seem reluctant to authorize even a simple IV, while others encourage an aggressive approach including paralysis for intubation and surgical airways. What skills should an EMS system use? This question has never been well studied. With more direct physician supervision, the opportunity exists to tailor the system to the local needs, without regard to artificially described levels. The medical director should consider the needs of the patients, the skills of the paramedics, the cost of training and equipment, and the likelihood of success within the individual system. This chapter provides some guidance and background regarding the selection of procedures currently available.

The procedures a medical director authorizes must be related to the individual region.[17] Considerations here include the patient mix, travel times, and the availability of backup services. A service that treats a high volume of urban trauma might place greater emphasis on immobilization and airway control and minimize time spent on the scene. Rural systems may require procedures that would be precluded by the short transport times of a municipal system. The availability of backup is another consideration.

DAVID P. THOMSON, MS, MD, FACEP

In a rural setting, the nearest hospital may not be equipped, either in staffing or facilities, to care for a severely injured patient.[18] Although air-medical services have alleviated some of this problem, they are not always available. The rural EMT will need the training and authorization to perform highly "advanced" procedures if he or she is to have any hope of keeping certain patients alive until he or she can transport the patient to an appropriate facility.[19]

The difference between ALS and BLS providers is primarily in the procedures they are allowed to perform. Each state has developed its own terminology corresponding to advanced-, intermediate-, and basic-level providers. Within each of these categories are often several subgroups of providers. Even within a state or region there may be little uniformity in which procedures are authorized. A basic unit in one region may be authorized to perform some procedure that advanced units in another area are prohibited from using. There is frequently little correlation between the needs of the local region and the level of training of the paramedics serving there. This chapter will use the generic term EMT to refer to any prehospital care provider capable of performing ALS procedures.

Two myths seem to guide this decision: ALS is more expensive and a high call volume is necessary to maintain ALS skills. The idea that more advanced procedures should cost significantly more appeals to intuition, but investigation proves this incorrect. Ornato et al. performed a brief analysis of the cost differential between a mixed BLS/ALS system and an all ALS system.[20] In their system, there was a difference of only $2.88 per run! This analysis did not factor in any increased risk of litigation in a mixed or BLS-only system, nor did it evaluate the potential savings in hospital costs that early intervention may provide. In the West German EMS system, which uses physicians to provide prehospital care, it was estimated that early intervention with trauma patients in one region alone saved $28 million yearly due to prevention of death, $15.5 million due to preventing disability, and $800,000 yearly in ICU costs.[15] For this last figure it is important to note that they estimated an ICU charge of $160 per day. This is ten to twenty times less than the cost of an ICU bed in most U.S. hospitals. While to some it is evident that providing ALS in the field is cost effective, we have only recently begun to look at the cost effectiveness of the individual procedures. Garrison has done an excellent job of looking at the cost effectiveness of pediatric intraosseous infusion, providing a solid model for systems to use when assessing cost-benefit ratios.[21] As health-care funds become tighter and the number of prehospital modalities expands, medical directors will need to show that the therapies chosen are cost effective. Certainly costs of providing ALS must consider the initial cost difference involved in training and skill maintenance.

Skill retention has been cited as a reason for not permitting rural and suburban paramedics to perform some ALS procedures. In 1977, Skelton and McSwain looked at skill degradation among Kansas City EMT-paramedics.[22] Their results indicated that the basic skills of short board immobilization and Hare traction splint application degraded at a faster rate than the "advanced" skills of intubation and IV access. They suggested that this was an effect of a continuing education program that placed an increased emphasis on the advanced skills. An investigation of English ambulance staff concluded that, regardless of the effectiveness of the training, skill retention can only be ensured by providing an adequate monitoring system.[23] The skills taught in the Basic Trauma Life Support (BTLS) course degrade with time, in spite of frequent field experience with trauma patients.[24] Regardless of the technical difficulty of the procedure or the setting in which it is performed, skill maintenance among prehospital care providers requires careful education and ongoing quality assurance. If these are provided, the overall frequency of performance of a procedure for the individual provider becomes largely irrelevant.

The comments of McSwain and Pepe regarding endotracheal intubation provide some insight into the role of the medical director regarding procedures: "prehospital personnel with *inadequate training and inadequate supervision* should not use the ET tube."[25] "Key to predictable success in the performance of endotracheal tube placement is the *quality of initial training, the frequency of performance, and the close scrutiny by supervisors expert in emergency* endotracheal intubation techniques."[26] Medical directors who cannot ensure this sort of supervision should seriously reconsider their role.

Patient Assessment Procedures

The most fundamental procedures a prehospital care provider performs are those related to patient assessment. These skills are often afforded relatively little time in the initial training of health-care providers, and it is a rare system that reviews these skills in a rigorous fashion. Yet these procedures are the cornerstone of any treatment.

History and Physical Assessment

The prehospital care provider must be able to gather a concise and accurate history and physical in a minimal amount of time. This provides the basis for any treatment rendered in the field and may help guide the treatment in the emergency department. The need to rapidly assess and treat trauma victims has been the impetus for the creation of the BTLS and Pre-Hospital Trauma Life Support (PHTLS) courses, but the assessment principles taught in these courses may be applied to any patient, regardless of the illness. When used for all patients, these assessment procedures ensure that the information needed to provide good patient care is gathered. BTLS and PHTLS help direct the EMT to the critical problems, which are frequently overlooked in a less systematic evaluation. EMTs should be encouraged to use these tools as part of their assessment of every patient they see.

Vital Signs

EMTs are expected to take vital signs on every patient they care for. As with every procedure, though, vital sign assessment should have an indication and a proper sequence. BTLS has placed the vital sign assessment in the secondary survey, where it will not interfere with the identification and treatment of life-threatening problems. In patients without obvious life-threatening problems, vital signs are thought to help unmask a previously hidden injury.

Although vital signs are expected to be taken with each patient encounter, often they are not obtained. Spaite et al. prospectively studied the frequency with which vital signs were omitted.[27] Even with an observer present, blood pressure or pulse were not taken in 37% of patients. While this was an urban study, and it could be argued that short transport times precluded vital sign assessment in some cases, Moss has reviewed the data for nonurban areas of Arizona.[28] He found that optically scanned charts were missing either systolic blood pressure, diastolic blood pressure, pulse rate, or respiratory rate between 15%-18% of the time. Many of these transports involved long distances, which should have provided the paramedics adequate time to assess vital signs. A study of the Los Angeles County system showed that as patient age

decreased, so did the frequency of vital sign assessment.[29] Vital signs were rarely obtained on patients less than 2 years old. The EMTs surveyed felt significantly less confident in their ability to assess vital signs in the pediatric age group than in their ability with adults.

In 1978, Cayten attempted to look at the ability of basic EMTs, paramedics, and emergency department nurses to correctly assess a variety of physical parameters.[30] Their research showed that there was consistent error by all groups, with systolic blood pressures being most accurately assessed. Diastolic blood pressure readings taken by the EMTs and paramedics were accurate only 54% of the time. They note that there was significant error among the nursing personnel and that the level of training of both the nurses (which included registered, graduate, and licensed practical nurses) and the EMTs did not affect the performance. Although they tried to set tolerance limits for errors that would reflect clinical significance, they suggest that perhaps the accuracy they demanded is not necessary in emergency care. Another source of error may be related to the tools one uses. One paper has noted that a significant number of ambulance sphygmomanometers are inaccurate.[31] Medical directors must provide methods to ensure the accuracy of these measurements as part of their quality management plan. These plans must address both the equipment and the skills involved.

A recent study using a standardized blood pressure model showed a very large difference in the accuracy of blood pressures obtained in a quiet environment versus a moving ambulance.[32] Thus it must always be remembered that in treating patients there may be a significant error in the vital signs as relayed by the EMT, particularly in a moving ambulance.

No one has ever looked at the specific utility of the various measures that are obtained in the field. Until this research is performed, medical directors should insist that EMTs attempt to obtain the pulse, blood pressure, and respiration of every patient and repeat these readings as frequently as the clinical situation warrants or allows. Although the individual reading may in itself be less than perfectly accurate, development of a trend may help guide the course of treatment.

Most systems also use some rating scales to rank the case severity. These rating scales can take on major importance for an EMS system because they often form the basis for decisions about destination hospitals and the mode of transport. Because these measures have subjective components, medical directors must clearly define the terms and ensure that their personnel understand the parameter being assessed. In Cayten's study, he noted better than 95% agreement in assessing level of consciousness.[30] Menegazzi has found excellent agreement between paramedics and emergency physicians in assessing patients with the Glasgow Coma Scale[33], a commonly used rating tool. Similar studies have been conducted on global case severity rating systems.[34] Although the nature of these overall ratings requires more subjective judgment, the authors found excellent reliability. Although some may view these types of numerical ratings as research tools, the ability to support a triage decision with a concise number may help the medical director in both the political and medico-legal arenas if questions arise.

Airway Management

Effective management of the patient's airway is the most essential skill in the care for critically ill and injured patients. Many devices are available for field airway care; however, few were thoroughly investigated before use in prehospital care.

Supplemental Oxygen Administration

The nasal cannula and oxygen mask have long been accepted as part of the repertoire of the EMT-B. Oxygen administration is frequently considered a benign procedure, and many services provide some form of supplemental oxygen to all of their patients. The standard teaching for EMTs was expressed by Nancy Caroline: "When in doubt, give oxygen."[35]

While oxygen is freely dispensed by many BLS providers, not to mention athletic teams, it should be viewed as a drug. Although it has an extremely high therapeutic-to-toxic ratio, its use should be supervised. As most third year medical students will tell you, giving oxygen to a COPD patient who is dependent of hypoxic drive may result in apnea. However, too often paramedics err on the side of hypoxia in these patients, which may produce ischemia and other serious side effects.

Oxygen serves to promote combustion, and in an environment surrounded by gasoline, diesel, or jet fuel, increases the risk of fire. The fittings of tanks can be sheared off, turning the body of the tank into a projectile. These risks can be minimized by ensuring that the tanks are secured properly. Finally, the cost of administering a

medication unnecessarily should be factored into this decision. This needs to include both the cost of the drug (oxygen) and the materials to administer it (cannula or mask). Written protocols and medical command help eliminate unnecessary oxygen use.

As a practical matter, the determination of hypoxia in the field historically has been difficult, prompting Dr. Caroline's statement. In spite of all the hazards listed above, unless the service has access to pulse oximetry (see page 40), oxygen administration for most patients is still the safest practice. In patients with a history of COPD, the protocol should encourage incremental increases in oxygen supplementation, rather than immediate high flow oxygen. If the paramedic finds that the patient loses respiratory drive, he or she should be prepared to assist ventilation. Protocols may be devised that restrict oxygen use in otherwise healthy individuals without systemic involvement, but medical directors should err on the side of supplemental oxygen whenever there is any question, particularly if pulse oximetry is not available.

Aiding Ventilation

The Bag-Valve-Mask

Classically, prehospital care providers have been taught to use the bag-valve-mask, which was felt to provide an improvement over mouth-to-mouth ventilation by allowing supplemental oxygenation. This technique was borrowed from the operating room, where it had met with great success. The primary problem that anesthesiologists found was gastric insufflation, which they solved in the operating room by the use of cricoid pressure (Sellick maneuver). Unfortunately, the application of the bag-valve-mask in the moving ambulance has brought less satisfactory results.[36,37] In the operating room the most common use of the bag-valve-mask is preoxygenation before intubation. It is not routinely used for more than a few minutes in this setting. For many "basic" systems, the bag-valve-mask is the only device available for assisting ventilation. As such, it is often used for long periods. When used by a single rescuer in the back of a moving ambulance, the actual volume delivered to the patient may be small. This is because the bag-valve-mask requires the provider to perform an airway maneuver and mask seal with one hand, while squeezing the bag with the other hand. Significant volumes may be lost from around the mask. When a resuscitation bag is squeezed with one hand, the volume may be as small as 500 cc.[38] Several authors have suggested that two providers be used whenever bag-valve-mask ventilation is attempted, one to provide the airway maneuver and mask seal and another to squeeze the bag.[34,39] The new EMT curriculum recommends that this is ideally a two-person procedure and with only one basic EMT managing the airway that the order of priority of airway management is 1) mouth-to-mask, 2) two-person bag-valve-mask, 3) flow-restricted oxygen powered ventilation device, and finally 4) one-person bag-valve-mask ventilation.[40] When combined with an additional crew member to perform chest compressions, this can lead to a very tight fit in an ambulance. Unfortunately, many EMS systems budget for only one patient caregiver in the back of the ambulance, with that person frequently feeling like a "one-armed paperhanger."

Mask design and size may have a significant impact on the ability to ventilate the patient.[41-43] Facial trauma, dentition, and congenital anomalies may all present problems for the prehospital rescuer who attempts to ventilate a patient with a bag-valve-mask. Some paramedics have abandoned the bag-valve-mask in favor of using a bag with the EOA™, but studies do not support this practice.[44] An investigation by Rhee demonstrated that the bag-valve-mask, combined with aggressive management of secretions, can provide an adequate airway for patients whose mental status is slightly depressed but not sufficiently so as to allow direct endotracheal intubation.[45] This suggests that the EOA™ provides no advantage over the bag-valve-mask in the management of airway secretions.

Oxygen content of the bag-valve-mask may vary, depending on the ventilatory frequency and the reservoir used. To ensure an FiO_2 level of 1.0, the bag must have a reservoir consisting of either a demand valve or a 2.5 liter reservoir (for a 1500 cc adult bag).[46] Other reservoirs, such as tubes, may provide significantly lower FiO_2 levels.

The Demand Valve

Some systems allow the use of a demand valve, or oxygen powered resuscitator. This device connects directly to the oxygen tank and allows the paramedic to deliver a breath by pressing a trigger. Since it is actuated by a finger, it allows the paramedic to use both hands to provide the airway maneuver and seal, while delivering the breath with only one finger. This solves the problem of ensuring volume delivery but deprives the rescuer of any sense of lung compliance. Many of these devices have a pressure relief valve, which may provide some protection against barotrauma, although studies proving this are lacking.

Mouth-to-Mask Ventilation

In an effort to devise a simple compromise between mouth-to-mouth and bag-valve-mask ventilation, mouth-to-mask ventilation was invented. This procedure allows the use of supplemental oxygen by connecting a tube to the mask. It prevents direct rescuer-to-patient contact, which can be important for both aesthetic[47] and infection control reasons.[48] Because no additional hands are needed to squeeze the resuscitation bag, both hands can be used to effect the airway maneuver and mask seal. The use of the rescuer's lungs to power the device allows larger tidal volumes to be delivered[37], and the rescuer may be able to overcome decreases in compliance by exerting greater force with his or her breathing. Unfortunately, greater gastric insufflation occurs with increases in airway pressures[49], potentially increasing the risk of regurgitation and aspiration. Because expired air is used to drive the ventilation, it is impossible to achieve 100% oxygen concentrations, but concentrations up to 50% may be possible.[50]

In a study using infant mannequins, Terndrup and Warner demonstrated that use of mouth-to-mask ventilation in this age group has significant advantages over the mouth-to-mouth or bag-valve-mask methods.[51] They found that there were higher peak airway pressures using pediatric bags. When they used a pediatric bag, the FiO_2 level was 0.8 at a flow rate of 10 liters per minute. With the mouth-to-mask technique, they achieved an FiO_2 level of 0.9.

Recent concerns regarding infections, especially with HIV, have led to increased awareness of these devices as a substitute for mouth-to-mouth ventilation. A variety of devices are now available, including both masks and foil sheets. The former have the advantage of distancing the patient from the rescuer, while the latter have been made small enough to attach to a key chain. In spite of their small size, the foils appear to provide good protection, so long as care is taken to avoid cutting them with the patient's or rescuer's teeth.[52] Medical directors may wish to recommend these devices for those individuals who may need to respond while off duty.

Procedures for Active Airway Management

The gold standard for airway management has long been the endotracheal tube. Because this device has traditionally been reserved for physicians, alternative airways, most

| Table 3-1 | Comparison of Airway Management Devices | | | | | |

Device	Difficulty of use	Likelihood of complications	Cost	Definitive treatment?	Medication administration	Pediatric use
BVM	++++	++	+	No	No	Yes
ET tube	+++	++	++	Yes	Yes	Yes
EOA™	++	++++	+++	No	No	No
PtL™	+	+++	++++	No	No	No
ETC	+	+++	++++	No	No	No

Difficulty of use: How difficult it would be for a single paramedic to initiate and maintain the airway.
Likelihood of complications: The possibility of hypoxia, airway trauma, aspiration, or unrecognized esophageal ventilation.
Cost: All these assume a resuscitation bag will be used.
Note: These ratings are subjective judgments of the author based on the information in the following text.

notably the Esophageal Obturator Airway (EOA™), Pharyngeal Tracheal Lumen (PtL™) airway, and the Esophageal Tracheal Combitube™ (ETC) have been advocated by some for prehospital airway management (Table 3-1).

Endotracheal Intubation

Endotracheal intubation is the optimal method of managing the unstable airway. Its use in prehospital care has been controversial, with proponents citing its efficacy and critics claiming that it is a difficult technical skill that should be reserved for highly trained physicians.

The endotracheal tube has many advantages. It isolates the airway from secretions or gastric contents. When connected to a bag-valve-mask, a prehospital care provider can supplement both the oxygenation and ventilation of a patient without having to worry about airway maneuvers. Gastric insufflation, a major problem in the patient who is being mask ventilated, is eliminated. If the patient has significant pulmonary pathology, positive end-expiratory pressure (PEEP) can be applied by way of the endotracheal tube, improving oxygenation in patients who might otherwise remain hypoxic. Medications can be administered through the endotracheal tube, providing a route when IV access is not possible. Endotracheal tubes are inexpensive, usually costing less than five dollars. The tube may be placed using several different techniques, which adds to its versatility in the prehospital setting.

When compared to the EOA™ and oropharyngeal airways, patients who received an endotracheal tube during prehospital cardiac arrest had an improved survival rate.[53] These patients also appeared to have good neurological recovery and experienced a quality of life similar to patients with coronary artery disease.

Criticism of endotracheal intubation by non-physicians in the prehospital setting has focused on the concern that it is a very difficult procedure, potentially fraught with complications. Stewart et al. looked at methods to train paramedics in endotracheal intubation.[54] Their study found that paramedics could be trained to intubate using a variety of methods, including operating room, mannequin, and animal laboratory experience. The success rates for field intubation ranged from 76%-92%, depending upon the seniority of the operator. This suggests that even if mannequins alone are used for training, paramedics can be taught to correctly intubate more than 75% of the time. Stratton et al. performed a similar study with like results.[55] In their study comparing endotracheal intubation to esophageal airways, Shea et al. found that training paramedics to perform endotracheal intubation took approximately 7 hours, while training with the EOA™ took 4 hours[56], an insignificant difference given the clear superiority of the endotracheal tube. In a study of skill retention by medical students who were trained in intubation as part of an ACLS course, 70% of students were able to successfully intubate 2 to 3 months after initial training, despite the lack of any reinforcement in the interim.[57] Finally, paramedics have been shown to be superior to physicians in performance of selected motor skills.[59] Clearly, the difficulty of this manual procedure has been greatly exaggerated.

Complications, primarily unrecognized esophageal intubation, have led some systems away from allowing their paramedics to intubate. The complication rate appears to vary greatly from system to system and is probably related to the protocol used for patient selection. In the Alameda County, California system, Pointer had a relatively high rate of unrecognized esophageal intubation, 5 in 383 attempts (1.3%).[60] Stewart demonstrated a rate of 0.4% for this complication[61], while Jacobs in Boston and Guss in San Diego had no complications.[62,63] In Stewart's study, he concluded that all of the unrecognized esophageal intubations resulted from protocol violations (inadequate auscultation of the lung fields and epigastrium). Pointer reached this same conclusion.

A review of methods for detecting esophageal intubation among anesthesia patients suggests that auscultation may be insufficient.[64] Birmingham et al. indicated that even with careful chest and epigastric auscultation, presumably performed in a quiet operating room, a significant rate of unrecognized esophageal intubations could occur. They noted in their introduction that this has been a significant cause for malpractice actions against anesthesia personnel. Their conclusion was that prevention of esophageal intubation requires capnometry, which will be discussed later.

Endobronchial tube placement, primarily in the right mainstem bronchus, is another potential hazard. Bissinger noted a 7% rate of endobronchial tube placement, with another 13% of emergency patients having endotracheal tubes positioned near the carina.[65] He recommended that tubes be placed to 21 cm in women and 23 cm in men and that tubes be shortened before placement. His series did not describe any actual harm that occurred from endobronchial tube placement, but several theoretical concerns were addressed.

Intubation of the pediatric population has been another area of concern. This was addressed by a study of the Fresno, California system, where a 64% success rate was seen.[66] The authors found, though, that intubation was attempted on only 67% of eligible patients. This may have been secondary to the EMT's lack of experience with intubation in general (it had only recently been authorized in this system) and with pediatric intubation in particular. Given that the bag-valve-mask and endotracheal tubes are the only available pediatric airways, and that most pediatric arrests have respiratory causes, clearly EMTs need to possess the skills and equipment to expertly manage children's airways.

Cervical spine movement during endotracheal intubation has always been a significant concern because many of the patients who require intubation are at high risk for cervical spine injuries. A recent study indicates intubation, regardless of technique, results in less cervical spine displacement than bag-valve-mask ventilation.[67]

Endotracheal intubation may mean the difference between adequate and inadequate care in the back of an ambulance. No other method of airway management will permit a single attendant to control ventilation, monitor lung compliance, remove secretions, prevent aspiration, and perform the myriad other tasks often asked of the lone patient attendant EMT. In air-medical transport, endotracheal intubation is especially critical, because the patient care crew is unable to monitor many of the signs that signal airway compromise, and it is not always possible to land to re-check the breath sounds or assess stridor.

In addition, in some rotor craft adequate space is not available to optimally perform endotracheal intubation while the patient is in flight.

Methods of Endotracheal Intubation

Several methods of endotracheal intubation are available; these include direct oral intubation, nasotracheal intubation, digital intubation, and lighted stylet intubation.

DIRECT ORAL INTUBATION (LARYNGOSCOPIC INTUBATION)

Direct oral intubation is the most common method of intubation. There are several advantages to this method of intubation: Because the operator sees the pathway of the endotracheal tube, placement is felt to be more sure, although some have questioned this reasoning.[57] Direct laryngoscopy allows the removal of any foreign bodies that may be obstructing the airway. This method also appears more efficient because the route is visualized and the tube placed without searching for the airway.

Disadvantages of this technique include the need for the patient to be able to tolerate the laryngoscope, which requires either sufficient depression of the mental status or pharmacological adjuncts. Trismus, not uncommon in the head-injured patient, also prevents this route of intubation. Although paralytic agents, such as succinylcholine, have been used by prehospital care providers[48,68], this practice is not common. Generally, the patient must be supine, which places significant limitations on the paramedic whose patients are not always conveniently positioned. Several authors have raised concerns regarding this intubation route in the patient with potential cervical spine injuries. The ATLS manual advocates oral endotracheal intubation with "in-line manual cervical immobilization" as the means to intubate apneic trauma patients, but only if they do not have maxillofacial injuries.[69] Bivins et al. feel that patients with potential cervical spine injuries should have their airway managed by either nasotracheal intubation or cricothyrotomy because of the risk of worsening an injury with manual traction and direct laryngoscopy.[70] Other authors have produced conflicting studies.[71,72] Walls encourages the use of oral endotracheal intubation in the trauma patient, but only if the technique can be performed in a "gentle... manner."[73] He suggests that the best method is probably rapid sequence induction using succinylcholine or rapid tranquilization. For those medical directors who feel uncomfortable having their paramedics use succinylcholine, sedation with an opioid (reversible with naloxone) or with a benzodiazepine (reversible with flumazenil) could be considered. Etomidate is a nonopioid, nonbarbiturate that is capable of inducing the rapid onset of hypnosis, allowing for intubation to be facilitated. Its major advantage is its lack of cardiovascular depression.[74,75] It is an agent that has many potentially useful properties for field use.

Probably the most realistic statement regarding this question was by Joyce, who warns that any airway maneuver may affect the cervical spine, no matter what modality is used.[76] Therefore in any patient with a potential cervical spine injury rescuers must aggressively manage the ABC's while paying as much attention as possible to minimizing cervical spine motion.

NASOTRACHEAL INTUBATION

Another commonly used route for tracheal intubation is by way of the nasal passages. This generally requires that the person have some respiratory effort to guide the tube into the trachea, although adjuncts, such as the flexible lighted stylet, may facilitate this route in the apneic patient.[77] It is ideal for the patient who cannot be placed recumbent, either because of entrapment or because of their clinical condition (e.g., congestive heart failure). Nasotracheal intubation is well-tolerated by the awake patient. Since it does not require jaw opening, the patient with trismus may be intubated without pharmacological adjuncts. Although there are no good models for teaching the technique, when prehospital personnel have not received specialized training in this modality it has still been applied with a low complication rate.[58]

In the Louisville EMS system, paramedics who had been trained in endotracheal intubation were authorized to perform nasotracheal intubation.[58] They achieved a 71% success rate with this intubation modality without receiving any hands-on training in humans before performing the procedure.

This success rate compares favorably with the 75%-98% success rates for direct oral intubation. Another study showed no difference in success rates between the orotracheal and nasotracheal routes.[78] Some authors feel the nasotracheal technique may involve less manipulation of the cervical spine than laryngoscopic intubation, concluding that nasotracheal intubation is the only non-surgical airway maneuver to use in blunt trauma victims.[61]

Concerns regarding this method of intubation have come from several areas. Passage of a tube through the nose tends to make the very friable mucosa bleed. Even if the nares are prepared with a vasoconstrictor and lubricant, bleeding may become a problem. Most adults can tolerate a tube larger than 4 mm, the minimum need for ventilation. Sinusitis has also been cited as a complication, but this is related to the duration of intubation. Should tube size or sinusitis become concerns, the tube can be replaced when the patient is stable in the hospital. There is considerable concern over perforation of the cribriform plate with subsequent intracranial placement[79], although the incidence of this appears to be exceedingly rare. Many caregivers have difficulty in locating the trachea, but use of the Endotrol™ directable tube or flexible lighted stylet may aid in this problem.

In the noise of the prehospital environment, it may be difficult to hear the breathing of the patient to help guide the tube. The bell of the stethoscope can be placed over the open tube to facilitate this. Commercial devices, such as the Beck Airway Airflow Monitor (BAAM™) (Great Plains Ballistics, Inc., Donaldsonville, LA) can also be used to amplify the breath sound.[80]

Because this technique is used only on spontaneously breathing patients, concerns regarding esophageal intubation should be minimal. End-tidal CO_2 detectors can be used to eliminate any shred of doubt.

DIGITAL INTUBATION

Digital intubation is the original method of endotracheal intubation. It is an excellent way to orally intubate the unresponsive patient who is entrapped or is otherwise in an awkward position for laryngoscopy.[81] When batteries fail, digital intubation may be the only method available. Like direct oral intubation the tube is placed under guidance, but unlike the laryngoscopic method, the landmarks are palpated, not seen. Because visualization is not necessary, this modality is useful when there are copious secretions or bleeding.

The primary disadvantage of the digital technique involves the risk one incurs when one places the fingers into another person's mouth. Of course, gloves should always be worn. A dental prod or mouth gag is used to keep the mouth open during the procedure. The prod should be used regardless of mental status in case the patient awakens during the procedure.

LIGHTED STYLET INTUBATION

A rigid stylet, tipped with a light, can be used to intubate a patient without laryngoscopy.[82] It has many of the advantages of the digital technique but is safer in that the operator need not reach into the patient's mouth. The paramedic holds the tip of the patient's tongue with a gauze square, thus opening the airway and raising the epiglottis. The endotracheal tube, with the stylet in place, is formed into a hockey-stick shape. It is inserted into the mouth and trachea by watching the passage of the light in the end of the stylet. This technique is best performed in a partially darkened room or ambulance, because bright sunlight may limit the ability of the operator to visualize the glow the stylet produces. This method offers the additional advantage that tube placement can be easily verified simply by reinserting the stylet.[83] The lighted stylet technique has also been described to assist nasotracheal intubation.[84,85]

Due to the diameter of the stylet, it can only be applied to patients able to tolerate tubes of more than 7 mm. No large studies have been reported yet from the prehospital environment, but the Laerdal Co. has just introduced a technologically advanced version of this device that may have field indications.

ESOPHAGEAL OBTURATOR AIRWAY (EOA™)/ ESOPHAGEAL GASTRIC TUBE AIRWAY (EGTA)

The EOA™ was first described by T.A. Don Michael in 1968.[86] The original design was invented for use in the coronary care unit. It was later refined and promoted primarily as a tool to allow prehospital personnel to control the airway when they are unable to provide endotracheal intubation.[87] It gained amazingly widespread use despite a dearth of clinical studies.

The American Heart Association classifies this technique as II b, which they define as "A therapeutic option that is not well established by evidence but may be helpful and probably not harmful."[88] The primary advantage of this device is that it allows the paramedic to ventilate the patient without being concerned over gastric distention or regurgitation. An improvement, the EGTA, features a lumen in the esophageal tube through which a nasogastric tube can be placed to evacuate the stomach. Advocates report blood gas results equivalent to those obtained with endotracheal intubation.[89-91] Several other authors agree that EOA™ are useful when the patient cannot be endotracheally intubated or if the patient has such copious gastric contents that aspiration is a hazard.[54,92,93]

Esophageal airways essentially are a bag-valve-mask with an obturator; as such, they suffer from some of the same problems as the bag-valve-mask. The operator must still provide both a mask seal and an airway maneuver, so ideally the device should be used with two paramedics to perform ventilation. It is difficult to effect a seal on edentulous patients[42], and its use is contraindicated in patients who are less than 15 years of age. Caustic ingestion or esophageal pathology are also contraindications to the use of this device. Esophageal perforation has been described[94], as has unrecognized tracheal intubation[95] and gastric rupture due to cuff failure.[96] Esophageal tube placement with an EOA™ has been suggested to help aid in endotracheal intubation, but Gatrell cites two instances where both the esophageal obturator and endotracheal tubes were placed in the esophagus, and this error was not recognized.[97]

Most of the studies mentioned thus far were performed in the hospital setting. In an early prehospital study, Schofferman found adequate blood gas levels in a series of 18 patients ventilated with the EOA™ by paramedics.[98] Twelve of these patients had a spontaneous supraventricular rhythm; six were undergoing CPR. The mean $PaCO_2$ level in the arrested patients was 62 mmHg, while those with a rhythm had a $PaCo_2$ level of 40 mmHg. The patients all underwent endotracheal intubation in the emergency department, and subsequent blood gas levels were obtained, but no comparisons were made. This is the only prehospital study in which the EOA™ was seen in a favorable light. Auerbach and Geehr looked at the prehospital setting in two prospective studies.[99,100] In the first of these they obtained blood gas levels from patients who had undergone EGTA intubation in the field. The patients were then endotracheally intubated, and the gas levels were redrawn 5 minutes after the new airway was established. Their results demonstrated a significant improvement in both oxygenation and ventilation following endotracheal intubation in the emergency department. The follow-up study was performed after paramedics were trained in endotracheal intubation. They compared a group of patients who were treated using an endotracheal tube with a group of patients treated in the field with the EGTA. There was a substantial difference in age between the two groups, the EGTA group being younger. No difference was detected in downtime or field times. Oxygenation, ventilation, and pH level were all significantly better among those patients who had received endotracheal intubation. Similar results were reported by Smith et al.[101] They found the EOA™ could not be passed in 18% of patients, which is worse than the rates quoted for endotracheal intubation failures in many systems. Bass et al. concluded that the complication rate of the EGTA, when compared with the reported successes with endotracheal intubation, made the EGTA an airway of last resort for use only when endotracheal intubation could not be achieved.[102] Smith, Bodai, et al. reviewed the literature in 1983 and concluded that the EOA™ was a poor substitute for endotracheal intubation in the prehospital setting.[103] This conclusion was reaffirmed in a more recent paper by Hankins.[104]

THE PHARYNGO-TRACHEAL LUMEN AIRWAY (PtL™) AND THE ESOPHAGEAL TRACHEAL COMBITUBE™ (ETC)

The tracheoesophageal airway, a precursor of the PtL™ and the ETC, was developed because of the incidence of endotracheal placement of the esophageal obturator. This device allowed the patient to be ventilated through the mask if the tube passed into the esophagus or by way of the tube should it enter the trachea.[105,106] Difficulties with mask ventilation prompted the creation of two other devices, the Pharyngo-Tracheal Lumen Airway (PtL™) and the Esophageal Tracheal Combitube™ (ETC). These devices are similar in design, both essentially being a double lumen tube with a distal and a proximal balloon. The distal balloon is inflated once the device is in place and is designed to occupy the trachea or esophagus. The proximal balloon is larger, designed to occupy the oropharynx when inflated. The inner lumen is similar to an endotracheal tube, while the outer lumen is truncated (PtL™) or perforated (ETC) to allow ventilation if the long tube is placed in the esophagus. Both of these devices are placed blindly. The operator then uses breath sounds and chest movement to determine whether the distal lumen is in the esophagus or trachea. Niemann's group at Harbor-UCLA initially tested the PtL™ in an animal study, with the device placed deliberately in the esophagus.[107] They were able to demonstrate ventilatory

efficiencies and blood gas levels equivalent to those seen with endotracheal tubes. Included in their report was a pilot study on six patients in cardiac arrest. They drew blood gas levels on patients who were endotracheally intubated, then replaced this device with the PtL™. After a stabilization period, gas levels were again collected. No difference in blood gas values was seen between the two devices. In a study of the ETC in patients undergoing anesthesia, it appeared to provide better oxygenation than conventional endotracheal airway management.[108] Frass then used the ETC on patients who suffered cardiac arrest in the hospital and noted that the ETC provided adequate oxygenation and ventilation in all of these patients. He concluded that the ETC was a useful device for airway management. Bartlett's group has demonstrated that the PtL™ can provide significant protection for the airway in the setting of upper airway hemorrhage.[109] Atherton looked at the use of the ETC in the field.[110] In this study the device was compared with the endotracheal tube using an alternate day design. The ETC was used as a backup airway on days when the endotracheal tube was primary. When the ETC was used as the primary airway, it was successfully placed 72% of the time. When used as a backup for failed endotracheal tube placement, successful placement occurred in 64% of patients. The endotracheal tube, as the primary airway, was placed 84% of the time. McMahan compared the PtL™ with the endotracheal tube and found no difference in the rate of successful intubation.[111]

The major concern regarding the use of these airways has been the need for the paramedic to discriminate between esophageal and endotracheal placement. The difficulty in making this determination has been one of the major stumbling blocks preventing paramedics from using the endotracheal tube. As noted previously, the use of breath sounds or chest rise to determine the placement of a tube is not foolproof, even in a quiet operating theater.[62] When paramedics were trained in the use of the PtL™ and then retested 6 weeks after training, they were unable to correctly determine the site of placement in over 40% of cases.[112] The authors concluded that paramedics using this device need extensive training in assessment of tube placement.

When these devices are placed in the esophagus (the most likely location) the trachea cannot be suctioned without deflating the oropharyngeal balloon. While resuscitation medications could potentially be administered, it is unlikely that any significant amount would reach the bronchial tree. Most would be deposited on the oropharynx.

Just like the EOA™, the ETC has a long list of contraindications. It should not be used in pediatric patients, patients with a gag reflex, or patients who have ingested caustic substances.[113]

Both the PtL™ and the ETC have been touted as airways that can be placed when endotracheal tubes cannot be inserted. Multiple attempts at endotracheal intubation without success might be an indication to use these devices. They have also been authorized for use in some states by paramedics who are not permitted to perform endotracheal intubation, although it appears they may be at least as difficult to correctly use as an endotracheal tube. While it is considered more difficult to train personnel in the use of the endotracheal tube, both Hunt[101] and Atherton[99] showed that the PtL™ and ETC both require significant ongoing training and supervision. Neither is superior to a correctly placed endotracheal tube. Paramedics should be trained in all the methods of endotracheal tube insertion, and significant amounts of ongoing education should be devoted to intubation skills. If the medical director elects to use other devices as backup, he or she needs to realize that their use will also require substantial training and supervision. Confirmation of placement with an end-tidal CO_2 detector or other method should still be performed. The Self-Inflating Bulf (SIB) has been used successfully to confirm proper placement of the ETC.[114] The training demands for these devices suggest that this time might be better spent instructing the paramedic in the correct use of intubation and invasive airway skills.

LARYNGEAL MASK AIRWAY (LMA)

The laryngeal mask airway (LMA) was first used as an alternative to endotracheal tube ventilation in operating rooms in Great Britain in 1983.[115] Because of its purported ease of use and efficacy, this device has appeal as a useful field airway adjunct.[116] A study comparing the LMA to endotracheal intubation in 19 patients undergoing elective surgery showed that paramedics and respiratory therapists were able to successfully ventilate the patients in less time and with less attempts at placement when using the LMA. There has been some suggestion that the LMA may also have the advantage of minimizing cervical spine motion when being placed.[117] Cases have been described of the field use of the LMA where patients are trapped with limited access preventing endotracheal intubation.[118]

One of the major disadvantages to this airway is that it does not protect against aspiration.[119]

Tools for Confirming Airway Placement

End-tidal CO_2 detectors/monitors

Medical directors should insist on the use of a CO_2 detection technique in any patient who has been intubated. This has been shown to be the most reliable method of determining endotracheal placement in a perfusing patient.[62] At the present time, both electronic and chemical devices are available for detection of exhaled CO_2. The device that has been studied most extensively in the acute-care setting is the EZCap colorimetric device, made by Nelcor. Recent studies have demonstrated the utility of this device in the prehospital[120,121] and emergency department settings.[122]

These devices are designed for single patient use. MSA has recently introduced the Mini-cap III™, an electronic device that features a sterilizable head and an LED readout. These devices should be used for all intubated patients, especially when the patient was intubated by a blind technique, such as digital intubation.

Quantitative monitoring of end-tidal CO_2 will probably be available for prehospital care in the near future, with several manufacturers offering smaller versions of their operating room capnometers. Use of these devices will allow the paramedic to accurately titrate the degree of ventilation to the patient's needs, preventing the severe hyperventilation that occasionally occurs due to the sympathetic arousal of the paramedic.

Other techniques

Aside from the devices described above, two other ways of confirming endotracheal tube placement deserve mention. Lighted stylets, both of the rigid and flexible type, can be used to confirm placement of a tube inserted by another method.

The use of a large syringe to aspirate the airway has also been advocated. This device is commercially available as the EID™—Esophageal Intubation Detector. In this situation the syringe is attached to the endotracheal tube and the plunger is rapidly withdrawn. If the tube is in the esophagus, it will collapse from the vacuum and the operator will not be able to withdraw air. In the trachea, because it will not collapse, the syringe will aspirate air. Several studies have demonstrated the utility of this device in the operating room, where all researchers noted it to be 100% accurate at detecting esophageal intubation in adults.[123-127] A study by Jenkins demonstrated the utility of this device in the prehospital and emergency department setting.[128] Although there were only two esophageal intubations in their series of 90 patients, they were both detected. The authors noted that there were no false negatives despite the presence of a large hemothorax in one patient and pulmonary edema in nine patients. Other aspiration devices have recently been introduced.

Airway Confirmation—A Summary

It is absolutely essential that medical directors choose a method for auxiliary confirmation of tube placement and insist on its use. The risk of an undetected esophageal intubation is minimized when one (or more) of these auxiliary techniques is used. Not using these tools or having protocols not properly performed risks not only the patient's life, it also jeopardizes the paramedic, the medical director, and the EMS system.

Invasive Airway Procedures

When endotracheal intubation has failed or when the anatomy of the face has been so distorted so as to prevent placement of an endotracheal tube, a surgical airway may be lifesaving. Cricothyroidotomy has usually been the route used in emergencies and by non-surgeons. Tracheotomy has been considered too difficult and too complicated to perform in the emergency situation. Alternatives to formal cricothyrotomy have included "minicricothyroidotomy" and translaryngeal needle ventilation.

Cricothyroidotomy

This procedure has a long history, but it fell into disfavor after Chevalier Jackson implicated it as a cause of airway stenosis in his 1921 article.[129] Like so many techniques, it was later resurrected as a method of emergency airway management. Some authors feel it is the method of choice for management of apneic patients with suspected cervical spine injuries.[61] McGill reviewed 3 years' data at Hennepin County Medical Center.[130] During this period, 38 cricothyroidotomies were performed in their department, primarily for failure of other airway management techniques. Twelve patients were long-term survivors. They had a 39% complication rate, which included placement of the tube through the thyrohyoid membrane, prolonged procedure times, and hemorrhage from the incision. Only one sur-

vivor had permanent dysphonia. They state that their complication rate is much higher than others have quoted, but this was due to the emergency nature of the procedures in their series. A series of 69 patients who underwent cricothyroidotomy by flight nurse/paramedics in the field was reviewed by Boyle.[131] He reported a complication rate of 8.7%, all of which occurred in patients who were in traumatic cardiac arrest at the time of the procedure. In another series of air-medical service patients, no complications were seen among 20 patients on whom the procedure was performed.[132] Their indications included maxillofacial or cervical trauma or the failure of other methods of airway management when patients were in arrest. None of the arrested patients survived, but seven of the maxillofacial trauma patients survived. Spaite and Joseph reviewed the records of 20 patients who presented to a Level 1 trauma center after undergoing prehospital cricothyroidotomy.[133] Their results were not encouraging in that only one patient survived without neurological complications. They concluded that many of the massively injured or arrested patients probably did not benefit from this procedure and that the indications for this procedure in the prehospital setting should be very narrowly defined. Other investigators have had better success. Nugent found that when flight nurses performed cricothyroidotomy, 27% of their patients survived to hospital discharge.[134] Their retrospective study also noted that during the first year the procedure was performed primarily on victims in cardiac arrest. In subsequent years, this population made up a minority of the patients. This suggests that as the flight nurses became more comfortable with the procedure, they began to use it earlier, which may explain their good results. The lesson here is that if paramedics are authorized to perform this procedure, they need to perform it as soon as the indications arise, rather than using it only on patients in cardiac arrest.

Minicricothyroidotomy

Several studies have looked at minimizing the amount of surgical expertise and the size of the device placed through the cricothyroid membrane. Yealy has shown that adequate tidal volumes can be delivered using a 4 mm catheter.[122,123] Campbell has used an 8.5 French (2.8 mm) central venous catheter to ventilate dogs with conventional bag-valve-mask techniques.[135] The Seldinger technique has been used to percutaneously place larger diameter devices.[136] These studies suggest that it may be possible to cannulate the trachea percutaneously with larger diameter devices, eliminating the need for a special high-pressure connection, without requiring a formal cricothyroidotomy.

Commercial devices are available for performing minicricothyroidotomy. One of these, the Pertrach™, consists of a needle, wire, dilator, and cannula. This procedure is performed by making a small skin incision, through which the needle is introduced into the cricothyroid membrane. Air is aspirated to confirm position, then a dilator is passed through the breakaway needle to spread the tissues. The tube is then placed into the airway. When compared to conventional cricothyroidotomy, paramedics found this technique to be just as successful as the conventional method but felt it was more difficult to perform.[137]

Transtracheal Jet Ventilation

Transtracheal jet ventilation, occasionally called needle cricothyroidotomy, is one of the simplest methods of invasive airway access, but unfortunately it is also one of the most underutilized. This is probably because of the perception that it can only be used for a very short time. The ATLS manual states that this technique can provide adequate oxygenation for only 30-45 minutes.[138] However, the technique they describe is not jet ventilation, but apneic oxygenation. Frame has been able to demonstrate adequate oxygenation when using 14 and 16 gauge catheters in cats with total airway obstruction, applying the ATLS technique. Use of an 18 gauge catheter did result in hypoventilation.[139] Ventilation requires that a 50 psi source, such as is available directly from a wall connection or oxygen tank regulator sidearm, be used in conjunction with a 14 or 16 gauge catheter. It can be performed indefinitely, since a 16 gauge catheter will allow flow rates in excess of 50 liters per minute.[140] If extrapolated to 20 breaths per minute, this is equivalent to a tidal volume of 950 cc[141], which is more than adequate to ventilate most adult patients. Aspiration has also been a concern with this method, because it, like the surgical cricothryroidotomy, is often used in patients with massive upper airway injury or hemorrhage. When Yealy looked at this problem using Gastrograffin™ as the marker, he found no evidence of aspiration when the head of the bed was at a 30 degree angle, noting mild aspiration only in two of six animals who were set at a 45 degree angle.[142] He concluded that at 30 degrees or less the jet ventilator provided sufficient airway protection. As most patients in critical condition are transported in the supine position, this should not be a problem. In patients with a totally obstructed airway there may be an increased risk of baro-

trauma. Stothert has shown that in these patients inspiration times greater than 1 second or expiration times of less than four times the inspiration time have a greatly increased risk of barotrauma or hemodynamic compromise.[143]

When assembled, the device consists of a connection for a high pressure (50 psi) source, a connecting line, a spring loaded trigger valve, and a tube with a Luer lock connection. This connects to the catheter. This is a high pressure system and will not work if it is fed from a 125 liter flow meter. The tubing must be the same as that used to connect a ventilator to a wall connection. Oxygen tubing, like that used for a mask or cannula, will not work. Supplies to make this device are usually available locally from the respiratory supply company or respiratory therapy departments of local hospitals. The medical director must ensure that the supplies are available and assembled well ahead of the time they are needed.

Ventilators

Some systems, especially air-medical systems and ground systems specializing in interhospital transfers, use portable mechanical ventilators. These devices are usually battery or oxygen powered, and they are produced by a variety of manufacturers.[144] Some are designed for transport only, while others are capable to be used during CPR. Some of these devices are designed as simple resuscitators, while others have many of the features of hospital ventilators, such as oxygen mixers, pressure gauges, and PEEP. They have the advantage of freeing the attendant from the task of manually ventilating the patient with a resuscitation bag. They also tend to produce a consistent volume, preventing the variation in ventilation that occurs with manual bagging. Costs vary.

Like any medical device, ventilators require some care to perform properly. Some have specialized cleaning requirements. The volume produced by the ventilator should be checked with a spirometer at the beginning of use and on a regular basis during transport. If the ventilator is pressure cycled, the volume may change as lung compliance changes. Paramedics using this type of ventilator should be aware of this effect. Some ventilators will continue to cycle even when their oxygen supply is cut off; the paramedic must be vigilant in this regard. Medical directors who permit their EMS service to use ventilators must be sure that there is a clear protocol governing their use. Frequent continuing education is also mandatory when using these devices.

Adjuncts for Airway Management

Pulse Oximetry

Oxygen is routinely given to most ambulance patients in the United States today. The public considers it to be lifegiving and without side effects. Paramedics are often of a similar mind. As mentioned before, oxygen is a drug with both benefits and side effects. In addition, increasing emphasis on cost-effective medical care discourages the use of a drug that may have no effect on the patient. Often, in spite of oxygen administration, unrecognized hypoxia may occur. However, until the advent of pulse oximetry, there was no method of assessing adequate oxygenation in the prehospital setting.

The arrival of pulse oximeters and their miniaturization in the 1980s provided medical caregivers with another parameter for assessing patients. One recent article described pulse oximetry as "the fifth vital sign."[145] Studies have demonstrated that pulse oximetry can be performed reliably in the prehospital setting. Aughey compared the pulse oximeter reading obtained in the field with the saturation of a simultaneously obtained blood gas level.[146] Her group demonstrated excellent correlation between the reading of the pulse oximeter and the co-oximeter. McGuire and Pointer found that paramedics were able to follow the patient's response to respiratory interventions more closely by use of oximetry.[147] In Silverton's series from England, he found that pulse oximetry was able to provide an early clue for finding developing pneumothorax, as well as helping to guide the caregivers in selection of appropriate airways.[148] When used during endotracheal intubation the pulse oximeter can help prevent unrecognized hypoxia from occurring.[149] Cydulka demonstrated that when a relatively conservative saturation of 97% was used, pulse oximetry could substantially decrease the unnecessary oxygen use.[150] This decrease in oxygen use was shown to produce substantial cost savings, without an apparent decrement in patient care.

In the air-medical setting, pulse oximetry has been proven valuable.[151,152] In helicopter transport the flight crew may be relatively isolated from the patient due to noise and packaging, making detection of hypoxemia difficult. The altitude changes associated with fixed wing (airplane) transport may rapidly produce hypoxemia. These changes are often detected by the pulse oximeter before there is clinical evidence.

As with any monitoring device, some control and education are necessary to guide the paramedic. Although both of the above authors demonstrated the device was reliable, it may give erroneous numbers due to local hypoperfusion, hypotension, movement of the probe, fingernail polish, bright lights, carboxyhemoglobinemia, anemia, or other patient or equipment problems.[153,154] Special probes may be needed for small children, adding to the expense of the device. As with all types of monitoring devices, paramedics must be cautioned to treat the patient, not the monitor.

There is a wide range of monitor types and prices, ranging from several hundred to several thousand dollars. Prices for these units have been rapidly dropping. The less expensive versions usually have a single digit probe and an LED readout. As one moves up in price the units display waveforms and may have interchangeable probes for digits, ears, noses, or other areas. Most pulse oximeters look at the oxygenation at the time of the arterial pulse and depend upon plethysmography for timing. Some of the high-end monitors are now able to synchronize with the EDG, allowing more accurate monitoring of the patient, who may have peripheral hypoperfusion or is on pressors.

When added to the signs already commonly assessed by paramedics, pulse oximetry can be a valuable adjunct, but only if its use is audited and the medical director provides ongoing guidance.

Nasogastric Tubes

Nasogastric tubes may be useful in selected adults at risk for vomiting and aspiration and in infants where gastric distention may cause respiratory compromise. In systems with short transport times nasogastric tube placement is probably not useful, but in long-distance transports it may decrease the chance of airway compromise. These tubes may be placed through the mouth or the nose in adults. Children tolerate the oral route better because of concern over adenoidal bleeding with nasal passage. When used for aspiration only and not for fluid or medication administration, they should enjoy a low complication rate. Even an endotracheal placement would be unlikely to cause much harm. Take care to avoid aspiration, and suction should be available during the procedure. Paramedics must be cautioned against placing nasogastric tubes in patients with craniofacial injuries because of the risk of cribriform plate disruption and intracranial placement.[69]

Techniques for Chest Decompression

The placement of a needle to relieve tension pneumothorax is often used in ground EMS systems. Some air-medical services have also authorized the placement of a formal tube thoracostomy by their crews.

Needle Thoracostomy

The placement of a needle in the midclavicular line, second intercostal space can produce dramatic results in a patient suffering from a tension pneumothorax. This procedure should be considered in any patient who suffers from rapid cardiopulmonary decompensation. Although tracheal deviation or decreased breath sounds are commonly accepted as signs of a tension pneumothorax, they may not always be accurate.[155] Paramedics should be encouraged to perform this procedure in any patient who has a precipitous course, especially if there is a history of COPD, asthma, or chest trauma. Trauma patients with obvious subcutaneous emphysema can benefit from the early application of this technique. The procedure appears to be safe and simple, but no studies have been performed in the prehospital setting to confirm this. If the catheter is placed into the lung parenchyma, the puncture will be small and should heal rapidly. The resultant pneumothorax is an open one, and therefore the patient should suffer little further compromise. Although inappropriate placement generally results in the considerable morbidity of a tube thoracostomy, patients who are candidates for this procedure usually have other injuries that will require a hospital stay.

If the patient is intubated, the catheter may be placed and left open to the air. If the patient is spontaneously breathing, a one-way valve must be created to prevent re-entry of air during inspiration. One-way valves, such as the Heimlich valve, are available. Condoms may be used by puncturing the condom with the catheter and then unrolling it after it is placed in the patient. Surgical gloves have been used, but when compared to condoms, they produce unacceptable air leakage. (Michael Sayre, MD: personal communication)

Tube Thoracostomy

This common surgical procedure is used to evacuate air or blood from the pleural space. Its use in the field has commonly been limited to air-medical services or military situations. The primary advantage of this technique is that it can rapidly evacuate a large amount of blood from the trauma patient's pleural space, converting a tension hemothorax into an open hemothorax. In some cases this may be lifesaving, but in others the patient can exsanguinate from the tube, depending upon the source of the bleed-

ing. If this occurs in the field, though, it is unlikely that the tube would have contributed to the patient's demise.

If the transport time is sufficiently long, tube thoracostomy may be a useful procedure. Some systems (especially air-medical services) place chest tubes as a last-ditch effort in blunt trauma arrest. Although there is no literature to support this practice, this should be viewed in light of the difficulty of doing research with these patients.

The tube must be placed under sterile conditions, and it is difficult to provide even a modicum of sterility at many scenes. This may lead to empyema, should the patient survive. The technique has several areas where the operator must be careful: placement in the wrong interspace can result in injury to the abdominal organs, especially the liver, or the heart and great vessels. Use of trocars or Kelly clamps to place the tube may cause injury to the lung parenchyma or other thoracic structures.

Once the tube has been secured, one must decide what to do with the free end of the tube. If the patient is intubated the tube may be left open, creating an open pneumothorax. For a patient who is not intubated, a one-way valve must be created to prevent entry of air into the thorax during inspiration. Historically water seals were used, but these are highly impractical outside the hospital. More recently, commercially manufactured chest tube drainage bottles have been manufactured, many of which do not require instillation of water to seal the system. Because of their bulk, they are difficult to use in the prehospital setting. The Heimlich valve, essentially a rubber flapper valve in a tube, is the most practical device for the paramedic. It may be connected to suction if that is required, and if there is a large amount of drainage, a urinary catheter bag may be attached to collect the drainage. The Cook Company of Bloomington, IN makes several kits with this device, including adapters to allow it to be connected to a needle thoracostomy catheter.

Other devices, such as the McSwain Dart, have also been used for chest decompression, but they seem to confer no advantage over a venous catheter and are mentioned here only to discourage their use. In addition, catheters are usually carried by prehospital care providers, so they are readily available if the patient suddenly decompensates.

For most EMS systems, needle thoracostomy is the safest, most rapid, and most effective way of providing pleural decompression. Tube thoracostomy should be reserved for those situations in which transport times are long or needle thoracostomy is unsuccessful.

Venous Access

General Considerations

When the primary purpose of ALS in prehospital care was cardiac care, it was obvious that IVs were needed for medication administration. Indeed, when combined with airway management and defibrillation skills, IV access has allowed the paramedic to provide care equivalent to that given in many emergency departments. However, when trauma patients became part of the paramedic's practice, considerably less agreement could be found regarding the benefits of IV fluids.

In an often quoted article, McSwain stated that prehospital IV starts added 12.2 minutes to the on-scene time.[156] He questioned whether this delay was beneficial to the patient in cardiac arrest. Similar times were found in a study of the Sacramento EMS system.[6] Given that the delay resulted in an average of less than 1 liter of fluid administered, Smith concluded that IVs were unwarranted in trauma victims, who would benefit more from earlier surgical intervention. The times these authors quote were not directly measured, so there may have been other activities that contributed to the times. Similar times for IV starts have also been reported in the South Carolina EMS system.[157] Blaisdell quoted these data in his 1984 address to the American Association for the Surgery of Trauma.[1] He concluded that in an urban system with short transport times, scoop-and-run techniques were preferable to IV access being obtained at the scene. The volume of fluid administered has also come into question. Kaweski's review of fluid administration in San Diego found there was no effect on survival with prehospital fluids.[4] However, computer modeling of prehospital hemorrhage suggests that fluid administration in the field provides an advantage in both blood pressure and survival.[158] Aprahamian has noted an improvement in survival for abdominal trauma patients when provided ALS.[159] The setting in which the prehospital IV is placed may engender a higher complication rate, and this also must be accounted for when evaluating the utility of IV therapy. Lawrence has noted a significantly higher rate of phlebitis and febrile illness when patients had IVs started in the field versus the ED.[160]

Numerous studies have been published that dispute the claim that paramedic-started IVs significantly delay transport. In one of the few studies to directly measure the time for procedures, Pons' group in Denver found that IV access required less than 3 minutes in all patients. This included time to draw blood, which prolonged the procedure. When a second IV line was required, it took only 1.25 minutes for placement.[161] Another study measuring IV start times found an average time of 2.8 minutes, with a 91% success rate. They also found a high success rate for lines placed while en route.[162] A 95% success rate for en-route IV starts in trauma patients was seen by Slovis, who also noted an 80% en-route IV success rate in medical patients.[163] O'Gorman also found that IV lines could be initiated while en route with as much success as at the scene, leading him to suggest that prehospital IVs could be performed in "zero-time."[164] In a study of penetrating cardiac wounds the Denver group found that their medics could perform several procedures on these patients and still have an average on-scene time of less than 11 minutes.[165] For major trauma patients in Tucson, the average on-scene time was 8.1 minutes, with the sicker patients receiving *more procedures and having a shorter scene time.*[166] Recently a study was done in both urban and nonurban settings measuring IV success rate and time.[167] In both the success rate was greater than 97% at establishing an IV. More than 94% of lines in both settings were established in less than 4 minutes.

There is considerable debate regarding the appropriate amounts and types of fluid for prehospital trauma resuscitation.[168] While it may turn out that vigorous fluid resuscitation in the field produces no improvement or is even harmful, at present the clinical data are unavailable. Medical directors should follow this controversy closely, as it is fundamental to the way in which we resuscitate trauma victims. The most recent study done in Houston of almost 600 patients who were hypotensive secondary to penetrating torso injuries, the group that had a delay in aggressive fluid resuscitation until operative intervention had improved outcomes.[169] Many authorities now believe that in uncontrolled hemorrhage, vigorous fluid resuscitation increases blood pressure resulting in an increase in blood loss. Accelerating the blood loss is the dilution of coagulation factors. Some patients, however, are so hypotensive as to need at least enough resuscitation to maintain a modicum of blood flow to vital organs to prevent cardiac arrest.

While speed is of paramount importance for the trauma patient, the effectiveness of field therapy may be more critical to the medical patient. In Sydney, Australia, Potter noted a decrease in early mortality among patients treated by ALS units, which included IV therapy.[13] No difference in overall mortality was seen, however. In contrast, a study of North Carolina intermediate EMTs[170], who were authorized to start IVs but not administer drugs, showed no advantage to prehospital IV placement. In reality, there was a significant delay in medication administration for patients with EMT-I started IVs. In medical patients, the only reason for IV access should be immediate drug therapy. If the paramedic is prohibited from medication administration, medical patients should not have an IV.

IV Summary

For trauma patients, IVs should be started while en route unless the patient has a prolonged extrication, in which case the IV may be started before transport. Medical directors should consider the use of large bore tubing and catheters to ensure that adequate volumes can be infused. Medical patients should receive an IV line in the field only if they are to receive medications. "Prophylactic" lines should be discouraged. Strong medical control is essential to evaluate the use and success rates and provide guidance for this procedure. Without proper supervision, IV access can change from a lifesaving to a lifetaking intervention.

Peripheral Lines

Traditionally paramedics have started IVs in the veins of the upper limbs. Some systems have also authorized the use of the external jugular vein as a "peripheral" site. The immediate complications appear to be limited to unsuccessful attempts and local infiltration. There is some risk of infection[142], so many hospitals require that "field" lines be changed soon after the patient arrives. One of the major difficulties with sites is the difficulty in finding a "good vein" in some patients, such as the chronically debilitated or intravenous drug abuser. Many paramedics have a low comfort level in obtaining vascular access in pediatric patients.

In adult patients, most systems use 14-20 gauge catheters, depending upon the nature of the patient's complaint and the caliber of the veins. For medical patients, catheter size makes little difference because flow rates for all of these are sufficient for drug administration. Most of these will also allow the administration of blood, although it may be rather slow when pushed through a 20 gauge tube. For patients requiring high fluid volumes, short (3.2 cm / 1.25 inch) 14 gauge catheters can provide high flow rates. Flow is directly proportional to the pressure gradient, inversely proportional to the length,

and proportional to the diameter of the tube to the fourth power (Poiseuille's Law). Guisto has demonstrated that 12 gauge catheters can be used, with his paramedics having an 84% success rate with this large IV.[171] This allows fluid rates as high as many 8.5 French central lines. When used with wide bore tubing and a pressure bag, this catheter achieved a flow of nearly 900 cc per minute. Kits have recently become available using the Seldinger wire technique to convert peripheral 14-18 gauge IVs to an 8.5 French diameter IV. No studies are available to assess the utility of this technique in the prehospital setting.

For infants and pediatric patients, EMTs should be encouraged to look for access in the lower limbs. The dorsal veins of the foot and the treater saphenous vein can be cannulated by percutaneous means, and this area is often less "pudgy" than the upper limbs.

Central Venous Access

Many flight programs, but few ground ambulances, allow EMTs to place central venous catheters. In systems with short transport times this prohibition may be warranted, but if transport times are prolonged and peripheral access cannot be obtained, central venous cannulation may be lifesaving. Central administration of medications in cardiac arrest may increase the likelihood that drugs will reach their target organs. Several sites are described: subclavian, internal jugular, and femoral veins. No studies are available to assess the utility or morbidity of those in the prehospital environment. Studies of in-hospital use of these techniques suggest that even subclavian catheterization, which many feel has the highest morbidity, can be performed successfully in over 90% of cases and has few complications.[172,173] Excellent reviews of the subclavian route[174], internal jugular, and femoral techniques[175] can be referred to for details regarding the technique.

Intraosseous (IO) Infusion

One of the most exciting rediscoveries of the past several years has been intraosseous (IO) infusion. This technique was originally used early in the twentieth century to administer fluids and medications, but advances in IV technology caused IO infusions to fall into disuse. IO access today is primarily used in young children, where peripheral vascular access is unobtainable. IO techniques are easily taught, using readily available chicken and turkey legs as the model.[176] In the hands of paramedics and flight nurses this method enjoys a good success rate[177] and is much easier to perform than percutaneous IV cannulation in small children. Although most individuals rarely use the technique, the skill does not seem to deteriorate substantially over time.[178] It appears that any fluid or drug that can be administered intravenously can be given by the IO route. The only absolute contraindication appears to be the presence of a fracture of the selected bone proximal to the site, and relative contraindications include congenital bone disease and going through an area of burned tissue. Complications include fractures at the site of the infusion, which is most likely due to selection of too large of a needle in a small child, and bone marrow emboli. The latter problem was studied by Orlowski, who concluded that although there were notable amounts of emboli in the lung after IO infusion, they did not appear to affect the resuscitation and should be of no concern to rescuers considering this route.[179]

Because of the difficulty with vascular access in many pediatric patients, all paramedics should be familiar with IO infusion. One excellent way to acquire this training is through the Pediatric Advanced Life Support (PALS) course offered by the American Heart Association.

Medication Administration Techniques

Numerous methods have been used to give medications to patients. Not all of these are suitable for the prehospital environment. Table 3-2 and discussion list some of the routes that have been used.

Oral Administration

Medication administered orally is rarely used in daily EMS procedures. Recently, many systems have begun using oral aspirin as an antiplatelet agent in cases of suspected acute myocardial infarction. Systems that respond for mass gatherings may wish to stock mild analgesics, such as acetaminophen, but the usual time constraints of ambulance transfer mean that few medications are likely to be effective in the prehospital setting. A possible exception to this rule is nifedipine, which may be given in a "bite the capsule and swallow" mode for the treatment of hypertensive emergencies recognizing that it is not easily titratable and may cause too great a drop in blood pressure on occasion. The prehospital use of nifedipine remains controversial.

Table 3-2   Medication Administration

Route	Utility	Situations	Medications	
Oral	+	Mass gatherings	Mild analgesics Patient's medications	
Sublingual	+++	Chest pain	Nitroglycerin	
Nebulizer	++++	Bronchospasm	Albuterol	
ET tube injection	++++	Cardiac arrest/ no IV access	Epinephrine Lidocaine Midazolam	Atropine Naloxone
Rectal	++	Seizures/ no IV access	Diazepam Midazolam	
Subcutaneous	+++	Bronchospasm Analgesia	Epinephrine Morphine	
Sublingual injection	++	Opioid OD/ Extreme obtundation	Naloxone	
IM	++	Opioid OD, Hypoglycemia	Naloxone	Glucagon
IV push	++++	Cardiac arrest, Dysrhythmias	ACLS drugs	
IV infusion	++	Hypotension	Crystalloid Pressors Lidocaine	

Sublingual Administration

Perhaps the most commonly administered sublingual medication is nitroglycerin. It is currently available in tablet and spray forms. This route is easy to use, although there is the difficulty of placing a tiny pill under a patient's tongue in a moving ambulance. Some systems favor the use of the spray, but some people have questioned whether using this with multiple patients is sanitary. (Paris P: *Personal Communication,* 1996.) Many systems are using much higher doses of nitroglycerin for the treatment of cardiac ischemia and congestive heart failure.

Hand-Held Nebulizers

Direct delivery of medications to the lungs has become increasingly popular over the past several years. Although many types of medications, including antibiotics, steroids, and surfactants, are given by this route, the most common use for this route in the prehospital setting is bronchodilator administration. The frequency with which EMS systems are called to care for patients with reactive airway disease (25% of the respiratory distress calls in one system could be attributed to reactive airway disease or COPD)[180] suggests this is an important technique. Several authors have investigated the use of b-agonist therapy in the prehospital setting.[181-183] All of these studies have demonstrated benefit from use of b-agonist aerosols; none have shown significant problems. It is important that these patients receive supplemental oxygen both during and after treatment. This is usually not a problem in the field, since the nebulizers are usually oxygen driven and prehospital care providers are conditioned to provide oxygen to their patients. Receiving facilities should be alerted when these medications have been used, though, because patients may demonstrate a significant decrease in oxygen saturation within 30 minutes of bronchodilator treatments.[184]

In children, reactive airway disease has classically been treated with subcutaneous epinephrine injections. While highly effective, they are uncomfortable. Inhaled bronchodilator therapy may provide a more comfortable alternative, with no decrease in effectiveness.[185] Prehospital providers should become familiar with this technique and have the equipment to be able to give these treatments to patients of all ages.

Endotracheal Tube Administration

Many of the drugs used in ACLS may be injected into the endotracheal tube. Naloxone is also acceptable for endotracheal tube administration. In cases of extreme bronchospasm, b-agonists, such as albuterol, can be injected directly into the tube. It is no longer generally recommended that diazepam be administered by this route. The most commonly used are epinephrine, atropine, and lidocaine.

Rectal Administration

One route that is underutilized in the prehospital setting is rectal administration. Traditionally, suppositories have been administered in this manner, and few of them have any use in the prehospital setting. However, liquid (injectable) diazepam or midazolam may be given by this method, which may be useful in patients in status epilepticus. Paramedics should be familiar with this technique and consider its use whenever they have difficulty in establishing an IV line in a seizure patient.

Subcutaneous (SQ) Injections

Subcutaneous (SQ) injections in prehospital care have primarily been used to treat anaphylaxis or bronchospasm with epinephrine. In Ohio, a special class of EMT (EMT-epinephrine) was established for just this purpose. While inhaled bronchodilator therapy is superior for isolated bronchospasm, prehospital caregivers should continue to use SQ epinephrine in patients with moderate anaphylactic reactions. Although morphine can be given by this route, the delay in absorption makes it unlikely to be useful in prehospital pain management.

Sublingual Injections

Naloxone has been given by sublingual injection, taking advantage of the venous plexus in that area. It may be useful in the opioid overdose patient who is in extremis and who has no IV access. It seems to offer little advantage in the normotensive patient, where the deltoid intramuscular route will suffice. As with any intramuscular injection, there is a risk of hematoma. In the tongue, this has the potential of airway occlusion, so paramedics should consider this a last resort. The provider also runs the risk of being bitten, should the patient awaken while the paramedic is administering the drug. Paramedics should be familiar with this route of naloxone administration but should be discouraged from using it except in the significantly moribund patient.

Intramuscular (IM) Injections

Intramuscular (IM) injections should be routinely used for naloxone injection. If the patient is hypotensive, IM medications will probably have an erratic absorption pattern, causing difficulty with titration. Although analgesics, such as meperidine, can be given IM, the need for rapid onset and titration of effect in the prehospital setting make IV administration preferable. Benzodiazepines, such as diazepam, lorazepam, or midazolam, may be given IM, although diazepam should be given only deep in large muscles. This might be useful in status epilepticus, where obtaining IV access can be difficult at best. The paramedic should be aware that the onset of these medications is slow and somewhat erratic when given by this route. Succinylcholine can also be administered by this method, but it should be a rare circumstance that requires a paramedic to paralyze a patient without having established an IV route. Lidocaine for dysrhythmia management has been given by this route, but the large volume (usually 5-10 cc) makes it exceedingly uncomfortable for the patient. Glucagon has been shown to be useful in the prehospital treatment of hypoglycemia in patients in whom IV access cannot be achieved.[186] Some have suggested that thiamine be given in the field, but it is not clear that a brief delay before hospital administration mandates field administration.

Intravenous Push (IVP)

The most common procedure for administering parenteral medications in the prehospital setting is IV push (IVP). This technique has numerous advantages: medication effects are easily titrated, it provides guaranteed medication access to the circulation, and medications requiring large volumes or that would damage tissues (e.g., bicarbonate) may be given. It also is less uncomfortable for the awake patient, because it only requires one stick (for the initial IV). The ability of the paramedic to administer the medication through a port that is remote from the patient may also have advantages in the seizing or unruly patient.

Both prehospital and in-hospital providers have a tendency to rapidly push all IVP medications. Most medications, other than adenosine, should be pushed slowly. For example, lidocaine, when pushed rapidly (by the paramedic who is pumped up by the successful defibrillation) has a higher likelihood of causing seizures than if it is given over a minute or so. Other medications, such as D_{50}, are very toxic when extravasated, and special care should be given to ensure the patency of the IV. Some medications, such as diazepam and nitroglycerin, are absorbed by the IV tubing, making titration less accu-

rate. It is important that all medications given by IV push be flushed before administering another drug. This is especially critical in the cardiac arrest patient, where sluggish flow in the vein may delay action of the drug.

Intravenous (IV) Infusion

Intravenous (IV) infusions are used in prehospital care primarily for the administration of lidocaine and dopamine. Aminophylline is also given by this route, but it has few indications in the emergency setting.[187] The main advantage of this method is in providing a steady state drug level. Unfortunately, varying heights of IV holders, as well as the swinging and bouncing experienced in an ambulance, may make flow rates variable. Any sort of infusion also requires vigilance on the part of the caregiver to make sure that the flow rate does not inadvertently change, giving the patient a potentially lethal bolus injection. In systems with short transport times, dopamine and dobutamine should be the only medications given by this method, since lidocaine can be given by intermittent IVP injection with equivalent results to an infusion. When lidocaine is given as an infusion, there is a significant risk that a runaway drip may provoke a life-threatening dysrhythmia. The caregiver who is running dopamine or dobutamine should be taking frequent blood pressures (or using an automated blood pressure measuring device) and titrating the infusion to this parameter. Too frequently dopamine is started at a low dose, but movement produces a runaway infusion, risking ischemia. If paramedics are allowed to run dopamine at any rate slower than wide open, they must frequently evaluate the patient.

Systems with longer transport times or where there are frequent interhospital transfers with multiple infusions, should consider the purchase of syringe pumps. These devices allow precise titration of medications but are smaller and lighter than the IV pumps commonly found in hospitals. Some of them will calculate the flow rate needed given the medication concentration, patient weight, and desired dose. Many air-medical services routinely use these pumps, and most have been durable enough for that type of prehospital service. They cost from several hundred to a few thousand dollars but are well worth the price, considering the morbidity of runaway drips.

Crystalloid and colloid infusions in the field should be run at either of two rates: keep vein open (KVO) or wide open. If KVO rates are frequently used, systems may wish to consider using heparin or saline locks, which save the cost of the IV fluid bag and tubing. When patients need a fluid challenge, the IV can be opened until a desired amount of fluid is delivered, then reduced to KVO. Running IVs at a specified rate, as is done in the hospital, makes no sense in the field. The order "run at 100 cc per hr" may translate into less than 25 cc delivered to the patient during the ambulance run and adds unnecessary complication.

Cardiac Procedures

Monitoring and Defibrillation

The original ALS service, Pantridge's Mobile Intensive Care Unit, was established to decrease the morbidity and mortality associated with cardiac events occurring outside the hospital.[188] Monitoring was performed by physicians from the coronary unit. Because of this there was no question about their ability to interpret arrhythmias. His success led to the establishment of other mobile coronary care units, eventually evolving into our present EMS systems. Most of these systems have employed physician-surrogates rather than doctors. The ability to train these providers to accurately determine and treat rhythms has been the subject of a number of studies.

Training paramedics to assess arrhythmias and defibrillate has been done in courses ranging from 4 to over 40 hours. Some systems have decreased their arrhythmia teaching to only that needed to treat ventricular fibrillation and ventricular tachycardia. Such a program was used in Stockholm.[189] In an 8-hour session, paramedics were trained to recognize ventricular fibrillation and tachycardia and to use a defibrillator. The initial testing found an 88% pass rate, with 58 of 59 applicants eventually passing the test. When applied in the field, this group demonstrated a 98% accuracy in their ability to diagnose and treat these rhythms. Follow-up studies have confirmed the efficacy of this system.[190-192] Members of a volunteer EMS unit in Connecticut were trained to recognize ventricular fibrillation in a 4-hour course, with a 10 hour "standard" course being given as a control.[193] No differences in the ability of these paramedics to recognize and treat fibrillation were seen.

Early defibrillation is clearly the key to treatment of prehospital cardiac arrest. A recent study in Wisconsin demonstrated a clear improvement in survival after implementation of the EMT-Defibrillation program when compared to historical controls.[194] This study also empha-

sized the importance of rapid defibrillation, since there were no survivors when the response was greater than 8 minutes. As Eisenberg demonstrated in 1980, time to definitive care is the critical determinant in cardiac arrest survival[10], and defibrillation is definitive care for most cardiac arrest.

The advance of microcomputing technology has provided an alternative to manual EMT-defibrillation in the form of the semi-automatic and automatic external defibrillators. These devices are placed on the patient with self-adhesive electrodes and are designed to recognize ventricular fibrillation and deliver an electrical countershock. The semi-automatic defibrillator requires the operator to press a button on the device to deliver the energy, while the automatic model requires only that the operator attach the leads, then stand away from the patient. These have the advantage of requiring no training in arrhythmia recognition and little training (less than 4 hours) in their use. The units attempt to be 100% specific for ventricular fibrillation and rapid ventricular tachycardia; they are not supposed to deliver a shock to patients with other rhythms. Their sensitivity is therefore somewhat diminished, and very fine ventricular fibrillation may not be treated because the unit may consider it to be asystole. This is probably not of great importance, because both patients with fine fibrillation and asystole have extremely poor chances of survival. The American Heart Association has endorsed the use of these devices.[195] When Seattle firefighters were trained to use automatic defibrillators, survival to discharge increased from 19% with CPR alone to 30% with the defibrillator.[196] The fully automatic versions are simple enough that laypersons with only CPR training have been taught their use.[197] A 1 year follow-up study demonstrated that these skills are easily retained.[198] Indeed, their application is so easy that some authors feel that correct assessment of vital signs may be the limiting factor in their use.[199]

No studies have been performed to assess the use of these devices in pediatric patients. It seems likely though that a device could be developed that would allow the paramedic to enter the patient's age or weight, and the machine would then calculate the correct dose. Because the incidence of primary fibrillatory arrest in children is low, the demand for such a defibrillator might make it prohibitively expensive.

Paramedic training programs require several hundred hours beyond basic EMT training, and much of this time is involved with rhythm analysis and treatment.

Cardiac rhythm determination is a difficult skill to teach and learn. Its application in the rear of a moving ambulance, with a 4-square-inch display, motion artifact, and the other demands of caring for a critical patient makes it an even more difficult skill to apply. It is likely that if full spectrum arrhythmia detection is desired, paramedics would need extensive initial training and frequent continuing education. The command physician should ask specific questions regarding rate, regularity, QRS duration, and relationship of the P wave to the QRS complex (see Chapter 9).

External Cardiac Pacing

The idea of cardiac pacing dates from 200 years ago, but it was not until the 1950s that the first transcutaneous pacemakers were developed. In the intervening years the technology of transvenous pacemakers overtook that of the transcutaneous pacemaker, which fell into disuse. During the past decade, transcutaneous pacemakers for use in the emergency setting have been rediscovered and greatly improved.

When used promptly in patients suffering from hemodynamically significant bradycardias, transcutaneous pacing appears effective in the prehospital setting. Vukov showed that transcutaneous pacing was an important procedure among patients transferred by helicopter for acute cardiac problems.[200] Eitel's group at York, Pennsylvania found transcutaneous pacing was easy for prehospital providers to learn and apply.[201] O'Toole's series demonstrated survival in all patients who had pacing initiated immediately on bradyasystolic arrest.[202] Emphasis here is placed on early initiation of pacing, since pacing is increasingly ineffective when delayed.[203] In the study from York, mentioned above, there were no differences in outcome, regardless of whether the patient was paced. The authors felt that this reflected the long down time of the patients. Hedges alternate-day control trial of prehospital transcutaneous pacing also reached a similar conclusion.[204] Despite his enthusiasm for transcutaneous pacing in the interhospital transfer environment, Vukov was not able to extend this endorsement to the use of this procedure in the treatment of prehospital bradyasystolic cardiac arrest.[205] The benefits clearly outweigh the complications, and the current American Heart Association guidelines advocate early transcutaneous pacing in conjunction with medications. The most prevalent problem with transcutaneous pacing currently is the tendency to delay initiation of pacing and in sometimes spending too long a period of time using an ineffective energy setting.

Although not currently commercially available, transcutaneous burst pacing at high pulse rates (200-280 bpm), has been shown to be effective in terminating supraventricular tachycardias.[206] This may prove to be an attractive modality for unstable patients with PSVT who might otherwise require cardioversion.

Today, transcutaneous cardiac pacing is an important modality in those patients suffering from symptomatic bradycardia unresponsive to pharmacological intervention. When the patient suffers from a bradyasystolic arrest, transcutaneous pacing must be initiated *immediately* to be effective. The use of combination pacing/defibrillation pads should be standard in any patient who appears to be suffering from a cardiac event. Having these pads in place early will allow the paramedic to either defibrillate or pace without delay, should the need arise. The lack of significant side effects and the safety of this treatment indicate that this modality should be available to all paramedics.[207]

Pericardiocentesis

Pericardiocentesis is described in the ACLS text as the procedure of choice for treating cardiac tamponade.[208] It may be a lifesaving intervention when an effusion results in hemodynamic compromise. Its use in the prehospital setting has not been investigated, and the ACLS text reserves its use for physicians because of concern regarding complications, such as myocardial or coronary artery injury. In the patient suffering from pulseless electrical activity (PEA) due to cardiac tamponade, pericardiocentesis may theoretically produce a perfusing rhythm. Given the poor prognosis of PEA, it seems unlikely that these patients could come to much more harm from this procedure. Although Callaham discourages the use of this technique in the patient with a traumatic tamponade, this is because it may delay the implementation of thoracotomy[209], which is not available in the prehospital setting.

Medical directors may wish to include pericardiocentesis as part of the protocol for PEA. However, its use is strictly reserved for patients in whom fluid challenge and needle thoracostomy have not produced pulses. The prehospital care provider should use the subxyphoid approach, placing the needle to the left of the xyphoid and aiming at the left shoulder at a shallow angle. This technique minimizes the likelihood of injuring other important structures. It must be emphasized that this procedure should only be used as a final resort, when all other therapies have failed.

Patient Packaging

Before the appearance of organized EMS services and paramedic training, accident victims were often extricated without the use of any form of spinal immobilization. Patients often presented to the hospital with completed spinal cord injuries.[210] Immobilization has since become one of the most fundamental interventions provided by EMTs.

Spinal Immobilization

Immobilization is important not only in victims of motor vehicle crashes, but also in patients who suffer falls and gunshot wounds. Even falls from the standing position, especially in the elderly, may result in spinal injuries. In some areas, gunshot wounds are the leading cause of spinal cord injuries, while nationwide they are the third most common source of spinal injury.[211] Occult spinal injuries are very difficult to reliably detect in the field. Because the potential morbidity and the legal liability are so great, paramedics must be encouraged to immobilize all patients whose mechanism or complaint suggests the possibility of spinal injury. Studies are currently being conducted testing the safety of "clearing" C-spines in the field.

Apart from its primary purpose, spinal immobilization permits the patient to be easily log rolled, should vomiting occur. When properly immobilized, the patient is secured in the ambulance, an important consideration should the ambulance be involved in an accident. For unruly patients, spinal immobilization may decrease the security risk, making the journey safer for both patient and provider.

Cervical Collars

The first step in immobilizing the blunt trauma victim is manual stabilization of the patient's head followed by placement of a rigid cervical collar. Numerous collars are available on the market, ranging from cloth covered foam rubber to stiff plastics of various designs. The soft collar provides no immobilization[212] and has no place in prehospital care. Perhaps the most commonly used collar is the Philadelphia™ collar, a two-piece device made

of rigid foam. McCabe compared cervical spine motion on radiographs with volunteers immobilized in Philadelphia™, hard extrication, and two versions of the Stifneck™ collar.[213] The Stifneck™ collars were better than either the Philadelphia™ or hard extrication collars in immobilizing the patient in all directions except extension. Thom Dick, in a review of all spinal immobilization devices, was also enthusiastic about the Stifneck™ collar, stating that it provided the best immobilization among all collars tested.[214] A number of similar plastic collars are currently available, but limited data are available regarding their effectiveness. Regardless of the collar used, the medical director must emphasize that this is only one part of complete cervical immobilization.

Spine Boards

The spine board is the optimal method of cervical immobilization. Minimal amounts of motion were seen by Podolsky when the board was combined with tape and sandbags.[192] Graziano[215] and Cline[216] state that the lack of movement associated with short board stabilization of the cervical spine makes this the standard of comparison for all other devices. Howell has demonstrated, though, that the use of a collar does make a difference in immobilization when combined with the short board or Kendrick Extrication Device.[217] The ideal method is to have the patient placed in a cervical collar, then have a short board placed behind the patient. The head of the board should be padded to prevent pulling the patient into extension.[218] Once the patient is secured to the short board, the patient is then extricated to a long spine board and strapped down. If the patient must be extricated rapidly, though, the patient is placed in a collar and removed directly to a long board. This procedure provides an adequate compromise between spinal protection and other considerations, such as cardiopulmonary status and scene safety. Care must be taken to manually support the spine when this technique is used. Since no studies have demonstrated the safety of the latter technique, paramedics should be instructed to use this only when rapid extrication is indicated.

Although immobilization protects the spine from further injury, it may compromise ventilation. Even in children, who would be unlikely to suffer from COPD, spinal immobilization produced a significant decrease in forced vital capacity.[219] Providers must be ready to assist with ventilation, should immobilization result in compromise.

Cervical Immobilizers

Just as there are many different collars, so too are there many different devices to immobilize the head to the board. The only study that looked at these devices found that the two commercially available immobilizers tested did not control the pediatric patients well in flexion and extension when used without a collar. When a collar was used, the immobilization was as effective as that of a short board with tape, but not as good as a long board with sandbags and tape.[220] Sandbags are no longer routinely recommended however. The mass of the sandbag in a moving ambulance, especially with pediatric patients, would seem to pose a danger if the taping is less than optimal. Logrolling a vomiting patient can also be a difficult proposition when heavy sandbags are used. For these reasons, as well as because of the unaesthetic nature of tape residue, Dick advocates the use of commercially available head immobilizers.[221]

When an immobilizer is added to the Philadelphia collar (Philadelphia Red E.M. Collar with Head Immobilizer/Stabilizer™), the stability of the cervical spine was as good or better than that found with a short spine board.[222] The spine board was used without a collar, which is not the usual method of immobilization. These results once again point out the importance of a cervical immobilizer and collar combination.

Extremity Splints

Splinting of limbs in the prehospital setting today is primarily performed to control pain and to protect neurovascular structures. It is often forgotten that the major impetus for splinting of limbs came from the significant decrease in mortality that occurred with the use of the Thomas traction splint during the First World War.[223] Today several types of splints are available to paramedics.

Traction Splints

The Thomas splint and its variations are commonly used for fractures of the femur. Patients with these injuries can be afforded significant relief when traction is properly applied. Although these are simple devices, it is just as important to review their indications and use on a regular basis, as Skelton demonstrated in Kansas City.[21] Paramedics must be cautioned not to focus on splint placement while ignoring other aspects of the patient's care, such as spinal immobilization or cardiopulmonary status.

Vacuum and Pneumatic Splints

The development of these splinting devices in the past 20 years has changed the management of fractures in the prehospital setting. Much of the original teaching regarding fractures was to "splint it where it lies." Usually board splints were used and served well. The appearance of pneumatic splints in the early 1970s required the paramedic to reposition the limb to conform to the splint. The extent to which a paramedic repositions limbs in the field must be delineated in the system's procedure manual. One popular EMT text suggests that angulated long bone fractures be splinted in anatomic position, unless resistance is encountered.[224] They recommend any dislocation be splinted without reduction.

Both pneumatic and vacuum splints seem to work well, barring leaks. Most are radiolucent to a sufficient extent to allow X-ray assessment. Pneumatic splints are usually made of clear plastics, which allow some visual inspection of wounds and skin color. Vacuum splints are made of a rubberized cloth bladder filled with beads. Both types of devices will provide some degree of tamponade if there is an open wound. The major drawback with this type of splinting device is the possibility of failure if the splint is damaged. Just as with traction splints, paramedics must be warned against caring so much for the limb that they lose sight of the patient.

The prehospital care provider should be encouraged to use extremity splints only when the mechanism involves only one or two limbs and is not likely to involve multiple organ systems. For most patients the long board will provide adequate limb immobilization and is much quicker to apply. On occasion, paramedics become involved in placing traction splints for femur fractures, while the pelvic or abdominal injuries are relatively neglected. Medical directors must be vigilant in both their education and quality improvement programs to prevent this from occurring. With multiple trauma, time is of the essence and life threats take precedence over limb threats.

Pneumatic Anti-Shock Garments (PASG or MAST Suits)

McSwain has called the pneumatic anti-shock garment (PASG) "...the most controversial device in prehospital care of the 1980s."[225] Originally developed as a device to control hemorrhage, the pneumatic garment evolved into the G-suit of military aviators and astronauts. This device was then returned to its original use during the Vietnam War, where it was felt to dramatically improve survival from wounds. This experience was brought back from Vietnam by the combat medics, many of whom became paramedics. In a report from 1976, Civetta et al. described PASG use with the Miami, Florida Fire Rescue service. They felt the PASG was a significant device and advocated its incorporation into civilian EMS service.[226] By 1983, however, questions had arisen about its efficacy in the urban environment.[227] A 1985 study from Houston found there to be no difference in the trauma score on presentation to the emergency department with or without the PASG.[228] When this group looked only at penetrating abdominal trauma, their results again showed no improvement over controls.[229] Despite these investigations, McSwain argues in favor of the use of the PASG.[205] He cites laboratory investigations indicating that the PASG has an effect on blood pressure and that it controls hemorrhage in the area beneath it. He goes on to state that the complication rate is low and that at the worst the clinical trials have demonstrated no harm. When ventilatory compromise was investigated in healthy volunteers, no compromise was seen.[230] These authors caution that this might not be the case with patients in a shock state. Cayten has shown a higher-than-predicted survival rate among profoundly hypotensive (BP </= 50 mmHg) patients when the PASG was used.[231] There appears to be no likelihood of an early ceasefire in this conflict. Lloyd has proposed a multicenter trial of PASG[232], but no one has developed this study. At present, it would seem prudent to use the PASG under the following circumstances: 1) pelvic fractures, 2) lower limb fractures, where it would function as an air splint, 3) in penetrating trauma with hypotension where the wound appears to lie in the area covered by the PASG, 4) suspected abdominal aortic aneurysms with profound hypotension, 5) blunt trauma with hypotension where

its use does not prolong the scene time. 6) To increase peripheral vascular resistance when indicated, such as in cases of adrenergic resistant anaphylaxis. If they are going to use the garment, paramedics should be encouraged to place the PASG on the long board before extricating the patient, rather than attempting to place it while en route. Rural systems need to take a different look at the suit since prolonged transport time studies have not been conducted. The contraindications to PASG suit use include pulmonary edema, penetrating trauma above the suit, third trimester pregnancy, and abdominal evisceration or with suspected diaphragmatic rupture.

Summary

What should be the basic repertoire for the paramedic? Aside from rendering basic first aid for minor injuries, he or she should be able to rapidly assess the patient for life-threatening problems and have the tools to begin the patient resuscitation. Suggested procedures are listed in Table 3-3.

The selection of procedures a medical director will authorize his paramedics to perform determines much of the system's ability to respond to its patients. Procedures should be based on the needs of the population the system serves, not on arbitrary distinctions between provider levels. The repertoire may be limited by the amount of time available to the medical director and paramedics for continuing education and skills practice. Safe and effective prehospital procedures require an effective quality improvement program.

The medical director must provide the oversight, guidance, and discipline to ensure the procedures meet the patients' and system's needs.

Table 3-3   ALS Procedures

Procedure	Indication	Teaching	Difficulty of use	Comments
History and physical	Patient encounter	2	3	Basic to all other procedures; Requires training to be accurate and fast
Vital signs	Patient encounter — no other more important procedures pending	3	3	Should be attempted with each patient, but should not interfere with lifesaving procedures
Supplemental oxygen	Hypoxia; All patients when pulse oximetry is not available or not functioning	1	1	Not a benign drug, but should be applied liberally in the absence of pulse oximetry
Bag-valve-mask	Hypoventilation; Preoxygenation prior to intubation	3	5	Most difficult skill to perform properly under prehospital conditions; Should be viewed as precursor to intubation
Demand valve	Hypoventilation; Preoxygenation prior to intubation	2	4	Alternative to BVM; May allow a better mask seal than the BVM; No sense of compliance changes
Mouth-to-mask	Hypoventilation; Preoxygenation prior to intubation	1	3	Underutilized technique
Endotracheal intubation	**Hypoventilation; Airway compromise; Hypoxia**			
Direct oral intubation	No trismus; Tolerates laryngoscope	4	4	Most common; Requires patient to be supine; alternatives should be taught
Nasotracheal intubation	Breathing; Unable to lie supine	3	4	Safe; easy to teach
Digital intubation	Unresponsive	4	4	Use a mouth gag or bite block
Lighted stylet	Unresponsive	3	3	Requires a dark area
EOA® / EGTA	Excessive vomitus (obturator only); No indication as a primary airway management tool	2	3	Obsolete for ventilation; may be useful for controlling vomitus during intubation
PtL® / ETC	Legal restrictions barring use of ET intubation	4	4	Poor substitutes for endotracheal intubation
Cricothyrotomy	Need for airway management but unable to place ET tube	5	5	Should be performed rarely if intubation skills are good; should be practiced frequently
Transtracheal jet ventilation	Need for airway management but unable to place ET tube	3	4	Relatively easy alternate airway; Requires special equipment; Misplacement can cause massive subcutaneous emphysema
Minicricothyrotomy	Need for airway management but unable to place ET tube	4	4	Several manufacturers and devices
End-tidal CO_2 detection	Intubation	1	1	Mandatory after any intubation or cricothyrotomy
Pulse oximetry	Assessment for hypoxia	2	3	May be useful in titrating oxygen therapy; Benefits for COPD patients, multiple casualty incidents (where oxygen is limited)
NG tubes	Vomiting with risk of aspiration; Gastric decompression	3	4	Useful for long transport; Use only for aspiration of gastric contents; Not recommended for medication administration in the field
Needle thoracostomy	Tension pneumothorax; EMD	2	2	Should be performed promptly for tension pneumothorax

1 = easy, 5 = very difficult.

Procedure	Indication	Teaching	Difficulty of use	Comments
Tube thoracostomy	Pneumothorax; Hemothorax	5	5	Limited use in long transports, hemothorax
Medication administration				
Oral	Nifedipine; Nonemergent medications	1	1	Nifedipine is the only oral emergency medication; Mild analgesics in wilderness, mass gathering settings
Sublingual	Nitroglycerin	1	1	Nitroglycerin only
Nebulized aerosol	Bronchodilator delivery	2	2	Use in preference to epinephrine in all ages
Subcutaneous injection	Epinephrine	2	2	For moderate anaphylaxis (mild = no tx; severe = IV therapy, early intubation
Sublingual injection	Naloxone in moribund patient	2	3	Only when the patient is in extremis
Intramuscular injection	Rare; Use for naloxone; Possibly lorazepam, lidocaine, succinylcholine	2	2	Drugs other than naloxone only under exceptional circumstances
IV push	Most parenteral prehospital medications (not dopamine)	1	2	Route of choice
Intravenous infusion	Dopamine; Lidocaine (with extreme caution)	2	3	Drips must be watched with extreme care
Peripheral intravenous access	Fluid or medication administration prior to arrival at hospital	3	2	Most common; should have clear access indications; overused for "prophylactic access"
Central intravenous access	High volume fluid or critical medication administration; lack of peripheral access	4	4	Not as difficult or risky as some believe; may be lifesaving in severe trauma patients with long transports
Intraosseous access	Fluid or medication administration in a critical pediatric patient	3	3	Line of choice in critical pediatric patients
Cardiac monitoring	Patients at risk for dysrhythmias	5	4	Requires continual education to maintain dysrhythmia recognition skills
Defibrillation	Ventricular tachycardia or fibrillation	2	2	Automated defibrillators decrease the amount of training required
External cardiac pacing	Symptomatic bradycardia	2	2	Only successful if initiated early
Pericardiocentesis	EMD after failure of fluid resuscitation and bilateral needle thoracostomy	3	4	Should be available as a last resort
Spinal immobilization	All patients at risk for spinal injury (significant blunt force; Penetrating injuries of the trunk	2	3	Basic skill, but high risk; should receive more continuing education time
Traction splints	Isolated femur fractures and hemodynamic stability	3	4	Few indications except long distance transports; other techniques more efficient for urban/suburban setting
Vacuum/pneumatic splints	Isolated limb fractures and hemodynamic stability	2	2	Use in preference to traction splints
Pneumatic shock garments	Penetrating wound under area of device; Pelvic or lower limb fractures	2	3	Use much more limited than in past

References

1. Blaisdell FW: Trauma myths and magic: 1984 Fitts lecture, *J Trauma* 25(9):856-863, 1985.

2. Cales RH: Advanced life support in prehospital trauma care: an intervention in search of an indication? (editorial), *Ann Emerg Med* 17(6):651-653, 1988.

3. Gold CR: Prehospital advanced life support vs "scoop and run" in trauma management, *Ann Emerg Med* 16(7):797-801, 1987.

4. Kaweski SM, Sise MJ, Virgilio RW: The effect of prehospital fluids on survival in trauma patients, *J Trauma* 30(10):1215-1219, 1990.

5. Reines HD, Bartlett RL, Chudy NE, et al.: Is advanced life support appropriate for victims of motor vehicle accidents: the South Carolina highway trauma project, *J Trauma* 28(5):563-570, 1988.

6. Smith JP, Bodai BI, Hill AS, et al.: Prehospital stabilization of critically injured patients: a failed concept, *J Trauma* 25(1):65-70, 1985.

7. Trunkey DD: Is ALS necessary for pre-hospital trauma care? (editorial), *J Trauma* 24(1):86-87, 1984.

8. Aprahamian C, Thompson BM, Towne JB, et al.: The effect of a paramedic system on mortality of major open intra-abdominal vascular trauma, *J Trauma* 23(8):687-690, 1983.

9. Baxt WG, Moody P: The impact of advanced prehospital emergency care on the mortality of severely brain-injured patients, *J Trauma* 27(4):365-369, 1987.

10. Eisenberg MS, Copass MK, Hallstrom A, et al.: Management of out-of-hospital cardiac arrest: failure of basic emergency medical technician services, *JAMA* 243(10):1049-1051, 1980.

11. Hearne TR, Cummins RO: Improved survival from cardiac arrest in the community, *PACE* 11(2):1968-1973, 1988.

12. Honigman B, Rohweder K, Moore EE, et al.: Prehospital advanced trauma life support for penetrating cardiac wounds, *Ann Emerg Med* 19(2):145-150, 1990.

13. Potter D, Goldstein G, Fung SC, et al.: A controlled trial of prehospital advanced life support in trauma, *Ann Emerg Med* 17(6):582-588, 1988.

14. Pressley JC, Severance HW, Raney MP, et al.: A comparison of paramedic versus basic emergency medical care of patients at high and low risk during acute myocardial infarction, *J Am Coll Cardiol* 12(6):1555-1561, 1988.

15. Riediger G, Fleischmann-Sperber T: Efficiency and cost-effectiveness of advanced EMS in West Germany, *Am J Emerg Med* 8:76-80, 1990.

16. EMT: B National Standard Curriculum. Washington, D.C., U.S. Department of Transportation, National Highway Traffic Safety Administration, 1995.

17. Smith JP, Bodai BI: The urban paramedic's scope of practice, *JAMA* 253(4):544-548, 1985.

18. Waller JA: Urban-oriented methods: Failure to solve rural emergency care problems, *JAMA* 226(12):1441-1446, 1973.

19. Hedges JR: *Load and go — where?: The non-urban perspective of scoop and run,* Unpublished paper, 1989.

20. Ornato JP, Racht EM, Fitch JJ, et al.: The need for ALS in urban and suburban EMS systems (editorial), *Ann Emerg Med* 19(12):1469-1470, 1990.

21. Garrison HG, Downs SM, McNutt RA, et al.: A cost-effectiveness analysis of pediatric intraosseous infusion as a prehospital skill, *Prehosp Disaster Med* 7(3):221-227, 1992.

22. Skelton MB, McSwain NE: A study of cognitive and technical skill deterioration among trained paramedics, *JACEP* 6(10):436-438, 1977.

23. Walters G, Blucksman E: Retention of skills by advanced trained ambulance staff: implications for monitoring and retraining, *BMJ* 298:649-650, 1989.

24. Werman HA, Keseg DR, Glimcher M, et al.: Retention of basic trauma life support skills, *Prehosp Disaster Med* 5(2):137-144, 1990.

25. McSwain NE: Editorial comment on: Hankins DG, Carruthers N, Frascone RJ, et al.: Complication rates for the esophageal obturator airway and endotracheal tube in the prehospital setting, *Prehosp Disaster Med* 8(2):117-121, 1993.

26. Pepe P, Zachariah BS, Chandra NC: Invasive airway techniques in resuscitation, *Ann Emerg Med* 22(2 pt 2):393-403, 1993.

27. Spaite DW, Criss EA, Valenzuela TD, et al.: A prospective evaluation of prehospital patient assessment by direct in-field observation: failure of ALS personnel to measure vital signs, *Prehosp Disaster Med* 5(4):325-334, 1990.

28. Moss RL: Vital signs records omissions on prehospital patient encounter forms, *Prehosp Disaster Med* 8(1):21-27, 1993.

29. Gausche M, Henderson DP, Seidel JS: Vital signs as part of the prehospital assessment of the pediatric patient: a survey of paramedics, *Ann Emerg Med* 19(2):173-178, 1990.

30. Cayten CG, Herrmann N, Cole LW, et al.: Assessing the validity of EMS data, *JACEP* 7(11):390-396, 1978.

31. Jones JS, Ramsey W, Hetrick T: Accuracy of prehospital sphygmomanometers, *J Emerg Med* 5:23-27, 1987.

32. Prasad NH, Brown LH, Ausband SC, et al.: Prehospital blood pressures: inaccuracies caused by ambulance noise? *Am J Emerg Med* 12:617-620, 1994.

33. Menegazzi JJ, Davis EA, Sucov AN, et al.: Reliability of the Glasgow coma scale when used by emergency physicians and paramedics, *J Trauma* 34(1):46-48, 1993.

34. Keeler JL, Shuster M, Rowe BH: Reliability of pre-hospital rating scales for case severity and status change, *Am J Emerg Med* 11(2):115-121, 1993.

35. Caroline N: *Emergency medical treatment: a text for EMT-As and EMT-Intermediates,* Boston, 1987, Little, Brown, p. 133.

36. Elling R, Politis J: An evaluation of emergency medical technicians' ability to use manual ventilation devices, *Ann Emerg Med* 12(12):765-768, 1983.

37. Lande S: EMT ventilation skills (letter), *Ann Emerg Med* 17(1):107, 1988.

38. Harrison RR, Maull KI, Kennan RL, et al.: Mouth-to-mask ventilation: a superior method of rescue breathing, *Ann Emerg Med* 11(2):74-76, 1982.

39. Jesudian MCS, Harrison RR, Keenan RL, et al.: Bag-valve-mask ventilation; two rescuers are better than one: preliminary report, *Crit Care Med* 13(2):122-123, 1985.

40. Samuels DJ, Maull KI, Bock HC, et al.: *Emergency Medical Technician: Basic, National Standard Curriculum, U.S. Department of Transportation, DOT HS 808 149,* August 1994.

41. Stewart RD, Kaplan RM, Pennock B, et al.: Influence of mask design on bag-mask ventilation, *Ann Emerg Med* 14(5):403-406, 1985.

42. Palme C, Nystrom B, Tunnell R: An evaluation of the efficiency of face masks in the resuscitation of newborn infants, *Lancet* 1:207-210, 1985.

43. Terndrup TE, Kanter RK, Cherry RA: A comparison of infant ventilation methods performed by prehospital personnel, *Ann Emerg Med* 18(6):607-611, 1989.

44. Bryson TK, Benumof JL, Ward CF: The esophageal obturator airway: a clinical comparison to ventilation with a mask and oropharyngeal airway, *Chest* 74(5):537-539, 1978.

45. Rhee KJ, O'Malley RJ, Turner JE, et al.: Field airway management of the trauma patient: the efficacy of bag mask ventilation, *Am J Emerg Med* 6(4):333-336, 1988.

46. Campbell TP, Stewart RD, Kaplan RM, et al.: Oxygen enrichment of bag-valve-mask units during positive-pressure ventilation: a comparison of various techniques, *Ann Emerg Med* 17(3):232-235, 1988.

47. McCormack AP, Damon SK, Eisenberg MS: Disagreeable physical characteristics affecting bystander CPR, *Ann Emerg Med* 18(3):283-285, 1989.

48. Cydulka RK, Connor PJ, Myers TF, et al.: Prevention of oral bacterial flora transmission by using mouth-to-mask ventilation during CPR, *J Emerg Med* 9:317-321, 1991.

49. Johannigman JA, Branson RD, Davis K, et al.: Techniques of emergency ventilation: a model to evaluate tidal volume, airway pressure, and gastric insufflation, *J Trauma* 31(1):93-98, 1991.

50. Caroline N: *Emergency medical treatment: a text for EMT-As and EMT-Intermediates,* Boston, 1987, Little, Brown, p. 140.

51. Terndrup TE, Warner DA: Infant ventilation and oxygenation by basic life support providers: comparison of methods, *Prehosp Disaster Med* 7(1):35-40, 1992.

52. Rossi R, Linder KH, Ahnefeld FW: Devices for expired air resuscitation, *Prehosp Disaster Med* 8(2):123-126, 1993.

53. Hillis M, Sinclair D, Butler G, et al.: Prehospital cardiac arrest survival and neurologic recovery, *J Emerg Med* 11:245-252, 1993.

54. Stewart RD, Paris PM, Pelton GH, et al.: Effect of varied training techniques on field endotracheal intubation success rates, *Ann Emerg Med* 13(11):1032-1054, 1984.

55. Stratton SJ, Kane G, Wheeler NC, et al.: Prospective study of manikin-only versus manikin and human subject endotracheal intubation training of paramedics, *Ann Emerg Med* 20(12):1314-1318, 1991.

56. Shea SR, MacDonald JR, Gruzinski G: Prehospital endotracheal tube airway or esophageal gastric tube airway: a critical comparison, *Ann Emerg Med* 14(2):102-112, 1985.

57. Nelson MS: Medical student retention of intubation skills, *Ann Emerg Med* 18(10):1059-1061, 1989.

58. O'Brien DJ, Danzl DF, Hooker EA, et al.: Prehospital blind nasotracheal intubation by paramedics, *Ann Emerg Med* 18(6):612-617, 1989.

59. Pepe PE, Copass MK, Joyce TH: Prehospital endotracheal intubation: rationale for training emergency medical personnel, *Ann Emerg Med* 14(11):1085-1092, 1985.

60. Pointer JE: Clinical characteristics of paramedics' performance of endotracheal intubation, *J Emerg Med* 6:505-509, 1988.

61. Stewart RD, Paris PM, Winter PM, et al.: Field endotracheal intubation by paramedical personnel, *Chest* 85(3):341-345, 1984.

62. Jacobs LM, Berrizbeitia LD, Bennett B, et al.: Endotracheal intubation in the prehospital phase of emergency medical care, *JAMA* 250(16):2175-2177, 1983.

63. Guss DA, Posluszny M: Paramedic orotracheal intubation: a feasibility study, *Am J Emerg Med* 2:399-401, 1984.

64. Birmingham PK, Chesney FW, Ward RJ: Esophageal intubation: a review of detection techniques, *Anesth Analg* 65:886-891, 1986.

65. Bissinger U, Lenz G, Kuhn W: Unrecognized endobronchial intubation of emergency patients, *Ann Emerg Med* 18(8):853-855, 1989.

66. Aijan P, Tsai A, Knopp R, et al.: Endotracheal intubation of pediatric patients by paramedics, *Ann Emerg Med* 18(5):489-494, 1989.

67. Hauswald M, Sklar DP, Tandberg D, et al.: Cervical spine movement during airway management: cinefluoroscopic appraisal in human cadavers, *Am J Emerg Med* 9(6):535-538, 1991.

68. Dronen SC, Merigian KS, Hedges JR, et al.: A comparison of blind nasotracheal and succinylcholine-assisted intubation in the poisoned patient, *Ann Emerg Med* 16(6):650-652, 1987.

69. Advanced Trauma Life Support Program for Physicians: ed 5, Chicago, 1993, American College of Surgeons.

70. Bivins HG, Ford S, Bezmalinovic Z, et al.: The effect of axial traction during orotracheal intubation of the trauma victim with an unstable cervical spine, *Ann Emerg Med* 17(1):25-29, 1988.

71. Rhee KJ, Green W, Holcroft JW, et al.: Oral intubation in the multiply injured patient: the risk of exacerbating spinal cord damage, *Ann Emerg Med* 19(5):511-514, 1990.

72. Holley J, Jorden R: Airway management in patients with unstable cervical spine fractures, *Ann Emerg Med* 18(11):1237-1239, 1989.

73. Walls RM: Airway management, *Emerg Med Clin NA* 11(1):53-60, 1993.

74. Levine RL: Pharmacology of intravenous sedatives and opioids in critically illl patients, *Crit Care Clinics* 10:709-731, 1994.

75. Mendel PR, White PF: Sedation of the critically ill patient, *Int Anesthesiol Clinics* 10:185-200, 1993.

76. Joyce SM: Cervical immobilization during orotracheal intubation in trauma victims (editorial), *Ann Emerg Med* 17(1):88, 1988.

77. Verdile VP, Chiang J-L, Bedger R, et al.: Nasotracheal intubation using a flexible lighted stylet, *Ann Emerg Med* 19(5):506-510, 1990.

78. Krisanda TJ, Eitel DR, Hess D, et al.: An analysis of invasive airway management in a suburban emergency medical services system, *Prehosp Disaster Med* 7(2):121-126, 1992.

79. Kastendieck JG: Airway management. In Rosen P, Baker FJ, Barkin RM, et al.: *Emergency medicine: Concepts and clinical practice,* ed 2, St Louis, 1988, pp 41-68, Mosby.

80. Krishel S, Jackimczyk, Balazs K: Endotracheal tube whistle: an adjunct to blind nasotracheal intubation, *Ann Emerg Med* 21:33- 36, 1992.

81. Stewart RD: Tactile orotracheal intubation, *Ann Emerg Med* 13:175-178, 1984.

82. Ellis DG, Jakymec A, Kaplan RM, et al.: Guided orotracheal intubation in the operating room using a lighted stylet: a comparison with direct laryngoscopic technique, *Anesthesiology* 64:823-826, 1986.

83. Stewart RD, LaRosee A, Kaplan RM, et al.: Correct positioning of an endotracheal tube using a flexible lighted stylet, *Crit Care Med* 18:97-99, 1990.

84. Verdile VP, Heller MB, Paris PM, et al.: Nasotracheal intubation in traumatic craniofacial dislocation: use of the lighted stylet, *Am J Emerg Med* 6:39-41, 1988.

85. Hung OR, Lung KE, Multari J, et al.: *Clinical trial of a new light-wand device for nasotracheal intubation in surgical patients,* Presented at the Canadian Anesthesiologists Society, 1993.

86. Don Michael TA, Lambert EH, Mehran A: "Mouth-to-lung" airway for cardiac resuscitation, *Lancet* 2:1329, 1968.

87. Don Micheal TA, Gordon AS: The oesophageal obturator airway: a new device in emergency cardiopulmonary resuscitation, *BMJ* 281:1531-1534, 1980.

88. Cummins RO, editor: *Advanced cardiac life support,* 1994, pp. 1-17.

89. Don Michael TA: The esophageal obturator airway: a critique, *JAMA* 246(10):1098-1101, 1981.

90. Hammargren Y, Clinton JE, Ruiz E: A standard comparison of esophageal obturator airway and endotracheal tube ventilation in cardiac arrest, *Ann Emerg Med* 14(10):953-958, 1985.

91. Meislin HW: The esophageal obturator airway: a study of respiratory effectiveness, *Ann Emerg Med* 9(2):54-59, 1980.

92. Johnson KR, Genovesi MG, Lassar KH: Esophageal obturator airway: use and complications, *JACEP* 5(1):36-39, 1976.

93. Smock SN: Esophageal obturator airway: preferred CPR technique, *JACEP* 4(3):232-233, 1975.

94. Harrison EE, Nord HJ, Beeman RW: Esophageal perforation following use of the esophageal obturator airway, *Ann Emerg Med* 9(1):21-25, 1980.

95. Yancey W, Wears R, Kamajian G, et al.: Unrecognized tracheal intubation: a complication of the esophageal obturator airway, *Ann Emerg Med* 9(1):18-20, 1980.

96. Crippen D, Olvey S, Graffis R: Gastric rupture: an esophageal obturator airway complication, *Ann Emerg Med* 10(7):370-373, 1981.

97. Gatrell CB: Unrecognized esophageal intubation with both esophageal obturator airway and endotracheal tube, *Ann Emerg Med* 13(8):624-626, 1984.

98. Schofferman J, Oill P, Lewis AJ: The esophageal obturator airway: a clinical evaluation, *Chest* 69(1):67-71, 1976.

99. Auerbach PS, Geehr EC: Inadequate oxygenation and ventilation using the esophageal gastric tube airway in the prehospital setting, *JAMA* 250(22):3067-3071, 1983.

100. Geehr EC, Bogetz MS, Auerbach PS: Prehospital tracheal intubation versus esophageal gastric tube airway use: a prospective study, *Am J Emerg Med* 3:381-385, 1985.

101. Smith JP, Bodai BI, Aubourg R, et al.: A field evaluation of the esophageal obturator airway, *J Trauma* 23(4):317-321, 1983.

102. Bass RR, Allison EJ, Hunt RC: The esophageal obturator airway: a reassessment of use by paramedics, *Ann Emerg Med* 11(7):358-360, 1982.

103. Smith JP, Bodai BJ, Seifkin A, et al.: The esophageal obturator airway: a review, *JAMA* 250(8):1081-1084, 1983.

104. Hankins DG, Carruthers N, Frascone RJ, et al: Complication rates for the esophageal obturator airway and endotracheal tube in the prehospital setting, *Prehosp Disaster Med* 8(2):117-121, 1993.

105. Berdeen TN: One-year experience with the tracheoesophageal airway, *Ann Emerg Med* 10(1):25-27, 1981.

106. Eisenberg RS: A new airway for tracheal or esophageal insertion: description and field experience, *Ann Emerg Med* 9(5):270-272, 1980.

107. Niemann JT, Rosborough JP, Myers R, et al.: The pharyngeo-tracheal lumen airway: preliminary investigation of a new adjunct, *Ann Emerg Med* 13(8):591-596, 1984.

108. Frass M, Franzer R, Zhrahal F, et al.: The esophageal tracheal combitube: preliminary results with a new airway for CPR, *Ann Emerg Med* 16(7):768-772, 1987.

109. Bartlett RL, Martin SD, Perina D, et al.: The pharyngeotracheal lumen airway: an assessment of airway control in the setting of upper airway hemorrhage, *Ann Emerg Med* 16(3):343-346, 1987.

110. Atherton GL, Johnson JC: Ability of paramedics to use the Combitube™ in prehospital cardiac arrest, *Ann Emerg Med* 22(8):1263-1268, 1993.

111. McMahan S, Ornato JP, Racht EM, et al.: Multi-agency, prehospital evaluation of the pharyngeo-tracheal lumen (PTL) airway, *Prehosp Disaster Med* 7(1):13-18, 1992.

112. Hunt RC, Sheets CA, Whitley TW: Pharyngeal tracheal lumen airway training: failure to discriminate between esophageal and endotracheal modes and failure to confirm ventilation, *Ann Emerg Med* 18(9):947-952, 1989.

113. Johnson JC, Atherton GL: The esophageal tracheal combitube: an alternate route to airway management, *JEMS* 16(5):29-35, 1991.

114. Wafai Y, Salem MR, Baraka A, et al.: Effectiveness of the self-inflating bulb for verification of proper placement of the Esophageal Tracheal Combitube™, *Anesth Analg* 80:122-126, 1995.

115. Brain ALJ: The laryngeal mask airway: a new concept in airway management, *Br J Anaesth* 55:801-805, 1983.

116. Davies PRF, Tighe SQM, Greenslade GL, et al.: Laryngeal mask airway tube insertion by unskilled personnel, *Lancet* 336:977-979, 1990.

117. Pennant JH, Pace NA, Gajraj NM: Role of the laryngeal mask airway in the immobile cervical spine, *J Clin Anesth* 5:226-230, 1993.

118. Greene MK, Roden R, Hinchley G: The laryngeal mask airway: two cases of prehospital trauma care, *Anaesthesia* 47:688-689, 1992.

119. Reinhart DJ, Simmons G: Comparison of placement of the laryngeal mask airway with endotracheal tube by paramedics and respiratory therapists, *Ann Emerg Med* 24:260-263, 1994.

120. MacLeod BA, Heller MB, Gerard J, et al.: Verification of endotracheal tube placement with colorimetric end-tidal CO_2 detection, *Ann Emerg Med* 20(3):267-270, 1991.

121. Ornato JP, Shipley JB, Racht EM, et al.: Multicenter study of a portable, hand size, colorimetric end-tidal carbon dioxide detection device, *Ann Emerg Med* 21(5):518-523, 1992.

122. Anton WR, Gordon RW, Jordan TM, et al.: A disposable end-tidal CO2 detector to verify endotracheal intubation, *Ann Emerg Med* 20(3):271-275, 1991.

123. Wee MYK: The oesophageal detector device: assessment of a new method to distinguish oesophageal from tracheal intubation, *Anaesthesia* 43:27-29, 1988.

124. O'Leary JJ, Pollard BJ, Ryan MJ: A method of detecting oesophageal intubation or confirming tracheal intubation, *Anaesth Intens Care* 16:299-301, 1988.

125. Anderson KH, Hald A: Assessing the position of the tracheal tube: the reliability of different methods, *Anaesthesia* 44:984-985, 1989.

126. Williams KN, Nunn JF: The oesophageal detector device: a prospective trial on 100 patients, *Anaesthesia* 44:412, 1989.

127. Zaleski L, Abello D, Gold MI: The esophageal detector device: does it work? *Anesthesiology* 79(2):244-247, 1993.

128. Jenkins WA, Verdile VP, Paris PM: The syringe aspiration technique to verify endotracheal tube position, *Am J Emerg Med* 12:413-416, 1994.

129. Jackson C: High tracheostomy and other errors: the chief causes of chronic laryngeal stenosis, *Surg Gynecol Obstet* 32:392-395, 1921.

130. McGill J, Clinton JE, Ruiz E: Cricothyroidotomy in the emergency department, *Ann Emerg Med* 11(7):361-364, 1982.

131. Boyle MF, Hatton D, Sheets C: Surgical cricothyroidotomy performed by air ambulance flight nurses: a 5-year experience, *Am J Emerg Med* 11:41-45, 1993.

132. Miklus RM, Elliott C, Snow N: Surgical cricothyroidotomy in the field: experience of a helicopter transport team, *J Trauma* 29(4):506-508, 1989.

133. Spaite DW, Joseph M: Prehospital cricothyroidotomy: an investigation of indications, technique, complica-

tions, and patient outcome, *Ann Emerg Med* 19(3):279-285, 1990.

134. Nugent WL, Rhee KJ, Wisner DH: Can nurses perform surgical cricothyroidotomy with acceptable success and complication rates? *Ann Emerg Med* 20(4):367-370, 1991.

135. Campbell CT, Harris RC, Cook MH, et al.: A new device for emergency percutaneous transtracheal ventilation in partial and complete airway obstruction, *Ann Emerg Med* 17(9):927-931, 1988.

136. Corke C, Cranswick P: A Seldinger technique for mini-tracheostomy insertion, *Anaesth Intens Care* 16:206-207, 1988.

137. Johnson DR, Dunlap A, McFeeley P, et al.: Circothyroidotomy performed by prehospital personnel: a comparison of two techniques in a human cadaver model, *Am J Emerg Med* 11(3):207-209, 1993.

138. Advanced Trauma Life Support Program for Physicians: ed 5, Chicago, 1993, American College of Surgeons, p. 54.

139. Frame SB, Timberlake GA, Kerstein MD, et al.: Transtracheal needle catheter ventilation in complete airway obstruction: an animal model, *Ann Emerg Med* 18(2):127-133, 1989.

140. Yealy DM, Stewart RD, Kaplan RM: Myths and pitfalls in emergency translaryngeal ventilation: correcting misimpressions, *Ann Emerg Med* 17(7):690-692, 1988.

141. Yealy DM, Stewart RD, Kaplan MS: Clarifications on translaryngeal ventilation (letter), *Ann Emerg Med* 17(10):1130, 1988.

142. Yealy DM, Plewa MC, Reed JJ, et al.: Manual translaryngeal jet ventilation and the risk of aspiration in a canine model, *Ann Emerg Med* 19(11):1238-1241, 1990.

143. Stothert JC, Stout MJ, Lewis LM, et al.: High pressure percutaneous transtracheal ventilation: the use of large gauge intravenous-type catheters in the totally obstructed airway, *Am J Emerg Med* 8(3):184-189, 1990.

144. Nolan JP, Baskett PJF: Gas-powered and portable ventilators: an evaluation of six models, *Prehosp Disaster Med* 7(1):25-34, 1992.

145. Porter RS, Merlin MA, Heller MB: The fifth vital sign, *Emergency* 22(3):37-41, 1990.

146. Aughey K, Hess D, Eitel D, et al.: An evaluation of pulse oximetry in prehospital care, *Ann Emerg Med* 20(8):887-891, 1991.

147. McGuire TJ, Pointer JE: Evaluation of a pulse oximeter in the prehospital setting, *Ann Emerg Med* 17(10):1058-1062, 1988.

148. Silverston P: Pulse oximetry at the roadside: a study of pulse oximetry in immediate care, *BMJ* 298:711-713, 1989.

149. Mateer JR, Olson DW, Stueven HA, et al.: Continuous pulse oximetry during emergency endotracheal intubation, *Ann Emerg Med* 22(4):675-679, 1993.

150. Cydulka RK, Shade B, Emerman CL, et al.: Prehospital pulse oximetry: useful or misused? *Ann Emerg Med* 21(6):675-679, 1992.

151. Melton JD, Heller MB, Kaplan R, et al.: Occult hypoxemia during aeromedical transport: detection by pulse oximetry, *Prehosp Disaster Med* 4(2):115-121, 1989.

152. Valko PC, Campbell JP, McCarty DL, et al.: Prehospital use of pulse oximetry in rotary wing aircraft, *Prehosp Disaster Med* 6(4):421-428, 1991.

153. Craft TM, Blogg CE: Pulse oximetry at the roadside (letter), *BMJ* 298:1096, 1989.

154. Cockroft S, Dodd P: Pulse oximetry at the roadside (letter), *BMJ* 298:1096, 1989.

155. Ross DS: Thoracentesis. In Roberts JR, Hedges JR, editors: *Clinical procedures in emergency medicine*, Philadelphia, 1985, WB Saunders, p. 85.

156. McSwain GR, Garrison WB, Artz CP: Evaluation of resuscitation from cardio-pulmonary arrest by paramedics, *Ann Emerg Med* 9:341-345, 1980.

157. Border JR, Lewis FR, Aprahamian C, et al.: Panel: prehospital trauma care—stabilize or scoop and run, *J Trauma* 23(8):708-711, 1983.

158. Wears RL, Winton CN: Load and go versus stay and play: analysis of prehospital IV fluid therapy by computer simulation, *Ann Emerg Med* 19(2):163-168, 1990.

159. Aprahamian C, Thompson BM, Towne JB, et al.: The effect of a paramedic system on mortality of major open intra-abdominal vascular trauma, *J Trauma* 23(8):687-690, 1983.

160. Lawrence DW, Lauro AJ: Complications from IV therapy: results from field-started and emergency department-started IVs compared, *Ann Emerg Med* 17(4):314-317, 1988.

161. Pons PT, Moore EE, Cusick JM, et al.: Prehospital venous access in an urban paramedic system—a prospective on-scene analysis, *J Trauma* 28(10):1460-1463, 1988.

162. Jones SE, Nesper TP, Alcouloumre E: Prehospital intravenous line placement: a prospective study, *Ann Emerg Med* 18:244-246, 1989.

163. Slovis CM, Herr EW, Londorf D, et al.: Success rates for initiation of intravenous therapy en route by prehospital care providers, *Am J Emerg Med* 8:305-307, 1990.

164. O'Gorman M, Trabulsy P, Pilcher DB: Zero-time prehospital IV, *J Trauma* 29(1):84-86, 1989.

165. Honigman B, Rohweder K, Moore EE, et al.: Prehospital advanced trauma life support for penetrating cardiac wounds, *Ann Emerg Med* 19(2):145-150, 1990.

166. Spaite DW, Tse DJ, Valenzuela TD, et al.: The impact of injury severity and prehospital procedures on scene time in victims of major trauma, *Ann Emerg Med* 20(12):1299-1305, 1991.

167. Spaite DW, Valenzuela TD, Criss EA, et al.: A prospective in-field comparison of intravenous line placement by urban and nonurban emergency medical services personnel, *Ann Emerg Med* 24:209-214, 1994.

168. Pollack CV: Prehospital fluid resuscitation of the trauma patient: an update on the controversies, *Emerg Med Clin NA* 11(1):61-70, 1993.

169. Bickell WH, Wall MJ, Pepe PE, et al.: Immediate versus delayed resuscitation for hypotensive patients with penetrating torso injuries, *N Engl J Med* 331:1105-1109, 1994.

170. Donovan PJ, Cline DM, Whitley TW, et al.: Prehospital care by EMTs and EMT-Is in a rural setting: prolongation of scene times by ALS procedures, *Ann Emerg Med* 18(5):495-500, 1989.

171. Guisto JA, Iserson KV: The feasibility of 12-gauge intravenous catheter use in the prehospital setting, *J Emerg Med* 8:173-176, 1990.

172. Emerman CL, Bellon EM, Lukens TW, et al.: A prospective study of femoral versus subclavian vein catheterization during cardiac arrest, *Ann Emerg Med* 19(1):26-30, 1990.

173. Arrighi DA, Farnell MB, Mucha P, et al.: Prospective, randomized trial of rapid venous access for patients in hypovolemic shock, *Ann Emerg Med* 18(9):927-930, 1989.

174. Dronen SC: Subclavian venipuncture. In Roberts JR, Hedges JR, editors: *Clinical procedures in emergency medicine,* Philadelphia, 1985, pp. 304-321, WB Saunders.

175. Wyte SR, Barker WJ: Central venous catheterization: internal jugular approach and alternatives. In Roberts JR, Hedges JR, editors: *Clinical procedures in emergency medicine,* Philadelphia, 1985, pp. 321-332, WB Saunders.

176. Fuchs S, LaCovey D, Paris P: A prehospital model of intraosseous infusion, *Ann Emerg Med* 20(4):371-374, 1991.

177. Smith RJ, Keseg DP, Maney LK, et al.: Intraosseous infusions by prehospital personnel in critically ill pediatric patients, *Ann Emerg Med* 17(5):491-495, 1988.

178. Glaeser PW, Hellmich TR, Szewczuga D, et al.: Five-year experience in prehospital intraosseous infusions in children and adults, *Ann Emerg Med* 22(7):1119-1124, 1993.

179. Orlowski JP, Julius CJ, Petras RE, et al.: The safety of intraosseous infusions: risks of fat and bone marrow emboli to the lungs, *Ann Emerg Med* 18(10):1062-1067, 1989.

180. Eitel DR, Meador SA, Drawbaugh R, et al.: Prehospital administration of inhaled metaproterenol, *Ann Emerg Med* 19(12):1412-1417, 1990.

181. Hawkins J, Hakala K, Heller MB, et al.: Metered-dose aerosolized bronchodilator in prehospital care: a feasibility study, *J Emerg Med* 4:273-277, 1986.

182. Emerman CL, Shade B, Kubincanek J: A controlled trial of nebulized isoetharine in the prehospital treatment of acute asthma, *Am J Emerg Med* 8(6):512-514, 1990.

183. Vonderohe EA, Jones JH, McGrath RB, et al.: The prehospital use of albuterol inhalation treatments, *Prehosp Disaster Med* 6(3):327-330, 1991.

184. Hedges JR, Cionni DJ, Amsterdam JT, et al.: Oxygen desaturation in adults following inhaled metaproterenol therapy, *J Emerg Med* 5:77-81, 1987.

185. Ben-Zvi Z, Lam C, Hoffman J, et al.: An evaluation of the initial treatment of acute asthma, *Pediatrics* 70(3):348-353, 1982.

186. Vukmir RB, Paris PM, Yealy DM: Glucagon: prehospital therapy for hypoglycemia, *Ann Emerg Med* 20:375-379, 1991.

187. Lam A, Newhouse MT: Management of asthma and chronic airflow limitation: are methylxanthines obsolete? *Chest* 98:45-52, 1990.

188. Pantridge JF, Geddes JS: A mobile intensive-care unit in the management of myocardial infarction, *Lancet* 2:271-273, 1967.

189. Jakobsson J, Nyquist O, Rehnqvist N: Concise education of ambulance personnel in CG interpretation and out of hospital defibrillation, *Eur Heart J* 8:229-233, 1987.

190. Jakobsson J, Nyquist O, Rehnqvist N, et al.: Prognosis and clinical follow-up of patients resuscitated from out-of-hospital cardiac arrest, *Acta Med Scand* 222:123-132, 1987.

191. Jakobsson J, Nyquist O, Rehnqvist N: Cardiac arrest in Stockholm with special reference to the ambulance organization, *Acta Med Scand* 222:117-122, 1987.

192. Jakobsson J, Nyquist O, Rehnqvist N: Effects of early defibrillation of out-of-hospital cardiac arrest patients by ambulance personnel, *Eur Heart J* 8:1189-1194, 1987.

193. Bradley K, Sokolow AE, Wright KJ, McCullough WJ: A comparison of an innovative four-hour EMT-D course with a 'standard' ten-hour course, *Ann Emerg Med* 17(6):613-619, 1988.

194. Olson DW, LaRochelle J, Fark D, et al.: EMT-Defibrillation: the Wisconsin experience, *Ann Emerg Med* 18(8):806-811, 1989.

195. Cummins RO, Thies W: Encouraging early defibrillation: the American Heart Association and automated external defibrillators, *Ann Emerg Med* 19(11):1245-1248, 1990.

196. Weaver WD, Hill D, Fahrenbruch CE, et al.: Use of the automatic external defibrillator in the management of out-of-hospital cardiac arrest, *N Engl J Med* 319(11):661-666, 1988.

197. Moore JE, Eisenberg MS, Cummins RO, et al.: Lay person use of automatic external defibrillation, *Ann Emerg Med* 16(6):669-672, 1987.

198. Cummins RO, Schubach JA, Litwin PE, et al.: Training lay persons to use automatic external defibrillators: success of initial training and one year retention of skills, *Am J Emerg Med* 7:143-149, 1989.

199. Hunt RC, McCabe JB, Hamilton GC, et al.: Influence of emergency medical systems and prehospital defibrillation on survival of sudden cardiac death victims, *Am J Emerg Med* 7(1):68-82, 1989.

200. Vukov LF, Johnson DQ: External transcutaneous pacemakers in interhospital transport of cardiac patients, *Ann Emerg Med* 18(7):738-740, 1989.

201. Eitel DR, Guzzardi LJ, Stein SE, et al.: Noninvasive transcutaneous cardiac pacing in prehospital cardiac arrest, *Ann Emerg Med* 16(50):531-534, 1987.

202. O'Toole KS, Paris PM, Heller MB: Emergency transcutaneous pacing in the management of patients with bradyasystolic rhythms, *J Emerg Med* 5:267-273, 1987.

203. Syverud SA, Dalsey WC, Hedges JR: Transcutaneous and transvenous cardiac pacing for early bradyasystole cardiac arrest, *Ann Emerg Med* 15:121-124, 1986.

204. Hedges JR, Syverud SA, Dalsey WC, et al.: Prehospital trial of emergency transcutaneous cardiac pacing, *Circulation* 76(6):1337-1343, 1987.

205. Vukov LF, White RD: External transcutaneous pacemakers in prehospital cardiac arrest (letter), *Ann Emerg Med* 17(5):554-555, 1988.

206. Grubb BP, Samoil D, Temesy-Armos P, et al.: The use of external noninvasive pacing for the termination of supraventricular tachycardia in the emergency department setting, *Ann Emerg Med* 22(4):714-717, 1993.

207. Vukmir RB: Emergency cardiac pacing, *Am J Emerg Med* 11(2):166-176, 1993.

208. Cummins, RO, editor: *Advanced cardiac life support textbook,* Dallas, 1994, American Heart Association, Chapter 13.

209. Calliham M: Pericardiocentesis. In Roberts JR, Hedges JR, editors: *Clinical procedures in emergency medicine,* Philadelphia, 1985, pp. 208-225, WB Saunders.

210. Green BA, Eismont FJ, O'Heir JT: Pre-hospital management of spinal cord injuries, *Paraplegia* 25:229-238, 1987.

211. Kihtir T, Ivatury RR, Simon R, et al.: Management of transperitoneal gunshot wounds of the spine, *J Trauma* 31(12):1579-1583, 1991.

212. Podolsky S, Baraff LJ, Simon RR, et al.: Efficacy of cervical spine immobilization methods, *J Trauma* 23(6):461-465, 1983.

213. McCabe JB, Nolan DJ: Comparison of the effectiveness of different cervical immobilization collars, *Ann Emerg Med* 15(1):50-53, 1986.

214. Dick T, Land R: Spinal immobilization devices; Part 1: cervical extrication collars, *J Emerg Med* Serv 12:26-32, 1982.

215. Graziano AF, Scheidel EA, Cline JR, et al.: A radiographic comparison of prehospital cervical immobilization devices, *Ann Emerg Med* 16(10):1127-1131, 1987.

216. Cline JR, Scheidel E, Bigsby EF: A comparison of methods of cervical immobilization used in patient extrication and transport, *J Trauma* 25(7):649-653, 1985.

217. Howell JM, Burrow R, Dumontier C, et al.: A practical radiographic comparison of short board technique and Kendrick Extrication Device, *Ann Emerg Med* 18(9):943-946, 1989.

218. Schriger DL, Larmon B, LeGassick T, et al.: Spinal immobilization on a flat backboard: does it result in neutral position of the cervical spine? *Ann Emerg Med* 20(8):878-881, 1991.

219. Schafermeyer RW, Ribbeck BM, Gaskins J, et al.: Respiratory effects of spinal immobilization in children, *Ann Emerg Med* 20(9):1017-1019, 1991.

220. Huerta C, Griffith R, Joyce SM: Cervical spine stabilization in pediatric patients: evaluation of current techniques, *Ann Emerg Med* 169(10):1121-1126, 1987.

221. Dick T, Land R: Spinal immobilization devices; Part 3: full spinal immobilizers, *J Emerg Med Serv* 2:34-43, 1983.

222. Joyce SM, Moser CS: Evaluation of a new cervical immobilization/extrication device, *Prehosp Disaster Med* 7(1):61-64, 1992.

223. Dick T: Prehospital splinting. In Roberts JR, Hedges JR, editors: *Clinical procedures in emergency medicine,* Philadelphia, 1985, pp. 576-597, WB Saunders.

224. Grant HD, Murray RH, Bergeron JD: *Emergency care,* ed 5, Englewood Cliffs, NJ, 1990, pp. 251-253, Prentice Hall.

225. McSwain NE: Pneumatic anti-shock garment: state of the art, *Ann Emerg Med* 17(5):506-525, 1988.

226. Civetta JM, Nussenfeld SR, Rowe TR, et al.: Prehospital use of the military anti-shock trouser (MAST), *JACEP* 5(8):581-587, 1976.

227. Mackersie RC, Christensen JM, Lewis FR: The prehospital use of external counterpressure: does MAST make a difference? *J Trauma* 24(10):882-888, 1984.

228. Bickell WH, Pepe PE, Wyatt CH, et al.: Effect of anti-shock trousers on the trauma score: a prospective analysis in the urban setting, *Ann Emerg Med* 14(30):218-222, 1985.

229. Bickell WH, Pepe PE, Bailey ML, et al.: Randomized trial of pneumatic antishock garments in the prehospital management of penetrating abdominal injuries, *Ann Emerg Med* 16(6):653-658, 1987.

230. Riou B, Pansard J, Lazard T, et al.: Ventilatory effects of medical antishock trousers in healthy volunteers, *J Trauma* 31(11):1495-1502, 1991.

231. Cayten CG, Berendt BM, Byrne DW, et al.: A study of pneumatic antishock garments in severely hypotensive trauma patients, *J Trauma* 34(5):728-735, 1993.

232. Lloyd S: MAST and IV infusion: do they help in prehospital trauma and management? *Ann Emerg Med* 16(50):565-567, 1987.

Pharmacotherapy

Prehospital medical command requires prudent and expeditious use of pharmacological agents. This chapter provides an overview of the common principles regarding prehospital pharmacotherapy. In addition, common medications currently available to the prehospital care provider are reviewed. Pitfalls in pharmacotherapy will be discussed. Drug dosage recommendations will strictly follow the AHA guidelines[1] where appropriate. Newer agents that may become integral to future prehospital systems will be discussed.

All recommendations made in this chapter are simply guidelines for the medical director to use in his or her development of prehospital protocols and are not to be construed as standards of practice.

Early hospital clinicians recognized that many pharmacological agents garnered greater success when administered earlier in the evolution of certain acute illnesses. The logical consequence of improved survival with early administration of medications was the addition of many pharmacological maneuvers to the prehospital environment. Box 4-1 lists medications currently in use in the state of Pennsylvania.

The almost dizzying number of medications available within a typical EMS system demands strict medical control. The prehospital medical director is charged with the choice of drugs for prehospital use based on ACLS guidelines, local standards, and state-approved drug lists. Jurisdictions vary across the country as to the type and number of drugs carried by field providers.[3]

While it is desirable to carry a broad range of medications to meet a variety of patient requirements, the medical command physician must understand the real cost of stocking medications, developing protocols, providing initial training, and continuing education. Adding succinylcholine to a field drug list might require extensive provider training, protocol revision, and the development of procedures for dealing with the drug's short shelf life. Drugs should not be added to the prehospital armamentarium just because they are available and useful in the hospital setting. The command physician must consider potential risks and benefits over existing therapies. For example, although diltiazem is a useful drug for supraventricular tachycardia (SVT) in the hospital, the cost of adding this agent to the prehospital drug list may not be justified in a service that, in the past year, saw very few cases of SVT (Box 4-2).

ADRIAN D'AMICO, MD, FACEP

Box 4-1	**Medication List for State of Pennsylvania[2]**

Adenosine	Lactated Ringers
Albuterol	Normosol
Aminophylline	Isoproterenol
Atropine	Lidocaine
Bretylium	Magnesium
Calcium chloride	Meperidine
Dexamethasone	Morphine
Diazepam	Naloxone
Diphenhydramine	Nitroglycerin IV drip
Dobutamine	Nitroglycerin ointment
Dopamine	Nitroglycerin spray,
Epinephrine	tablets
Furosemide	Nitrous oxide
Glucagon	Oxytocin
Heparin lock flush	Procainamide
Hydrocortisone	Sodium bicarbonate
IV electrolyte solutions	Sterile water for injection
Dextrose	Terbutaline
Saline	Verapamil

Box 4-2	**Issues Related to the Addition of New Medications to a Prehospital Drug List**

- Cost
- Risk/Benefit ratio
- Stocking issues
- Legal
- Potential frequency of use
- Training issues
- Alternative drugs

Finally, little outcome data are available for the use of pharmacological agents in the prehospital setting.[4] The 1992 National Conference on CPR and ECC adopted a system of classifying cardiac interventions based on supporting scientific evidence (Box 4-3). Ideally, in the future, all prehospital interventions will be classified in a similar manner based on available scientific evidence.

Routes of Administration

The prehospital care provider must understand the available routes of administration of indicated drugs, as well as their proper doses. Providers must realize that numerous drugs have beneficial effects through a particular route of administration and might be detrimental if administered via an inappropriate route.[5]

Box 4-3	**Classification of Therapeutic Interventions in CPR and ECC[17]**

Class I	Therapeutic option that is usually indicated, always acceptable, and considered useful and effective.
Class II	Therapeutic option that is acceptable, is of uncertain efficacy, and may be controversial.
Class IIa	Therapeutic option for which the weight of evidence is in favor of its usefulness and efficacy.
Class IIb	Therapeutic option that is not well established by evidence but may be helpful and probably not harmful.
Class III	Therapeutic option that is inappropriate, is without scientific supporting data, and may be harmful.

In the prehospital environment, often the optimal route of administration is the parenteral route. The advantages include a rapid onset of action and clearly predictable effects. Parenteral drugs can be administered to the patient who is unable to orally ingest a necessary drug, as well as to deliver the medications into the patient's system more quickly and efficiently.

Subcutaneous

Certain medications can be administered into the subcutaneous layer of the skin where vascular networks promote efficient absorption of a drug. Epinephrine is the prototypical drug in this class administered for the treatment of allergic disorders. Because subcutaneous absorption is dependent on local blood flow, there may be a significant reduction in absorption in conditions that decrease local perfusion in skin, such as hypotension or shocklike states.

Sublingual

The sublingual route permits absorption of a drug into the systemic circulation via the vascular network of the mucous membranes in the floor of the mouth. Nitroglycerin is the prototypical drug in this class, exhibiting rapid and predictable absorption.

Intramuscular

The intramuscular route is a common route of drug administration but generally exhibits slow absorption in comparison to the IV route. The absorption of an IM medication is dependent upon the regional vascular supply and physiological states that diminish blood flow either acutely or chronically, which can have a dramatic impact on the absorption of an IM medication. For example, shocklike states can adversely affect IM absorption. Therefore it is not the recommended route of administration for patients with decreased blood flow to the skin or muscle beds. For example, in a patient with unstable ventricular tachycardia, the use of IM lidocaine would result in delayed absorption of the drug with delayed onset of drug action.

Intraosseous

In children less than two years old, the IO route can be used for many medications when IV access is not readily available.[6-9] Most medications that are administered parenterally can be administered via the IO route, including the common cardiac drugs given during advanced resuscitation, with the exception of sodium bicarbonate. This route of administration requires specific training of prehospital personnel, since the technique requires specialized equipment and expertise not normally found in most prehospital training programs. The cost of initiating this training and continuing education is significant and must be considered in the context of other programs that may be more cost effective.[10] Potential complications of the procedure include tibial fracture, injury of the epiphyseal plate, and infection at the access site.[6-9] These complications, albeit rare, require the medical director to closely monitor the performance of this type of invasive procedure in the pediatric patient.

Inhalational

Some medications, such as metaproterenol, albuterol, and atropine, can be aerosolized and administered into the tracheobronchial tree in the awake patient. This is especially true for patients with reversible airway obstruction, such as asthma or COPD. These inhalational medications are commonly used in the field and have simplified the treatment of spontaneously breathing patients and have virtually eliminated the dangerous practice of administration of aminophylline, which is fraught with complications.

Intravenous

Most drugs used in the field are intended to be administered via the IV route. The rate of absorption of an IV administered drug is generally immediate and predictable. Unfortunately, the IV route is also fraught with risks inherent in the rapid delivery of a drug directly into the peripheral or central circulation.

The rate of drug administration varies dependent upon the drug type, class, and patient condition. Drugs may be administered via rapid IV push (adenosine), slow IV push (furosemide), repeated boluses (lidocaine) or via drip infusion titrated to effect (dopamine). To be effective, adenosine must be administered via rapid IV push due to its short half life in the peripheral circulation. Likewise, epinephrine during cardiac arrest is ideally administered via rapid IV push, since the desired effect generally is immediate. To enhance delivery of drugs to the central circulation during cardiac arrest, the dose of epinephrine should be followed by a 20-30 ml fluid bolus and the extremity should be elevated.[1]

Certain drugs are to be given by slow IV push, such as furosemide or morphine sulfate, whose anticipated effects are slower in onset. Several medications are to be given by slow infusion, such as dopamine or dobutamine. Medications given by slow infusion generally have potent hemodynamic effects and must be titrated slowly to achieve the desired effect. Drug infusions are often difficult to maintain in a moving ambulance, since administration pumps are not universally available in the prehospital setting.

Endotracheal

When IV access is delayed or unavailable, certain drugs can be given directly into the tracheobronchial tree via an endotracheal tube. The rate of absorption is essentially equal to the IV route. The dose of endotracheal drugs is typically 2 to 2.5 times the IV dose per ACLS recommendations.[1] The specific drugs administered endotracheally include lidocaine, epinephrine, atropine, and naloxone.[1] A common mnemonic for these agents is LEAN, representing the four listed medications: L(lidocaine)E(epinephrine)A(atropine)N(naloxone).

Rectal

The rectal route has been studied as a route of administration for certain drugs readily absorbed from the rectal mucosa.[11,12] This is of special benefit in the pediatric patient. Clinical studies have demonstrated the reliable results and ease of administration of diazepam in the control of seizures in the pediatric population.[11,12] Rectal administration usually results in a slower onset of action than the IV route but is of benefit in children, such as when IV access may be technically difficult to obtain in an actively seizing child.

A recent study has demonstrated the efficacy of rectally administered diazepam to a prehospital pediatric population.[12] Diazepam was administered rectally by a syringe containing 0.5 mg/kg as the initial dose in a seizing child to a 14G plastic IV catheter (with needle removed) and advancing the catheter assembly 4-6 cm to the rectum. Diazepam administered in this manner should be flushed with 5 cc of saline fluid. Rectally administered diazepam may cause respiratory depression, and appropriate precautions should be undertaken.

ACLS Medications

Epinephrine

Epinephrine is the most important and well-studied cardiac resuscitation drug. The beneficial effects of epinephrine during cardiopulmonary resuscitation arise primarily from alpha-adrenergic stimulation, which increases the myocardial and cerebral blood flow. Until clinical research suggests otherwise, epinephrine is the prehospital catecholamine of choice in cardiac arrest.[1]

The standard dose of epinephrine (1 mg) is not based on body mass but stemmed from the anecdotal use of intracardiac epinephrine in the operating room.[13] The dose became 1 mg without clinical research to determine an effective dosing regimen based on mass.

Several studies[14] were performed to determine the dose-response curve of epinephrine and suggested that the optimal dosing range was 0.045-0.20 mg/kg. A review of these trials did not demonstrate statistically significant improvement in survival rates to hospital discharge when compared with standard dose epinephrine.[15] The clinical trials that investigated the utility of high-dose epinephrine in cardiac arrest were not sufficiently convincing to modify the AHA recommendations in 1992 regarding epinephrine dosing.[16] However, most of the high-dose epinephrine trials administered the higher dose late in the cardiac arrest. The utility of high-dose epinephrine administered very early after the arrest has not been established. The recommended adult dose of epinephrine remains 1 mg

IV of the 1:10,000 concentration repeated every 3-5 minutes per the AHA guidelines. Higher doses are considered Class IIB per AHA/ACLS guidelines and are included in current treatment algorithms as a therapeutic option.[1] Class IIB dosing regimens can be considered including intermediate dosing, 2-5 mg IV every 3-5 minutes; or escalating dosing, 1- 3- 5 mg IV push, 3 minutes apart; or high dosing, 0.1 mg/kg IV push every 3-5 minutes.[1]

Epinephrine exhibits excellent bioavailability after endotracheal administration. And therefore the endotracheal route of administration should be used promptly in the absence of venous access. A dose of 2-2.5 mg as per AHA recommendations in the ACLS curriculum is required.[1]

Epinephrine can also be given by continuous infusion, although the utility of such infusions must be tailored to the particular EMS system. An infusion can be prepared by placing epinephrine hydrochloride into 250 cc of NS and titrating to a specific hemodynamic endpoint.[1]

Acute anaphylaxis may also require epinephrine administration. Epinephrine 1:1000 is administered subcutaneously at a dose of 0.01 mg/kg (0.01 cc/kg) maximum 0.5 mg in adults.[17] For adult patients refractory to subcutaneous epinephrine or into acute cardiovascular collapse, 0.3-0.5 mg (3-5 ml) epinephrine 1:10,000 is administered slowly, over 3-5 minutes via the IV route.[17]

Pitfalls

Epinephrine is a potent vasoactive catecholamine and can cause severe hypertension, tachycardia, and increased myocardial oxygen consumption. The on-line physician must be confident that the prehospital care provider has sufficiently established the "arrest" state before epinephrine is administered. Low-flow states with subsequent profound hypotension may mimic the "arrested" state in the noisy environment of a field resuscitation, and the use of epinephrine may be deleterious. EMS personnel must carefully assess vital signs and continuously monitor them.

Dopamine

Dopamine is a chemical precursor of norepinephrine and exerts its effects by stimulating adrenergic receptors in a dose-dependent fashion.[18] At dosage ranges from 1-2 mcg/kg/min, there is stimulation of dopaminergic receptors to produce renal and mesenteric vasodilatation. At this dosage range, there is also stimulation of alpha-adrenergic receptors, which produces an increase in venous tone. At a dosage range of 2-10 mcg/kg/min, dopamine stimulates both beta-1 adrenergic receptors, which causes increased cardiac output, as well as alpha-adrenergic receptors, which also affects cardiac output and results in a modest increase in systemic vascular resistance. At doses greater than 20 mcg/kg/min, dopamine exerts primarily prominent alpha-adrenergic effects, such as vasoconstriction, which results in an increase in systemic and peripheral vascular resistance, as well as preload.

Dopamine is indicated for hemodynamically significant hypotension without hypovolemia with a systolic blood pressure less than 90 mmHg with evidence of clinical shock.[1]

Pitfalls

Dopamine should be used cautiously if at all at doses greater than 20 mcg/kg/min because of the profound generalized vasoconstriction from the stimulation of alpha-adrenergic receptors. Dopamine can also induce a tachycardia and can result in various ventricular and supraventricular dysrhythmias. By increasing peripheral resistance, dopamine can worsen pulmonary congestion and increase myocardial lactate production.

Nausea and vomiting are frequent side effects. Extravasation of dopamine may cause tissue necrosis and sloughing of skin. Patients using MAO inhibitors should receive a much lower dose of dopamine because of the direct drug interaction.

Dobutamine

Dobutamine is a synthetic sympathomimetic amine that is a potent inotropic agent. It stimulates beta-1 and alpha-1 adrenergic receptors in the heart. Its effect on peripheral adrenergic receptors leads to a mild vasodilatory response, which leads to a direct rise in cardiac output. Dobutamine results in less tachycardia than dopamine at conventional doses and produces a beneficial rise in cardiac output without a concomitant rise in myocardial oxygen demand.[1]

Dobutamine is generally administered at a dosage range of 2-20 mcg/kg/min and is indicated in those patients with pulmonary congestion but a low cardiac output manifested clinically by hypotension.[1] Dobutamine may be superior to dopamine in those patients with mild-to-moderate hypotension and evidence of CHF where it is desirable to promote primarily inotropic effects in the

heart without the undesirable effects of tachycardia and peripheral vasoconstriction.[18] Studies of prehospital dobutamine use show that this agent may be useful in select cases of CHF.[19] Dobutamine may be combined with dopamine for additive effects to maintain arterial pressure in patients with pulmonary congestion and low cardiac output.

Pitfalls

Dobutamine can cause tachycardia and arrhythmias at higher doses and frequently results in headache, nausea and tremor. Prehospital care providers may not be familiar with dobutamine because of the traditional use of dopamine, but the benefits and pitfalls of dobutamine cannot be overstated. The medical director should carefully consider the addition of dobutamine to protocols.

Nitroglycerin

Nitroglycerin is a valuable prehospital drug, and familiarity with its drug profile is critical for the prehospital care provider. It is the cornerstone agent in the treatment of patients with suspected ischemic chest pain and signs and symptoms of CHF who present to the field provider.[20]

Nitroglycerin causes relaxation of vascular smooth muscle and relieves angina pectoris in part by producing peripheral venodilatation with reduction in preload volume to the heart. Nitroglycerin also dilates large coronary arteries and can antagonize coronary vasospasm.[1] It is available for prehospital use both in a tablet form and an aerosol spray for sublingual administration.[21]

Nitroglycerin is the drug of choice in the field for the treatment of chest pain of suspected ischemic origin and CHF. It offers significant benefits in the management of CHF, including ease of administration and rapid titratability. Tablets have been traditionally used, but the aerosol spray offers greater convenience of administration. The use of IV nitroglycerin is generally impractical in the field and will not be discussed. Certain prehospital care systems will perform interhospital transfers of patients receiving nitroglycerin infusions, but the online control in these instances should be individualized by the medical director.

The recommended sublingual dosage of nitroglycerin is 0.3-0.4 mg in either the tablet or aerosol form. Oral administration results in some deactivation of the drug in the liver, and patients with potential or real liver failure may require dosage adjustment. The use of rapid multiple doses of sublingual nitroglycerin is highly effective in the prehospital treatment of CHF when compared with treatment protocols using morphine and furosemide.[22]

Pitfalls

Typically, nitroglycerin can cause transient hypotension, especially in patients who are hypovolemic, and fluids should be cautiously administered to counteract changes in blood pressure. This is secondary to its potent hemodynamic effects primarily on the venous system, causing a drop in venous return to the heart. Headache is common after nitroglycerin administration, and patients receiving nitroglycerin in the field should be warned of this unpleasant side effect.

Not all chest pain encountered in the prehospital setting is cardiac in origin. Nitroglycerin administration should be limited to patients with chest pain suspected to be cardiac in origin. Administration of nitroglycerin to a patient with chest pain secondary to aortic dissection or pulmonary embolism may adversely impact the patient's hemodynamics.

Atropine

Atropine, which stimulates sinus node discharge and enhances atrioventricular node conduction, is the parasympatholytic agent of choice for symptomatic bradycardia.[1] While there are no randomized, controlled prehospital trials, atropine may be beneficial in nodal bradycardia. The data concerning the utility of atropine in pulseless idioventricular rhythm and asystole are inconclusive. A clinical trial of 21 patients was performed without improvement in mortality with the use of atropine in these specific dysrhythmias.[23]

The AHA-recommended initial dose is 0.5-1.0 mg IV in the adult patient.[25] The dose may be repeated at 5-minute intervals until the desired response is achieved. The total dose should be restricted to 2-3 mg if possible to avoid the adverse effects of an atropine-induced tachycardia.

Atropine may also be useful in patients with cholinesterase poisoning. The dose of atropine in this condition is titrated to effect.

Pitfalls

The administration of atropine should never delay the initiation of transcutaneous pacing (TCP). If the patient's condition is severe, the command physician should instruct the prehospital care providers to immediately begin TCP.

In less acute situations the physician must query the prehospital care provider regarding progressive bradycardic rhythms that exhibit ventricular escape activity. The

request for lidocaine in these circumstances must be rejected due to the potential suppressive effects on the ventricular myocardium that is manifesting a desirable physiological response. Atropine instead should be used to provide the desired chronotropic effect.

Atropine should also be used cautiously in patients exhibiting asymptomatic bradycardias, since an increase in heart rate may be deleterious in patients with underlying coronary artery disease, especially during myocardial ischemia. Atropine has been reported harmful in some patients with AV block at the His-Purkinje level (type II AV block) and third degree heart block.

Antidysrhythmic Drugs

Adenosine

Adenosine is the prehospital drug of choice for the treatment of paroxysmal SVT of the reentrant type. Its half life of 5 seconds makes this drug ideal for rapid conversion of supraventricular rhythms with minimal hemodynamic consequences.[24] Adenosine transiently interrupts cardiac impulse propagation through the AV node, thereby terminating AV nodal reentrant rhythms.[1]

Adenosine has earned a place in the ACLS treatment algorithms and is part of many standard prehospital protocols for the treatment of SVT.[25,26] Generally, the attempted conversion of atrial flutter and fibrillation will not be successful with adenosine, but the short-lived AV block that occurs may unmask the underlying mechanism of the tachycardia. The dosage of adenosine is 6 mg rapid IV bolus over 1-3 seconds. This should be accompanied by a 20 cc NS flush.[1] A 12 mg IV bolus should be given if termination of the SVT does not occur within 1-2 minutes. Although more expensive than verapamil[26], adenosine is probably a safer antiarrhythmic for prehospital use. The consequences of administering adenosine for a misinterpeted ventricular tachycardia are significantly less than those of inappropriate verapamil administration.[1]

Pitfalls

The most frequent side effects of IV adenosine administration are flushing and chest pain.[27] These effects usually abate promptly, but the patient should be warned before adenosine administration. Adenosine has minimal lasting hemodynamic effects because of its ultra short half life and rarely produces hypotension. Transient AV block may occur and may unmask underlying atrial arrhythmias such as atrial fibrillation or atrial flutter.

Several drugs interact with the action of adenosine. Theophylline and other methylxanthines block the receptor responsible for adenosine's action. Dipyridamole, on the other hand, blocks adenosine uptake and potentiates the drug's action.

Verapamil and Diltiazem

Verapamil and diltiazem are calcium antagonists that have great utility in the ED for the treatment of supraventricular tachycardias and in the control of ventricular response in rapid atrial flutter and fibrillation.[28] Both drugs exert negative chronotropic effects on the heart, while verapamil also exerts a strong negative inotropic effect. As a result, diltiazem produces less unwanted hemodynamic side effects, such as hypotension and decreased cardiac output.[28] Both drugs slow conduction and prolong the refractoriness of the AV node. Diltiazem may play a greater role for the treatment of hemodynamically significant atrial flutter or fibrillation.

Since diltiazem produces dose dependent depression of AV nodal conduction, it is effective in the treatment of paroxysmal SVT by interrupting reciprocation at the AV node. It also may be considered for patients in CHF because of its minimal depressant effects on the left ventricle.

For the prehospital care provider faced with a patient in an obvious atrial fibrillation with a rapid ventricular response and subsequent hemodynamic compromise, diltiazem appears to be an ideal agent before the use of electrical cardioversion.

The dosage of IV diltiazem is 0.25 mg/kg in a bolus fashion, typically 20 mg in an adult. A repeat bolus dose of 0.35 mg/kg may be given 15 minutes after the initial bolus if there is no observed effect. These dosages are recommended for both paroxysmal SVT and the slowing of a rapid atrial flutter and fibrillation.[1]

Verapamil remains a useful drug when used with caution. The dosage of verapamil is 2.5-5.0 mg IV over 1-2 minutes.[1] The dose should be administered over a longer period of time (3 minutes) in older patients. A repeat dose of 5-10 mg may be given in 15-30 minutes. The prehospital care provider should monitor the patient for rhythm change, hypotension, and worsening CHF.

Pitfalls

Both drugs, verapamil to a greater extent than diltiazem, may produce transient hypotension, especially in patients with left ventricular (LV) dysfunction. IV beta-blocking agents should not be used concomitantly with diltiazem because of the synergism of their hemodynamic effects and the risk of hypotension and depressed LV dysfunction. Patients on oral beta-blocking agents should receive diltiazem cautiously although this situation does not contraindicate the use of diltiazem. Patients exhibiting severe CHF should not receive diltiazem unless the underlying etiology is atrial fibrillation, in which case slowing of the ventricular rate may have immediate beneficial effects.

A major pitfall in the prehospital treatment of SVT is the variable ability of providers, paramedics, and base physicians to interpret tachydysrhythmias. One study found misinterpretation of tachydysrhythmias in 30 of 73 patients' 12-month prehospital chart review.[29] Inadvertent administration of either drug to a patient in ventricular tachycardia may produce severe hemodynamic compromise.[1]

Lidocaine

The antidysrhythmic agents used for the treatment of ventricular dysrhythmias in most prehospital systems are lidocaine and bretylium. While both agents have been studied extensively, conclusions about relative efficacy are difficult due to small sample sizes, overlapping treatments, and different dosing protocols. Lidocaine is recommended as the antidysrhythmic agent of choice for ventricular fibrillation and ventricular tachycardia.[1] In addition, lidocaine is recommended after termination of ventricular tachycardia or fibrillation. Lidocaine should be given to patients who are at risk for significant malignant ventricular dysrhythmias to prevent recurrence. Lidocaine is the drug of choice for the suppression of ventricular ectopy, but it should be reserved for patients with symptomatic ectopy in the acute setting, such as myocardial ischemia or after conversion of ventricular fibrillation or tachycardia. For refractory ventricular fibrillation and pulseless ventricular tachycardia, an initial dose of 1.0-1.5 mg/kg is recommended per AHA guidelines.[1] In addition to the initial dose, a subsequent dose of 1.0-1.5 mg/kg can be given for refractory ventricular rhythms to a total dose of 3 mg/kg.

It is of paramount importance to stress the need to administer lidocaine by the multiple bolus technique instead of continuous infusion. The pharmacokinetics of lidocaine are more predictable and reliable in the field when given by multiple boluses. Due to the altered pharmacokinetics in the arrested heart, only the multiple bolus technique is recommended. Since the clearance of lidocaine is decreased in the arrested heart, a single dose of lidocaine should produce therapeutic levels. After spontaneous circulation is restored, additional lidocaine should be administered. Lidocaine can also be given via the endotracheal route, and dosing should be 2-2.5 times the IV dose to obtain therapeutic levels.

Lidocaine is metabolized in the liver, and maintenance doses should be decreased in the setting of reduced hepatic blood flow, such as during acute myocardial infarction, CHF, or shock states. The initial loading dose of lidocaine remains the same in these conditions (1.0-1.5 mg/kg), however additional boluses should be reduced by 50% (0.25 mg/kg). The maintenance dose should also be reduced in patients over 70 years old.

Bretylium

Bretylium is an antifibrillatory agent effective for patients with refractory ventricular fibrillation. AHA guidelines list lidocaine as the drug of first choice for all ventricular ectopy, and bretylium has been reserved for cases of refractory ventricular arrhythmias.[1] Bretylium has potent adrenergic effects and tends to elevate the ventricular threshold as does lidocaine, although its mechanism of action differs in its electrophysiological site of action. It does not have first-line recommendations due to its adverse hemodynamic effects, especially during CPR. Bretylium should be included in prehospital algorithms for the treatment of ventricular fibrillation refractory to lidocaine and countershock or recurrent ventricular fibrillation despite lidocaine or procainamide therapy. The dose of bretylium is 5 mg/kg by rapid injection. The dose can be repeated for persistent ventricular fibrillation in a 10 mg/kg bolus. The conscious patient receiving bretylium for ventricular tachycardia may experience nausea or vomiting with rapid injection and hypotension may also occur.

Procainamide

Procainamide, which has ventricular and atrial stabilizing effects, is used in some prehospital systems for the treatment of arrhythmias. The clear advantage of procainamide is its combined antiarrhythmic effects for both atrial and ventricular arrhythmias. Procainamide is particularly useful in patients with arrhythmias secondary to Wolf-Parkinson-White syndrome (WPW).

However, the usefulness of procainamide is tempered by its potential hypotensive effects during its administration. The use of procainamide warrants close monitoring and careful titration, both of which are difficult to maintain during prehospital evaluation and treatment. In refractory ventricular tachycardia or fibrillation, the recommended IV dose is a total of 17 mg/kg administered at a rate of 30 mg/min by infusion.[1] Typically, the infusion rate is much faster but there are no substantiating clinical studies to support a higher rate of infusion.

Pitfalls

Probably the most aggressively used prehospital cardiac medication, lidocaine is fraught with potential toxicities that the on-line physician must be aware of and vigilant in its prehospital use. The on-line physician is often confronted with a prehospital report of "frequent PVCs" and a request for the administration of lidocaine. The on-line physician must query the field provider regarding the "clinical" significance and setting of the reported ectopy because that will predict the need for pharmacological treatment. Ventricular ectopy in the absence of significant risk factors or active symptomatology warrants only ongoing cardiac monitoring.

Lidocaine, bretylium, and procainamide should not be given to patients who exhibit high degree AV block, since these patients may be entirely dependent upon the spontaneous automaticity of the myocardium when the conduction system is failing. Currently, none of the above drugs are recommended for prophylactic use in the setting of chest pain since no recent clinical study has demonstrated clear benefit.

In the nonarrest state, the rate of administration and total dosage of lidocaine, bretylium, and procainamide must be monitored to prevent side effects and dysrhythmias.

Sodium Bicarbonate

Traditionally, sodium bicarbonate therapy has been used to buffer the acidemia that occurs in low-flow states, such as cardiac arrest, in the field. Traditional protocols, such as those from the AHA, required the use of sodium bicarbonate in the cardiac arrest patient and have now been abandoned in favor of specific recommendations in unique clinical circumstances. These unique clinical circumstances include preexisting metabolic acidoses, hyperkalemia, or tricyclic antidepressant overdose where the benefit of bicarbonate therapy has been demonstrated. The IV dosing recommendation of sodium bicarbonate is 1 mEq/kg.[1]

Pitfalls

There is evidence in animal models that the administration of sodium bicarbonate results in the generation of CO_2, which has been shown to produce intracellular acidosis and subsequently worsen central venous acidosis during CPR.[30] The administration of sodium bicarbonate can also result in hypernatremia and hyperosmolality.

Other Medications

Inhaled Bronchodilators

The prompt recognition and treatment of bronchospasm in the field is of paramount importance in the prevention of severe morbidity from unrecognized respiratory failure. Acute respiratory distress in whole or in part secondary to acute bronchospasm is one of the most common complaints presenting to prehospital care providers.

Once the diagnosis of acute bronchospasm is confirmed, the initial management includes supplemental oxygen and beta-agonist aerosolized agents. Beta-adrenergic agonists produce bronchodilation in airways by stimulation of $beta_2$ receptors and in addition, inhibit mediator release and promote mucociliary clearance.

Aerosol therapy has become the preferred route of administration of beta-adrenergic agonists. The aerosol route results in optimal local absorption of a relatively small dose of drug with minimal systemic absorption and few side effects.

Beta-adrenergic drugs are analogs of naturally occurring sympathetic-amines. The most commonly used bronchodilator agents are metaproterenol and albuterol. These drugs possess greater beta-receptor specificity than older agents such as isoproterenol or isoetharine.

The ability to administer aerosolized medications in the field has dramatically improved the acute management of bronchospasm. In the past, epinephrine and aminophylline were used primarily for acute bronchospasm with obvious adverse effects. These medications are still useful for bronchodilation but pose risks in the field, especially in patients susceptible to toxicity from increased sympathomimetic activity such as the very old or very young and those with comorbid illnesses. A study comparing metaproterenol alone with subcutaneous epinephrine and a combination of metaproterenol and epinephrine in the asthmatic prehospital patient suggested that metaproterenol alone was as effective in achieving bronchodilation as the other modalities studied.[31] This lends support to the notion that prehospital use of aerosolized medications alone is effective in the treatment of the bronchospastic patient. The use of multiple doses of aerosolized beta-agonists in the field is efficacious and demonstrates a safety profile well within acceptable limits.

Pitfalls

The potential pitfalls of aerosolized beta-adrenergic agonists in the field are minimal. There is little systemic absorption of aerosolized medications and therefore, systemic toxicity rarely occurs. To obtain maximum efficacy from the aerosolized route, the patient must be cooperative and understand the nature of the treatment that requires deep inspiratory efforts to promote efficient delivery of microscopic droplets. Prehospital care providers must be adequately trained in the delivery process of aerosolized medications and must be able to coach patients in the proper breathing techniques during the administration process.

Anticonvulsants

The appropriate prehospital pharmacological management of a seizure depends on the prompt recognition of tonic or clonic activity and a possible underlying etiology. A seizure may be a primary or idiopathic event or it may be secondary to multiple etiologies, such as metabolic derangements, inflammatory or infectious states, structural injury to the CNS, or generalized illness.

Before any pharmacological considerations, the prehospital care provider must address the airway and provide lifesaving measures to maintain ventilatory support, supply oxygen, and prevent aspiration. A seizure in and of itself is not typically life threatening and the first priority is the patient's respiratory status. The prehospital care provider must not be distracted by a seizure and therefore fail to search for a treatable etiology in the field. For example, a seizure in a child may be secondary to hyperpyrexia and therefore reassurance to the family and on-line communication may be sufficient, although transport is probably warranted in most cases.

One etiology of seizures is hypoglycemia and the prehospital care providers must search for evidence of hypoglycemia and treat the patient accordingly. Head injury with structural damage to the CNS may result in a seizure, and the treatment priorities are directed to the primary injury.

It is imperative to treat a seizure in the field when failure to do so might result in acute respiratory or cardiac compromise or place the patient in grave danger.

The most commonly used anticonvulsant is diazepam, a short-acting benzodiazepine with well-recognized and reliable properties. IV diazepam is administered 5 mg over 2 minutes, typically up to 10 mg in adults, watching for respiratory depression.[1] Diazepam has a rapid onset of action, achieving maximal CNS concentrations 1-2 minutes after IV administration.[1] The half-life of diazepam is 15-90 minutes. The rectal route of diazepam administration (0.2-0.5 mg/kg) has been shown to be very effective in the pediatric population when IV access is difficult and prolonged seizure activity warrants ablation of the event.[11,12] Lorazepam may also be used to control seizures (1-4 mg over 2-10 min).[1] Phenytoin and phenobarbital, two other commonly used anticonvulsants, are generally reserved for hospital administration. Midazolam will have an increased field role in many systems.

Pitfalls

The greatest pitfall in the pharmacological management of seizures is the potential to compromise respiratory and hemodynamic status. Since many idiopathic seizures stop spontaneously, aggressive treatment is not warranted. On the other hand, prolonged seizures and status epilepticus must be aggressively treated.[32]

A seizure is a dramatic event and the prehospital care providers may be dissuaded from the recognition of underlying causes, such as hypoglycemia, which is easily treated without resorting to benzodiazepines, for example. Failure to recognize a significant head injury manifesting a secondary seizure could delay the appropriate treatment for the patient's CNS injury.

Neuromuscular Blocking Agents

The use of intubation adjuncts, such as neuromuscular blocking agents, is a cornerstone in the management of the difficult airway in the ED. The medical director must evaluate the potential benefits of these agents in light of the risks associated with their use. These agents, if used in the field, require close scrutiny of the prehospital care provider and rigid adherence to protocols.[33,34]

Neuromuscular blocking agents are classified either as depolarizing or non-depolarizing agents depending on their interaction with the neuromuscular junction.[35] These agents are used for supplemental muscle relaxation. They can be of tremendous advantage in the uncooperative patient, especially when associated with a head injury. The potential risk of increased intracranial pressure with the stimulation of the airway reflex can be blunted by using these drugs.

The primary hazard in the use of a neuromuscular blocking agent is the inability to manage the airway when paralysis and subsequent apnea occur. The prehospital use of these agents must be tempered by the medical director's confidence in the airway skills of the prehospital care provider.

The prototypical agent in this class is succinylcholine, which depolarizes the postsynaptic junction and competitively inhibits the affects of acetylcholine. The duration of a single dose is 3-5 minutes. Potential vagal stimulation may require the concomitant use of atropine in the child or in adults receiving multiple doses. The recommended IV dose is 1.0-1.5 mg/kg.[35]

Nondepolarizing agents competitively block the effects of acetylcholine at the neuromuscular junction. In theory, this does not produce the fasciculations as seen with depolarizing agents. The two agents in this class in common use and of potential field use are pancuronium and vecuronium.

Pancuronium is a long-acting neuromuscular blocking agent with an onset of action of 2-5 minutes and a duration of action of approximately 60 minutes. The recommended IV dose is 0.1 mg/kg with repeated doses exhibiting a cumulative effect.[35] Reversal can be achieved with cholinesterase inhibitors, such as neostigmine, with concomitant use of atropine to minimize the cholinergic effects of neostigmine.

Vecuronium has few pitfalls in comparison with pancuronium, which is why it has been recommended as the ideal longer acting neuromuscular blocking agent for prehospital use. The use of priming doses; that is, the administration of a subparalytic dose before a smaller than usual "intubating" dose has been shown to have a more rapid onset of paralysis than a single dose of vecuronium. Unfortunately, the long interval between the priming and intubating dose, generally 4-6 minutes, has made this impractical for the emergent intubation in the field. Vecuronium has a shorter onset and duration of action than pancuronium and does not exhibit cumulative effects with repeated doses as does pancuronium. Vecuronium has an onset of action of approximately 3 minutes and a duration of action of 30-35 minutes. Its recommended IV dose is 0.1 mg/kg.[35]

Pitfalls

Succinylcholine may produce profound muscle fasciculations with resulting hyperkalemia, hyperthermia, or histamine release. In certain pathological states the hyperkalemic response may be profound, such as severe non-acute burns or severe muscle trauma.[36] Fasciculations may be prevented by preadministration of a subparalytic dose (0.01 mg/kg) of pancuronium.

Pancuronium may cause a rise in heart rate or blood pressure because of its vagolytic effects. Pancuronium may also cause release of histamine with the subsequent end organ effects of histamine.

Hypoglycemia

Hypoglycemia is a common cause of altered consciousness in the prehospital setting. In one series, 8.5% of patients with altered level of consciousness were found to be hypoglycemic.[37] Symptomatic hypoglycemia has been demonstrated in both diabetic and nondiabetic patients.[38] As a result many prehospital care protocols recommend the routine administration of 50% dextrose (D_{50}) as part of a "coma cocktail" to patients presenting with altered level of consciousness. Fifty percent dextrose, supplied in 50 ml prefilled syringes, is the drug of choice for the parenteral treatment of hypoglycemia in patients with IV access. In a series of 51 patients, one author documented a mean increase of serum glucose concentration from baseline of 166 mg/dl with a range of 37 to 379 mg/dl following the injection of 50 ml of D_{50} in hypoglycemic patients.[38] This study suggests that the magnitude of change of serum glucose level cannot be predicted from a single ampule of D_{50}.

Pitfalls

Recent literature has questioned the practice of routinely administering D_{50} in the patient with altered level of consciousness. Multiple studies in animals and humans have demonstrated increased neurological impairment and mortality in subjects with hyperglycemia after a neurological insult.[39,40] Hyperglycemia may produce its detrimental cerebral effect in the setting of hypoxia or ischemia due to an increase in the amount of substrate for anaerobic glycolysis and an accelerated accumulation of brain lactic acid.[39,40] This suggests that D_{50} and glucose containing IV solutions should be avoided in patients at risk for cerebral ischemia (i.e., acute stroke, cardiac arrest). The administration of D_{50} should be limited to patients with documented hypoglycemia.

Conveniently, the use of rapid glucose reagent strips in the prehospital setting provides an easy and reliable method for documenting hypoglycemia. Rapid glucose reagent strips require a drop of blood (via venepuncture or finger stick) applied to the strip. Estimation of serum

glucose level can then be read via strip in approximately 1-2 minutes. Hoyga found the Chemstrip bG to be 100% sensitive and 88% specific for the prehospital detection of hypoglycemia.[41] Reagent strips provide a rational means of detecting hypoglycemia in the field in patients with altered level of consciousness and provide a rational basis for D_{50} administration.[37,41] In addition, Hogya, at the time of his study, noted that the cost of a single Chemstrip bG (approximately $0.25) to be less than 1/10 the cost of an ampule of D_{50}.

Some systems include thiamine (vitamin B_1) as part of the series of drugs administered to the unconscious patient. Thiamine administration initiates the treatment of Wernicke's encephalopathy, a rare cause of unconsciousness. Although common wisdom suggests that a single bolus of hypertonic dextrose can precipitate such an event, the scientific evidence for this "wisdom" is lacking.[37] There is no evidence to support delaying the administration of dextrose until thiamine can be administered.

Glucagon

Unfortunately, D_{50} can only be administered via the IV route. Therefore D_{50} cannot be administered to the patient with altered level of consciousness without IV access. Glucagon, a naturally occurring polypeptide administered via the IM or SQ route, is useful in reversing hypoglycemia in patients without IV access. Glucagon acts on liver glycogen, converting it to glucose. Therefore patients must have liver glycogen stores for glucagon to work. Patients with hepatic glycogen depletion (starvation, chronic alcoholism, chronic illness, or impaired liver function) may not respond to glucagon.

Glucagon is packaged as a lyophilized powder and must be mixed with a diluent provided in the packaging. Glucagon administered in a dose of 1-5 mg has a slower onset of action than D_{50} (8-10 minutes for a 1 mg dose) with a duration of action of 10-30 minutes.[42,43] Side effects of glucagon include nausea and vomiting. Glucagon may cause extreme hypertension in pheochromocytoma and is therefore contraindicated in patients with this disorder. Glucagon produces a positive inotropic effect on the heart and may be useful in the reversal of hypotension associated with beta blocker overdose[44,45], calcium channel overdose[46], and anaphylactic shock.[47] For these indications, glucagon should be given IV in a dose titrated to effect.

Antihypertensives

Although it is rare for patients to engage EMS for the chief complaint of asymptomatic hypertension, prehospital care providers often encounter patients with hypertension. Hypertension may be part of the patient's primary problem (i.e., chest pain or CHF), secondary to pain or anxiety, or found unexpectedly during assessment of routine vital signs.

Hypertension is often treated in the field with nontraditional agents, such as morphine and nitroglycerin. Both agents will decrease blood pressure and may be appropriate for treatment of significant hypertension associated with chest pain of suspected cardiac origin or CHF.

Nifedipine, a calcium channel blocker, has also been used in the hospital[48-52] and prehospital settings[53] to decrease blood pressure. A 10 mg nifedipine capsule chewed and then swallowed by the patient has been effective in reducing blood pressure.[50] However, nifedipine administration has also been associated with symptomatic hypotension and heart block.[51] In addition the single oral dose cannot be accurately titrated or reversed. Hypovolemia and the concomitant use of other antihypertensive agents may predispose patients to complications. However, untoward reactions cannot always be predicted.

Pitfalls

Hypertension can be identified and options exist for its treatment in the prehospital setting. However, the rationale for treating hypertension in this setting has been questioned. There is probably no benefit to the short-term treatment of hypertension in the asymptomatic patient. To be effective, antihypertensive therapy must occur over the long term and must be monitored.

The treatment of hypertension associated with pain or anxiety should be corrected at the cause (i.e., administration of analgesics to control pain resulting from a fracture). The treatment of hypertension associated with an acute neurovascular or cardiovascular process is controversial and must be individualized. Patients probably benefit from mild blood pressure reductions in hypertensive emergencies, such as CHF, aortic dissection, subarachnoid hemorrhage, and hypertensive encephalopathy. These diagnoses can be suggested by patient presentation, but definitive diagnosis cannot be made in the prehospital setting.

Likewise, hypertension may be seen in the setting of an acute stroke. In the past, elevated blood pressure in the face of an acute neurological event was aggressively decreased to "normal ranges". Recently this practice has been called into question. Several authors have demonstrated that in patients with acute stroke and moderate hypertension (systolic blood pressures 170-220 or diastolic blood pressures from 90-120 mmHg), cerebral blood flow was negatively correlated with decreases in blood pressure.[54,55] In the setting of acute CVA, reduction of hypertension may reduce cerebral perfusion pressure and decrease cerebral blood flow in areas of viable tissue surrounding the ischemic cerebral brain. Therefore lowering the blood pressure may exacerbate ischemic brain injury.

In summary, the known risk (i.e, hypotension, heart block, exacerbation of ischemic brain injury) should be balanced with the unclear benefit of reducing blood pressure in the asymptomatic patient encountered in the prehospital setting. Should the command physician elect to initiate antihypertensive therapy, the physician must ensure adequate monitoring for decline in patient condition.

Opioid and Benzodiazepine Antagonists

The unconscious overdose patient provides a clinical and therapeutic challenge to the prehospital care provider and medical command physician. Ideally the etiology of the overdose can be rapidly identified and its toxidrome reversed.

Naloxone is commonly used in the "coma cocktail" administered to patients with decreased level of consciousness.[37,56] Naloxone, an opioid antagonist, reverses the effects of opioids including respiratory depression, sedation, and hypotension. Naloxone works faster when administered IV but also works when administered IM or subcutaneously. This is helpful in the prehospital setting, especially when dealing with chronic IV drug abusers who may lack venous access. The IM dose provides a more prolonged effect.

Basic resuscitative measures, including establishing the airway, breathing, circulation, and suctioning, should not be ignored while waiting for naloxone to take effect. Although providers should prepare for intubation of patients with profound respiratory depression, they might want to delay the procedure until the naloxone takes effect. There is a danger of narcotized patients traumatically self-extubating once the profound respiratory depression is reversed.

The initial dose of naloxone is 0.4-2 mg administered IM, IV, or subcutaneously. This dose may be repeated every 3-5 minutes. In the controlled, hospital setting, naloxone is often titrated to effect, however rapid opioid reversal is often desired in the prehospital setting. Although this may be appropriate in the patient unable to protect the airway, precipitation of acute opioid withdrawal and violent behavior has been demonstrated after rapid reversal.[57]

Pitfalls

Several opioids, including pentazocine, propoxyphene, and some synthetic designer opioids, may require high doses of naloxone to cause reversal (6-8 mg).[58] Therefore higher requirements of naloxone should be considered in selected patients with these overdoses.

Abrupt reversal of opioid intoxication, as mentioned above, may lead to acute opioid withdrawal, including nausea, vomiting, tachycardia, seizures, and violent behavior.[56,57] Hoffman has suggested the selective use of naloxone for patients with clinical evidence of opioid intoxication (i.e., decreased level of consciousness, myosis, and decreased respiratory rate).[37] Some have recommended that naloxone be administered only in patients with suspected opioid overdose and significant respiratory depression.

The mean serum half life of naloxone is 1½ hours with a duration of action of 2-3 hours.[58] Many opioids, including methadone, propoxyphene, and heroin, have a longer half life than naloxone. This suggests, but has not been thoroughly demonstrated, that patients given naloxone and released by prehospital care providers could lapse back into altered level of consciousness and respiratory depression.[59]

Another pitfall with the administration of naloxone is that the opioid overdose may be associated with the concomitant use of alcohol or other depressives. Naloxone may not adequately reverse the respiratory or cardiovascular depression in these patients.

Nalmefene, a relatively new opiate antagonist, is more potent than naloxone, has a longer serum half life (greater than 10 hours), and in the ED setting has been reported to be well tolerated.[59,60] Using a titrated dose 0.5-1 mg IV, nalmefene may be useful in the prehospital setting, especially in the opioid overdose patient that may refuse or not otherwise require hospital transport. Onset of action begins within 2 minutes and peaks within 5 minutes.[61] Nalmefene's higher cost, slower onset of action, and limited clinical studies in the field setting limit its usefulness at this time. In addition, nalmefene may cause a prolonged period of withdrawal in opioid-dependent patients.

Flumazenil is a selective benzodiazepine antagonist demonstrated to be effective in reversing coma secondary to benzodiazepine overdose. Flumazenil has been shown to increase level of consciousness, decrease PCO_2, and increase PO_2 in patients with benzodiazepine toxicity.[62-67] The activity of flumazenil is noted in 1-3 minutes after IV administration, and the drug has a serum half life of 60-90 minutes.[63] Flumazenil is administered in 0.1-0.2 mg incremental doses and titrated to effect.

Pitfalls

Similar to opioid reversal with naloxone, the half life of flumazenil might be shorter than the half life of the drug it is being used to reverse. Therefore patients released by the prehospital care provider may have a recurrence of symptoms. A major complication associated with flumazenil is seizures, especially in patients on chronic benzodiazepines or with concomitant tricyclic overdose. This serious side effect may be the most limiting factor in the prehospital use of flumazenil.

In conclusion, flumazenil should not be included in any routinely administered mixture (coma cocktail) but may be useful when administered in small, incremental doses in selective patients with respiratory depression secondary to benzodiazepine toxicity.[37]

Syrup of Ipecac

Inducing emesis has been a traditional treatment for ingested poisonings. The adult dose is 30 ml of syrup of ipecac followed by 300 ml of water. Children between 1 and 12 years of age should receive 15-30 ml of syrup of ipecac followed by 10-20 ml/kg of water. Infants between 6 months and 1 year should receive 5-10 ml syrup of ipecac followed by 10-20 ml/kg of water. Infants less than 6 months old should not receive ipecac.[68] The above doses may be repeated once if there is no vomiting in 30 minutes. Ipecac is contraindicated when there is ingestion of nontoxic substances, caustic agents (acids or bases), or hydrocarbons. Ipecac is also contraindicated in patients who are unable to protect their airway, who may have a rapidly changing mental status, or who have ongoing or imminent seizures.

Recently there have been several studies that indicate that inducing emesis contributes little to improving clinical outcome.[68,69] In addition, significant adverse reactions and complications may occur. In fact, studies have shown that the ED administration of syrup of ipecac resulted in longer ED stays, increased the delay before activated charcoal was given, and resulted in more complications.[69] Home use of ipecac resulted in lower serum levels of acetaminophen in children than in controls who did not receive ipecac. Most of these children had acetaminophen levels that were non-hepatotoxic.

Pitfalls

There is danger in the use of syrup of ipecac in patients who may lose their ability to protect their airways, for example, those who have ingested agents that may cause a rapid decrease in level of consciousness or seizures. Other potential complications of syrup of ipecac administration include prolonged vomiting, aspiration pneumonitis, abdominal pain, CNS depression, Mallory-Weiss esophageal tearing, pneumomediastinum, intracerebral hemorrhage in the elderly, and gastric rupture in children.[68]

In summary, the use of ipecac confers little advantage in the treatment of most ingestions in the prehospital setting and exposes the patient to potentially serious adverse reactions and complications.

Activated Charcoal

Activated charcoal has proven to be beneficial in a variety of poisonings. It is not absorbed from the gastrointestinal tract and has the property of adsorbing to many toxins, thus allowing them to pass through the gut and out of the body. The adsorption occurs within 1-2 minutes of contact with the toxin. Activated charcoal can adsorb to substances that have passed through the pylorus into the small bowel. Activated charcoal is equal to or more effective than syrup of ipecac for decontamination in awake overdose patients.[69,70] In patients with a decreased level of consciousness who present more than 1 hour after overdose, activated charcoal was more effective than gastric lavage followed by activated charcoal.[70]

Activated charcoal does not effectively bind to the following substances: acids, alkalis, arsenic, bromide, DDT, ethanol, ethylene glycol, heavy metals, iron, iodide, lithium, methanol, potassium, or tobramycin. Activated charcoal is indicated for nearly all significant poisons except those listed above. Activated charcoal is contraindicated in caustic ingestions and in the presence of an ileus or bowel obstruction.

The typical adult dose is 30-100 gm mixed with water as a slurry. Children up to 12 years old may receive 15-30 gm. Use 1-2 gm activated charcoal/kg in infants. Activated charcoal may be mixed with sorbitol to provide a more palatable flavor and to serve as a cathartic, speeding elimination from the body. Activated charcoal premixed with water or sorbitol is definitely easier for prehospital use.

Pitfalls

Potential complications of activated charcoal administration include vomiting, aspiration pneumonitis, constipation, and charcoal empyema when given through a lavage tube that has perforated the esophagus. Activated charcoal use in patients who have ingested caustic agents may limit the endoscopic evaluation of injury to the gastrointestinal tract.

Prehospital care providers may find patients to be reluctant to drink the black and gritty charcoal. The prehospital care provider can be instructed to place a towel over the glass and encourage the patient to drink without looking at the mixture. Activated charcoal tends to be very messy, especially when administered in the back of a moving ambulance.

In summary, activated charcoal is a rapidly effective agent with few or no serious side effects and may be useful for administration in the prehospital setting.

Magnesium

Over the past few years, magnesium has gained recognition as a clinically important electrolyte and effective therapeutic agent.[71] There are many articles and case reports documenting dramatic improvements in seriously ill patients after the administration of magnesium. Some of the conditions in which magnesium has been successfully used include severe asthma, cardiac arrhythmias, acute myocardial infarction, and eclampsia. These conditions are frequently seen in the prehospital environment, so it would be reasonable to include magnesium as another tool for EMS systems. One survey of state-approved drugs for EMS systems showed that five states suggested magnesium sulfate should be carried by prehospital care providers.[3] The specifics of different clinical settings in which magnesium could be helpful in the prehospital environment follow.

Magnesium has been successful in the treatment of ventricular tachycardia and ventricular fibrillation in cases where standard therapy (e.g., lidocaine and bretylium) have failed.[72,73] It is also considered to be the drug of choice for the treatment of Torsadas de Pointes.[74,75] Hypomagnesemia can exacerbate digitalis related arrhythmias even with therapeutic digitalis levels. In patients with suspected digitalis toxicity and cardiac arrhythmias, magnesium therapy should be considered.[76]

For cardiac arrhythmias in the prehospital environment, magnesium can be given as a slow IV bolus of 2 gm of magnesium sulfate diluted in 10 cc of NS or D_5W.[74]

The command physician should consider magnesium in the patient with refractory ventricular arrhythmias and history of risk factors for common causes of hypomagnesemia, such as alcoholism, malabsorption, and diuretics.

Several studies have suggested that magnesium may be useful in severe bronchospasm associated with asthma.[77-79] Although inhaled bronchodilator (beta-agonists) remain the mainstay of prehospital treatment for bronchospasm, magnesium may be administered in severe refractory cases. Magnesium has a bronchodilator effect and may improve ventilation in spontaneously breathing and intubated patients.[78-79]

For severe bronchospasm, magnesium can be given as a slow IV bolus of 2 gm of magnesium sulfate diluted in 10 cc of NS or D_5W.

Some authors have noted that serum magnesium levels fall transiently in the immediate postmyocardial infarction period.[80] This finding has prompted investigation into whether magnesium therapy may be beneficial in this setting. Several studies have provided evidence suggesting that magnesium may be of value in reducing arrhythmias and mortality following acute myocardial infarction.[81,82]

A loading dose of magnesium can be considered for patients with suspected acute myocardial infarction as a slow IV bolus of 2 gm of magnesium sulfate diluted in 10 cc of NS or D_5W.

In spite of some controversies, for decades IV magnesium has been considered the treatment of choice for the management of eclamptic seizures.[83,84] The recommended dose in the prehospital setting is a loading dose of 4-6 gm of IV magnesium sulfate.

Pitfalls

Magnesium is relatively contraindicated in patients with renal failure. In addition, patients may experience a burning sensation with IV administration. Toxic levels or rapid IV administration of magnesium may cause hypotension, weakness, decreased deep tendon reflexes (DTRs), and respiratory depression.

Prehospital care providers should monitor the patient for possibility of toxicity. However, toxicity is very rare with doses to be used in the prehospital setting, with the exception of the larger doses administered for preeclampsia/eclampsia.

Calcium

The therapeutic use of calcium in the prehospital environment is limited. Although calcium ions play a critical role in myocardial contractility and impulse formation, several studies in the cardiac arrest setting failed to show any benefit from calcium administration.[74] Calcium salts are available in two different preparations for IV administration. 1) Calcium chloride 10%, which contains 13.4 mEq of calcium; and 2) calcium gluconate 10%, which contains 4.6 mEq of calcium. This difference should be considered when specific doses of calcium need to be administered. The most common clinical situations in which calcium can be of benefit in prehospital emergency medicine are life-threatening arrhythmias associated with hyperkalemia and hemodynamic instability secondary to calcium channel blocker toxicity.

Patients with history of renal failure who present with sudden onset cardiac arrest or life-threatening arrhythmias should be considered at high risk for hyperkalemia. Calcium gluconate is usually given for severe hyperkalemia with level above 7.0 mEq/L. Calcium gluconate is administered in a 10-20 cc IV dose in a slow infusion over 10 minutes.[85] One ampule (10 ml) of calcium gluconate (10%) can be administered IV with an onset of action of 1-3 minutes.[85] Calcium antagonizes the toxic effects of hyperkalemia for approximately 30 minutes but does not alter the serum potassium levels.[86] Of course, other standard therapy to reduce the hyperkalemia and for life support should be used as needed.

The cardiovascular manifestations of calcium channel blocker toxicity can be treated with IV calcium. Calcium salts increase the concentration of extracellular calcium helping to overcome the blockade.[87] Initial calcium therapy is 1 amp (10 ml) of calcium chloride (10%) IV. Its effect is transient, and higher doses may be necessary in cases of refractory life-threatening toxicity. Unfortunately, treatment failure is not uncommon, and other life-supporting therapies should be initiated as necessary.

SAMPLE CASES

CASE #1

Paramedics are on scene with a 63-year-old male with a history of atherosclerotic heart disease and CHF who presents a profound respiratory distress and signs and symptoms of CHF. Medics note that he is complaining of chest pain similar to his typical angina, which was unrelieved by one of his nitroglycerin tablets before medics arrived. Paramedics found the patient's medications include digoxin and furosemide 40 mg per days and potassium. He has not taken his meds today. Vital signs are pulse 96, respirations 32, BP 210/110, pulse ox 89%.

The medic's physical exam reveals positive JVD, rales three quarters of the way up both lung fields, and marked peripheral edema. ECG is a sinus rhythm with a rate of 96. The paramedics have initiated a precautionary IV and place the patient on oxygen. Under protocol the paramedics have administered one sublingual nitroglycerin spray and administered 40 mg of furosemide IV.

What additional order would you provide?

Aggressive use of nitroglycerin in this case to both decrease preload and provide relief for chest pain. Even in the absence of chest pain, nitroglycerin could be administered as a prehospital treatment for CHF. As long as the patient's systolic blood pressure was maintained the patient could be aggressively treated by the prehospital crew with sublingual nitroglycerin sprays 2-3 sprays every 3-5 minutes.

CASE #2

Paramedics are on scene with a 75-year-old female with history of atherosclerotic heart disease, status post-coronary artery bypass who called EMS for generalized weakness. Upon arrival, the medics find an elderly female in no acute distress. Her meds include nitroglycerin patch and an anti-hypertensive Tenormin®. The patient shows no other symptoms other than weakness at this time.

Her pulse is 50, respirations 12, blood pressure 130/84, pulse ox 98%. The patient's lungs are clear. The rest of her physical exam is unremarkable. The cardiac monitor reveals a sinus bradycardia rate of 50 without ectopy. The paramedics have initiated a precautionary line of saline at KVO. They are requesting to administer 1 mg of atropine to increase the heart rate.

How would you proceed?

This patient is in a stable bradycardic rhythm possibly secondary to the beta blocker that she is taking on a regular basis. In addition, this patient is stable and asymptomatic and therefore does not require atropine at this time. An increase in this patient's heart rate may be deleterious secondary to her underlying coronary artery disease. An external pacemaker could be applied but not turned on as a precautionary measure.

CASE #3

The paramedics are on scene with an 84-year-old male with signs and symptoms consistent of CVA. The patient has a past history of hypertension and TIAs and now presents with right sided upper and lower extremity weakness. The onset of the symptoms was gradual, beginning approximately 2 hours prior to calling the field crew. The patient's medications include multiple unknown antihypertensives. On physical exam the patient's pulse is 70, respirations 14, blood pressure 220/108. Physical exam is remarkable for an awake, alert elderly male with obvious right, upper, and lower extremity weakness. The paramedics are requesting to administer several nitroglycerin sprays to lower the patient's blood pressure.

How would you proceed?

Although this patient is hypertensive and appears to be having a stroke, the risk of acutely treating this patient's probable chronic hypertension probably outweigh the unclear benefits. This patient is stable and does not appear to be having a hypertensive emergency. Medics should place the patient on oxygen, an ECG monitor, and initiate IV access. If available the paramedics could measure the patient's serum glucose level via Chemstrip and treat it appropriately.

CASE #4

The paramedics are on scene with a 25-year-old male found unresponsive in an alley way. Drug paraphernalia were found at the patient's side, although bystanders are not helpful in providing additional information about the patient's collapse. Upon examination, the medics find the following vital signs: pulse 90, respirations 6, BP 140/90, pulse ox 92%. The patient's pupils are pinpoint and minimally reactive. His lungs are clear and the patient has obvious track marks on both arms and in the neck. The medics note that they are assisting the patient's ventilations via bag-valve-mask and are unable to obtain IV access.

How would you proceed?

This patient appears to have opioid intoxication including pinpoint pupils, slow respirations, and decreased level of consciousness. Since IV access cannot be obtained, naloxone can be administered IM 1-2 mg. This dose could be repeated in 3-5 minutes should the patient not respond. The prehospital care provider should be prepared to intubate the patient having all the necessary equipment ready, including suction. The crew should be aware that occasionally patients under the influence of opioids become violent when reversed with naloxone.

References

1. Cummins RO, editor: Cardiovascular pharmacology 1. In: *Textbook of cardiac life support,* Dallas, 1994, American Heart Association.

2. Pennsylvania Department of Health, Division of Emergency Medical Services, 1994.

3. Delbridge TR, Verdile VP, Platt TE: Variability of state-approved emergency medical services drug formularies, *Prehosp Dis Med* 9:S55, 1994.

4. Shuster M, Chong J: Pharmacologic intervention in prehospital care: a critical appraisal, *Ann Emerg Med* 18:192-196, 1989.

5. Gilman AG, Rall T, Nies AS, et al., editors: *The pharmacologic basis of therapeutics,* ed 8, New York, 1990, Pergamon Press, pp. 9-11.

6. Chameides L, editor: Vascular access. In: *Textbook of pediatric life support,* Dallas, 1990, pp. 37-46, American Heart Association.

7. Glaeser PW, Losek JD: Emergency intraosseous infusion in children, *Am J Emerg Med* 4:34, 1986.

8. Iserson KV, Criss E: Intraosseous infusions: a usable technique, *Am J Emerg Med* 4:540, 1986.

9. Fiser DH: Intraosseous infusion, *N Engl J Med* 322:1579, 1990.

10. Garrison HG, Downs SM, McNutt RA, et al.: A cost-effective analysis of pediatric intraosseous infusion as a prehospital skill, *Prehosp Dis Med* 7:221-227, 1992.

11. Fuchs S: Managing seizures in children, *Emergency* Dec:47-52, 1990.

12. Dieckmann RA: Rectal diazepam for prehospital pediatric status epilepticus, *Ann Emerg Med* 23:216-219, 1994.

13. Beck C, Leighninger D: Reversal of death in good hearts, *J Cardiovasc Surg* 3:357-375, 1962.

14. Brown CG, Taylor RB, Werman HA, et al.: Effect of standard doses of epinephrine on myocardial oxygen delivery and utilization during CPR, *Crit Care Med* 16:536-539, 1988.

15. Brown CG, Werman HA, Davis EA, et al.: The effects of graded doses of epinephrine on regional myocardial blood flow during CPR in swine, *Circulation* 75:491-497, 1987.

16 Brown CG, Werman HA, et al.: Comparative effects of graded doses of epinephrine on regional brain blood flow during CPR in a swine model, *Ann Emerg Med* 15:1138-1141, 1986.

17. Bochner BS, Lichtenstein LM: Anaphylaxis, *N Engl J Med* 324:1785-1790, 1991.

18. Levy D, Lyons E: Pharmacology of antiarrythmic and vasoactive medications. In Tintinalli JE, editor: *Emergency medicine: a comprehensive study guide,* ed 4, New York, 1996, McGraw Hill, p 183.

19. Oberg B, Sorenson MB: Out of hospital treatment with dobutamine, *Prehosp Disaster Med* 8:247-249, 1992.

20. Bledsoe BE: *Out of hospital emergency pharmacology,* ed 3, Englewood Cliffs, NJ, 1992, Simon and Schuster, pp. 127-130.

21. Rottman SJ, et al.: Nitroglycerin lingual aerosol in prehospital emergency care, *Prehosp Disaster Med* 4:11, 1989.

22. Hoffman JR, Reynolds S: Comparison of nitroglycerin, morphine, and furosemide treatment of presumed prehospital pulmonary edema, *Chest* 92:586-593, 1987.

23. Coon GA, Clinton JE: Use of atropine for brady-asystolic out of hospital cardiac arrest, *Ann Emerg Med* 10:462-467, 1981.

24. Bertolet BD: Adenosine: diagnostic and therapeutic uses in cardiovascular medicine, *Chest* 104:1860-1871, 1993.

25. Gausche M, Persse DE, Sugarman T, et al.: Adenosine for the prehospital treatment of paroxysmal SVT, *Ann Emerg Med* 24:183, 1994.

26. Belhassen B, Viskin S: What is the drug of choice for the acute termination of paroxysmal supraventricular tachycardia: verapamil, adenosine triphosphate or adenosine? *PACE* 16:1735, 1993.

27. Camm AJ, Garrett CJ: Adenosine and supraventricular tachycardias, *N Engl J Med* 325:1621-1629, 1991.

28. Dougherty AH, Jackman WM, et al.: Acute conversion of paroxysmal supraventricular tachycardia with intravenous diltiazem, *Am J Card* 70:587-592, 1992.

29. Madsen CD, Pointer JE, Lynch TG: A comparison of adenosine and verapimil for the treatment of supraventricular tachycardia in the prehospital setting, *Ann Emerg Med* 25:649-655, 1995.

30. Weil MH, Rackow EC, Trevino R, et al.: Difference in acid base state between venous and arterial blood during cardiopulmonary resuscitation, *N Engl J Med* 315:153-156, 1986.

31. Quadrel M, Lavery RF, Jaker M, et al.: A prospective, random trial of epinephrine, metraproterenol and epinephrine and metaproterenol in the prehospital treatment of adult asthma, *Prehosp Disaster Med* 26(4):469-473, 1995.

32. Pellegrino TR: Seizures and status epilepticus in adults. In Tintinalli JE, editor: *Emergency medicine: a comprehensive study guide,* ed 4, New York, 1996, McGraw Hill, p. 1032.

33. Rhee KJ, O'Malley RJ: Neuromuscular blockade: assisted oral intubations versus nasotracheal intubation in the prehospital care of injured patients, *Ann Emerg Med* 23:37-42, 1994.

34. Hedges JR, Dronen SC, et al.: Succinylcholine-assisted intubations in prehospital care, *Ann Emerg Med* 17:469-472, 1988.

35. Savarese JJ: Pharmacology of muscle relaxants and their antagonists. In Miller RD, editor: *Anesthesia,* ed 4, New York, 1994, Churchill Livingston, pp. 1:417-487.

36. Roberts JR, Hedges JR: *Clinical procedures in emergency medicine,* ed 2, Philadelphia, 1991, WB Saunders, pp. 34-35.

37. Hoffman RS, Goldrank LR: The poisoned patient with altered level of consciousness: controversies in the use of a "coma cocktail", *JAMA* 274:562-569, 1995.

38. Adler PM: Serum glucose changes after the administration of 50% dextrose solution, *Am J Emerg Med* 4:504-506, 1986.

39. Browning RG, Olson DW, et al.: 50% dextrose: antidote or toxin? *Ann Emerg Med* 19:683, 1990.

40. deCourten-Myers G, et al.: Hyperglycemia enlarges infarct size in cerebrovascular occlusion in cats, *Stroke* 19:623, 1988.

41. Hogya P, Yealy DM, Paris PM, et al.: The rapid prehospital estimation of blood glucose using chemstrip bG, *Prehosp Dis Med* 4:109-113, 1989.

42. Hall-Boyer K, Zaloga GP, Chernow B: Glucagon: hormone or therapeutic agent? *Crit Care Med* 12:584, 1984.

43. Vukmir RB, Yealy DM: Glucagon: prehospital therapy for hypoglycemia (abstract), *Ann Emerg Med* 18:479, 1989.

44. Salzberg MR, Gallagher EJ: Propranolol overdose, *Ann Emerg Med* 9:26, 1980.

45. Weinstein RS: Recognition and management of poisoning with beta-adrenergic blocking agents, *Ann Emerg Med* 13:1123, 1984.

46. Ramoska EA, Spiller HA, et al.: A one year evaluation of calcium channel blocker overdoses: toxicity and treatment, *Ann Emerg Med* 22:196, 1993.

47. Zaloga GP, DeLacy W, Holmboe E, et al.: Glucagon reversal of hypotension in a case of anaphylactic shock, *Ann Int Med* 105:65, 1986.

48. Ellrodt AG, Ault MJ, Riedinger MS: Efficacy and safety of sublingual nifedipine in hypertensive emergencies, *Am J Med* 79:19-25, 1985.

49. Ellrodt AG, Ault MJ: Calcium channel blockers in acute hypertension, *Am J Emerg Med* 3:16-24, 1985.

50. Davidson RC, Bursten SC, Keeley PA: Oral nifedipine for the treatment of patients with severe hypertension, *Am J Med* 79:26-30, 1985.

51. Wachter RM: Symptomatic hypotension induced by nifedipine in the acute treatment of severe hypertension, *Arch Intern Med* 147:556, 1987.

52. Davidson RC, Bursten SL, Keeley PA: Oral nifedipine for the treatment of patients with severe hypertension, *Am J Med* 79:26, 1985.

53. Heller MB, Duda JR, Maha RJ, et al.: Use of nifedipine for field management of severe hypertension (abstract), *Ann Emerg Med* 16:520, 1987.

54. Lisk DR, Grotta JC, Lamki LM: Should hypertension be treated after stroke? *Arch Neurol* 50:855, 1993.

55. Powers WJ: Acute hypertension after stroke: the scientific basis for treatment decisions, *Neurology* 43:461, 1993.

56. Yealy DM, Paris PM, Kaplan RM: The safety of prehospital naloxone administration by paramedics, *Ann Emerg Med* 19:902-905, 1990.

57. Gaddis GM, Watson WA: Naloxone associated patient violence: an overlooked toxicity, *Ann Pharmoco* 26:196, 1992.

58. Smith JA, Stenbach GL: Narcotics. In Tintinalli JE, editor: *Emergency medicine: a comprehensive study guide,* ed 4, New York, 1996, McGraw Hill, pp. 772-773.

59. Kaplan JL, Marx JA: Effectiveness and safety of intravenous nalmefene for emergency department patients with suspected narcotic overdose: a pilot study, *Ann Emerg Med* 22:187-190, 1993.

60. Barsan WG, Seger D, Danzi DF: Duration of antagonist effects of nalmefene and naloxone in opiate induced sedation for emergency department patients, *Am J Emerg Med* 7:155-161, 1989.

61. Nalmefene: a long acting injectable opioid antagonist, *Medical Letter* 27:97-98, 1995.

62. Hojer J, Baehrendtz S, Matell G, et al.: Diagnostic utility of flumazenil in coma suspected poisoning: a double blind, randomized controlled study, *Br Med J* 301:1308-1311, 1990.

63. Weintraum M, Standish R: Flumazenil (RO-1788): a benzodiazepine antagonist, *Hosp Formul* 23:332, 1988.

64. Geller E: Flumazenil in clinical medicine: indications and precautions, *Eur J Anaesth* S2:325, 1988.

65. Spivey WH: Flumazenil and seizures: analysis of 43 cases, *Clin Ther* 14:292, 1992.

66. Winkler E, Almog S, Kriger D: Use of flumazenil in the diagnosis and treatment of patients with coma of unknown etiology, *Crit Care Med* 21:538, 1993.

67. Haverkos GP, DiSalvo RP, Imhoff TE: Fatal seizures after flumazenil administration in a patient with mixed overdose, *Ann Pharmacother* 28:1347, 1994.

68. Ipecac syrup and activated charcoal for treatment of poisoning in children, *Medical Letter* 21:70, 1979.

69. Albertson TE, Derlet RW, Foulke GE: Superiority of activated charcoal alone compared with ipecac and activated charcoal in the treatment of acute toxic ingestions, *Ann Emerg Med* 18:56-59, 1989.

70. Merigian KS, Woodard M, Hedges JR: Prospective evaluation of gastric emptying in the self poisoned patient, *Am J Emerg Med* 6:479-483, 1990.

71. Tso EL, Barish RA: Magnesium: clinical considerations, *J Emerg Med* 10:735-745, 1992.

72. Iseri LT: Magnesium and cardiac arrythmias, *Magnesium* 5:111-126, 1986.

73. Iseri LT, Chung P, Tobis J: Magnesium therapy for intractable ventricular tachyarrhythmias in normomagnesemic patients, *West J Med* 138:823-828, 1983.

74. American Heart Association: Guidelines for cardiopulmonary resuscitation and emergency cardiac care, *JAMA* 268:2135-2302, 1992.

75. Tzivoni D, Banai S, Schuger C, et al.: Treatment of Torsade de pointes with magnesium sulfate, *Circulation* 77:392-397, 1988.

76. Seller RH, Cangiano J, Kim KE, et al.: Digitalis toxicity and hypomagnesemia, *Am Heart J* 79:57-68, 1970.

77. Skobeloff E, Spivey WH, McNamara RM, et al.: Intravenous magnesium sulfate for the treatment of acute asthma in the emergency department, *JAMA* 262:1210-1213, 1989.

78. Dorn MR, Wrenn KD, Slovis CM, et al.: When asthma attack turns deadly: principles of aggressive effective interventions, *Emerg Med Rep* 12:179-186, 1991.

79. Rolla G, Bucca C, Bugiana M, et al.: Reduction of histamine induced bronchoconstriction by magnesium in asthmatic subjects, *Allergy* 42:186-188, 1987.

80. Rasmussen HS, Norregard P, Lindeneg O: Intravenous magnesium in acute myocardial infarction, *Lancet* 1:234-235, 1986.

81. Teo KK, Yusuf S, Collins R, et al.: Effects of intravenous magnesium in suspected acute myocardial infarction: overview of randomized trials, *Br Med J* 303:1499-1503, 1991.

82. Ceremuzynski L, Jurgiel R, Kulakowski P, et al.: Threatening arrythmias in acute myocardial infarction are prevented by intravenous magnesium sulfate, *Am Heart J* 118:1333-1334, 1989.

83. Sibai BM: Magnesium sulfate is the ideal anticonvulsant in preeclampsia-eclampsia, *Am J Obst Gynecol* 162:1141, 1990.

84. Jagoda A, Riggio S: Emergency department approach to managing seizures in pregnancy, *Ann Emerg Med* 20:80-85, 1991.

85. Wilson RF, Barton C: Fluids and electrolyte problems. In Tintinalli JE, editor: *Emergency medicine: a comprehensive study guide,* ed 4, 1996, McGraw Hill.

86. Janson CL, Marx JA: Fluid and electrolyte balance. In Rosen P, et al., editors: *Emergency medicine: concepts and clinical practice,* ed 3, St. Louis, 1992, Mosby, p. 113.

87. Smilkstein: Common cardiac medications. In Rosen P, et al., editors: ed 3, St Louis, 1992, Mosby, p. 131.

PART 2

Clinical Conditions

The following chapters deal with clinical conditions commonly seen in the practice of prehospital emergency care. These conditions include common entities such as chest pain and shortness of breath as well as less frequently encountered entities such as OB GYN and pediatrics. Each chapter includes discussion of the clinical condition along with potential pitfalls in dealing with patients with the prescribed clinical condition. In general the topics are arranged by symptom (i.e. shortness of breath) as opposed to specific diagnosis (i.e. pulmonary embolism) since often the underlying diagnosis cannot be made in the field. On the other hand there are several specific diagnoses which are easily made in the field (i.e. cardiac arrest, childbirth, hypoglycemia) and their prehospital treatment is relatively straightforward.

The prehospital medical command physician must be aware that often the clinical conditions may overlap, for example, a patient with altered level of consciousness may be short of breath and have dysrhythmias. The role of the prehospital medical command physician is to assist the prehospital care providers in identifying and treating the primary problem with the goal of improving the patient's overall condition.

5

Prehospital Analgesia

Pain and suffering are not confined within hospital boundaries. While prehospital personnel are usually focused on the ABC's, the treatment of moderate-to-severe pain should also be considered an important priority in the care of ill and injured patients.[1,2] The challenge of treating pain in the prehospital setting is to use agents and techniques that are not only effective but are safe and do not lead to physiological compromise or a delay in diagnosis upon arrival in the emergency department.[3,4] Because of inordinate fears of "masking the diagnosis" and the desire to prevent side effects, many EMS systems have opted for little or no use of pharmacological analgesics. Providing analgesia has been largely ignored in prehospital care education.[1] Few EMS texts devote any significant attention to this topic. Most systems do not even have protocols to treat pain and suffering other than ischemic chest pain. Prehospital providers are frustrated daily by not being able to offer patients more than the "bite the bullet" approach to providing relief from acute pain.

Very few clinical studies have examined the safety and efficacy of analgesics in the field. The time has come for all health-care providers to make the provision of relief of pain and suffering one of their most important responsibilities in both the hospital and prehospital settings. This philosophy recognizes that all clinicians must first be guided by the principle of "Do no harm" and that some patients seen in the field may be so physiologically compromised that pharmacological techniques of analgesia may need to be delayed. However, this group of patients is the minority of those seen in the field with moderate-to-severe pain. It should be stressed that there are many pathological consequences of untreated acute pain.[2] This philosophy was well summarized by Evans when he said "To allow a patient to suffer unnecessary pain does harm to the patient—a violation of the first ethical principle of medicine."[5]

PAUL M. PARIS, MD, FACEP

In choosing an analgesic for the field, desirable properties should be—

1. Safety.
2. Efficacy.
3. Ease of administration.
4. Rapid onset.
5. Short duration.
6. Low abuse potential for patient and staff.
7. Reversible.

Unfortunately, no ideal analgesic exists. However, to simply delay the administration of any agents until arrival at the hospital is inhumane in many cases. The classes of agents to be discussed in this chapter will be nitrous oxide, opioids, ketamine, and nonsteroidal anti-inflammatories. Another vital aspect of patient care for pain is use of proper communication techniques, which will also be discussed.

Nitrous Oxide

Nitrous oxide–oxygen mixtures fulfill many of the properties desired for a prehospital analgesic.[6] Most important is that several field studies in urban, suburban and rural systems have demonstrated the safety and efficacy of self-administered 50% nitrous oxide in prehospital care.[7-9] All studies have confirmed that the majority (80%-85%) of patients with moderate-to-severe pain from a variety of sources will achieve significant pain relief. In a 16-year study of over 2700 patients in the city of Pittsburgh, significant analgesia was achieved in over 80% of patients.[*] One of the major advantages of the use of nitrous oxide is that it is relatively devoid of serious side effects. In 1994, NIOSH published an alert entitled "Controlling exposure of nitrous oxide during anesthetic administration".[#] The alert provides guidelines to prevent environmental levels from exceeding their recommended standards. In a moving vehicle, or one with a fan, short term administration should be safe for the ambulance attendants. It is

*Kaplan RM, Yealy DM, Paris PM, et al: *Prehospital nitrous oxide: oxygen analgesia: A 16-year multicenter evaluation,* Submitted for publication, 1996.

#U.S. Department of Health and Human Services: *Controlling exposures to nitrous oxide during anesthetic administration,* NIOSH Alert. April, 1994.

important that well-designed protocols be written and followed in using this gas mixture. A prototype of a nitrous oxide use protocol is listed on page 87.[10]

Opioids

Opioid analgesics have been used in many EMS systems for over two decades. In many systems, morphine sulfate is the analgesic of choice for ischemic chest pain that is not relieved with administration of nitrates.[11] For noncardiac pain, most physicians have been reluctant to use opioids such as morphine because of exaggerated fears of producing side effects. For many types of pain, opioids can be titrated by the IV route to produce safe and effective analgesia.[12] One of the major benefits of opioids is that most side effects can be rapidly reversed with an opioid antagonist, such as naloxone, which is carried by all ALS systems.

Fentanyl (Sublimaze) is an opioid that is rarely available on ambulances but which has many advantages for field use. Fentanyl is 75 to 200 times more potent than morphine due to its lipid solubility and ability to cross the blood-brain barrier and bind to opiate receptors. The characteristics of fentanyl that are desirable include short half life and duration of action of 60 minutes or less, lack of histamine release, and lack of myocardial depression.[12] The lack of histamine release is important since other opioids release histamine, which results in vasodilation. Opioid-induced hypotension is rare with fentanyl, but in patients who are only able to maintain normal systemic pressure due to extreme sympathetic drive, fentanyl can blunt the sympathetic response and theoretically lower blood pressure. Should this occur, fluid administration or alpha-adrenergic agents should be used to restore blood pressure to an acceptable range.

Opioid Agonist-Antagonists

Some characteristics of the opioid agonist–antagonist class of analgesics make them ideally suited for prehospital use. Drugs in this group include nalbuphine (Nubain™) and butorphanol (Stadol™). The primary benefits of this class are the ceiling on respiratory depression, minimal euphoria and limited abuse potential, lack of biliary spasm, and minimal hemodynamic effects. Stene described the prehospital use of nalbuphine in 46 patients with moderate-to-severe pain due to multiple trauma, burns, fractures, and intraabdominal conditions.[13] The

SAMPLE STANDING ORDERS / PROTOCOLS

NITROUS OXIDE/NON-CARDIAC PAIN

The following standing orders and protocols for non-cardiac analgesia use nitrous oxide as the pharmacological cornerstone of therapy but still stress the psychological support that can be provided by prehospital caregivers.

1. Develop a rapport with the patient with appropriate reassurance and encouragement.
2. Properly prepare the equipment necessary to administer the gas.
3. Offer nitrous oxide to the patient if there are no contraindications to its use. The patient should self-administer the gas via a mask or mouthpiece.
   NOTE: When using nitrous oxide–oxygen mixtures, remember that it induces a trancelike state in patients, thereby making them particularly sensitive to suggestion. This can be used to increase the therapeutic effect of the gas, but caution must be taken since idle conversation may be misinterpreted by the patient and have detrimental effects. Sample instructions would be "We're going to give you some oxygen with pain-relieving medicine in it to help relieve your discomfort. To get the medicine, you have to hold the mask (or mouthpiece) firmly to your face and breathe normally. In a minute or two, you will feel calm and relaxed and you may feel a little drowsy. Your arms and legs may feel a little heavy as you begin to feel more comfortable. Just relax and let the medicine work for you."
4. Immobilization and splinting if necessary.
5. Gentle handling and movement.
6. Monitor the patient's vital signs every 5-10 minutes.

CONTRAINDICATIONS

1. Obvious intoxication
2. Altered level of consciousness
3. Pregnancy (except during labor)*
4. Suspected pneumothorax
5. Decompression sickness
6. Suspected bowel obstruction
7. Patients with blood pressure <90 mmHg or respirations <8
8. Chronic obstructive pulmonary disease (COPD)*

   *This is only a relative contraindication.

NOTES

1. All inflow ventilating fans must be operating in the patient compartment during administration of this agent.
2. Studies have shown that female dental assistants have a higher rate of spontaneous abortions if they work around nitrous oxide than a control group. The exact risk is not clear but it would seem to be a reasonable policy to have female prehospital providers who are considering pregnancy or may possibly be pregnant to limit their total time in the patient care compartment of the ambulance when nitrous oxide is being used. Finally, it is also desirable for EMS systems to monitor the use of the agent with a log and consider using a locking system to limit the temptation of providers to abuse the agent.

---

agent was partially to completely effective in 89% of patients and was without any major untoward effects. Nalbuphine also causes very minimal if any hemodynamic changes. One of the other advantages of this drug is that it is not a controlled substance, easing some of the paperwork required when using morphine. Butorphanol (Stadol™) is now available as a nasal spray.[14,15] This agent and route of administration have many theoretical benefits in the prehospital environment, but studies have yet to be reported on the field use of nasal butorphanol.

Ketamine

Ketamine is a dissociative anesthetic that is structurally related to phencyclidine, and it has some very unique properties. The dissociative state produced by ketamine is characterized by analgesia and amnesia, while preserving airway protective reflexes.[16] Since ketamine is a bronchodilator, it can be used to treat severe asthma.[17,18] While this agent has little indication for routine prehospital care, it can be used as a field anesthetic for unusual situations, such as field amputations.[19] Ketamine has also been described as a useful agent for field surgical procedures during disasters.[20]

Non-Steroidal Antiinflammatory (NSAIDs) Agents

Currently few EMS systems routinely use aspirin, acetaminophen, or other non-steroidal antiinflammatory (NSAID) agents. Aspirin use is now increasing as an antiplatelet agent to treat suspected acute myocardial infarction. Now that parenteral NSAIDs are available, this class will most likely have an expanded prehospital role as an analgesic. NSAIDs are particularly well-suited for treatment of uretheral and biliary colic.[21,22] These drugs may also potentiate the analgesic action of opiates.[23] While these agents do not work as quickly as opiates, if given at the scene they will frequently have beneficial effect before the patient arrives at the hospital. These agents should not be considered as a substitute for opiates and nitrous oxide but as another helpful adjunct with selected indications. The major side effects to consider with a single-dose use in the field would be allergic reactions and platelet inhibition. They should therefore be withheld in the field if the patient has known allergies to NSAIDs such as aspirin or if the antiplatelet effect may exacerbate the underlying problem.

Communication Techniques

The most ignored aspect of providing prehospital relief to those with pain and suffering is the powerful effects that can result from therapeutic communication techniques.[24] These techniques can be mastered by BLS providers and can bring a significant degree of comfort to patients without use of pharmacological agents. Jacobs points out that many patient responses to an injury or illness are occurring at an unconscious level and that "every word, phrase, sentence, pause, voice inflection and gesture can initiate automatic psycho-physiologic effects."[25] An example of a suggested dialogue for a patient with burns is as follows:

> "I'll bet you can imagine some place you'd rather be than here. As a matter of fact, go ahead and do that now while we get you bandaged up. Think of your favorite place. When you are there in your mind's eye, look around and notice all the things there are to notice. Listen to the sounds. Feel the good feelings. There might even be a special aroma you can smell. When you are really experiencing that place, let me know by raising your index finger. Good."

While many prehospital providers may feel uncomfortable with guided imagery techniques such as this they all should recognize the powerful implications of their verbal and non-verbal communication. Providers should be capable of engaging a patient in a way that distracts them from their injury or illness.

Distraction can also be very helpful while prehospital providers are performing potentially painful interventions, such as starting an IV line or splinting a fracture. Music has been shown to be effective in decreasing pain of laceration repair in emergency departments, and could be adapted for use on an ambulance.

Words should be chosen carefully when communicating with a patient. It is very important to use non-threatening terms, such as "mild discomfort," as opposed to terms such as "bee sting," "prick," or "shot".

Pitfalls

The major pitfall regarding analgesia is the attitude that it should not be provided in the field, instead wait for hospital evaluation. Safe and effective pharmacological and non-pharmacological techniques are available for the majority of patients. These techniques will not "mask" the diagnosis or worsen the patient's condition. Pain is subjective and should be measured by the patient's words and not our expectation of how much we think a patient should be suffering for a given condition.

Another pitfall is to believe that there is a "uniform" dose of analgesic that will bring elimination of pain when using pharmacological therapy. Particularly with the use of opioids there is tremendous interpatient variability. The best way to achieve the desired result is to slowly titrate, monitoring for side effects and efficacy.

A particularly common pitfall is the belief that the degree of a patient's pain can be gauged by a patient's vital signs or facial expressions. The pain literature has repeatedly documented the unreliability of either vital signs or facial expression in assessing the severity of a patient's pain. The only scale that should be used is the patient's verbal expression. A helpful technique to use is a 1-10 verbal analogue scale, with 10 representing the worst pain the patient has ever experienced.

Another pitfall is to fail to distract the patient while performing painful procedures. Just the opposite usually occurs where the provider calls attention to every step of the procedure using terms that are intended to soften the insult but usually actually magnify it.

Summary

Treating acute pain and relieving suffering should be one of the primary missions of all health-care providers. Unfortunately EMS providers have not been given the tools or training to satisfactorily accomplish this worthy mission. While patient "safety" and "doing no harm" must always be considered, these should not be used as excuses for "doing no good" for the majority of patients with acute pain treated in the field.

SAMPLE CASES

CASE # 1

The paramedics are called to see a 25-year-old male complaining of severe lumbar pain that started while lifting a refrigerator. The vital signs are blood pressure of 130/86, pulse 88, and respiration of 14. The neurological examination and remainder of examination are unremarkable.

How would you proceed?

The paramedics' appropriate treatment of this patient's pain should involve a kind, compassionate, caring approach combined with the use of nitrous oxide if available. The nitrous oxide should be started before any attempt is made to move the patient. The efficacy of the nitrous oxide will be improved if the paramedics present the benefits and efficacy of inhalational analgesia to the patient in a positive light. It also cannot be overemphasized how important gentle handling is in cases such as this. Patients are very quick to gauge how caring the providers are in terms of language, nonverbal communication, and patient handling.

CASE # 2

The paramedics call the base station to report that they are seeing a 70-year-old male complaining of severe abdominal pain radiating to his groin. The vital signs are a blood pressure of 70 by palpation with a pulse of 120 and a respiratory rate of 20. The patient has a past history of hypertension and coronary artery disease.

How would you proceed?

This is one of the few times where the axiom "First do no harm" precludes the initial use of a pharmacological analgesic. This presentation is very compatible with a ruptured abdominal aortic aneurysm. Because of the major hemodynamic instability that is occurring in this patient, the primary consideration should be very rapid transport to the hospital with communication with the receiving facility to allow the hospital to begin preparation for the staff and resources that may be necessary to save this patient's life. Patient communication techniques may actually be very calming. Even the presentation of oxygen in a positive reassuring way can allay some anxiety.

CASE # 3

You are asked to give orders on a 22-year-old female who was working in a restaurant and had hot oil spilled over both lower extremities with resultant 10% body surface second- and possibly third-degree burns.

How would you proceed?

This patient would be a candidate for use of 50% nitrous oxide or an IV opioid. If nitrous oxide was not available or was ineffective, there should be no reluctance to slowly titrate IV opioids such as morphine. The goal would not be total elimination of all pain but achieving the state where the patient is relatively comfortable and able to tolerate the pain.

References

1. Stewart RD: Pain control in prehospital care. In Paris PM, Stewart RD, editors: *Pain management in emergency medicine*, Norwalk, CT, 19:313-321, 1987, Appleton & Lange.

2. Clinical Practice Guideline: Acute pain management: Operative or medical procedures and trauma. Agency for Health Care Policy and Research, U.S. Department of Health and Human Services, AHCPR Pub. No. 92-0032. Rockville, MD, 1992.

3. Verdile VP, Stewart RD: The prehospital management of pain. In May HL, editor: *Emergency medicine*, ed 2, Boston, 1992:626-630, Little, Brown.

4. Stewart RD: Analgesia in the field, *Prehospital and Disaster Medicine* 1989; 4:31-35.

5. Evans WO: The undertreatment of pain, *Indiana Med* 81:848-850, 1988.

6. Stewart RD: Nitrous oxide. In Paris PM, Stewart RD, editors: *Pain management in emergency medicine*, Norwalk, CT, 1988:221-239, Appleton & Lange.

7. Johnson JC, Atherton GL: Effectiveness of nitrous oxide in a rural EMS system, *J Emerg Med* 9:45-53, 1991.

8. Yealy DM, Paris PM, Kaplan RM, et al.: The safety of prehospital naloxone administration by paramedics, *Ann Emerg Med* 19:902-905, 1990.

9. Donen N, Tweed WA, White D, et al.: Prehospital analgesia with Entonox, *Can Anaesth Soc J* 29:275-279, 1982.

10. Mossesso V, Stewart RD, Paris PM, et al.: City of Pittsburgh ALS Protocols (Adaptation), 1994.

11. Bruns BM, Dieckmann R, Shagoury C, et al.: Safety of pre-hospital therapy with morphine sulfate, *Am J Emerg Med* 10:53-57, 1992.

12. Paris PM, Weiss LD: Narcotic analgesics: The pure agonists. In Paris PM, Stewart RD, editors: *Pain management in emergency medicine*, Norwalk, CT, 1988, Appleton & Lange, pp. 125-156.

13. Stene JK, Stofberg L, MacDonald G, et al.: Nalbuphine analgesic in the prehospital setting, *Am J Emerg Med* 6:634-639, 1988.

14. Joyce TH, Kubicek MF, Skjonsby BS, et al.: Efficacy of transnasal butorphanol tartrate in postepisiotomy pain: a model to assess analgesia, *Clin Ther* 1993;15:160-167.

15. Diamond S, Freitag FG, Diamond ML, et al.: Transnasal butorphanol in the treatment of migraine headache pain, *Headache Quarterly, Cur Ther and Res* 3:164-170, 1992.

16. Bennett CR, Stewart RD: Ketamine. In Paris PM, Stewart RD, editors: *Pain management in emergency medicine*, Norwalk, CT, 1988:295-310, Appleton & Lange.

17. Sarma VJ: Use of ketamine in acute severe asthma, *Acta Anaesthesiol Scand* 36:106-107, 1992.

18. Jahangir WM, Islam L: Ketamine infusion for postoperative analgesia in asthmatics: a comparison with intermittent meperidine, *Anesth Analg* 76:45-49, 1993.

19. Bion JF: Infusion analgesia for acute war injuries: a comparison of pentazocine and ketamine, *Anaesthesia* 39:560-564, 1984.

20. Dick W, Hirlinger WK, Mehrkens HH: Intramuscular ketamine: an alternative pain treatment for use in disasters? In Manni C, Magnalini SI, editors: *Emergency and disaster medicine: proceedings of the Third World Congress in Rome, 1983*, Berlin, Springer-Verlag, 1985, 167-172.

21. Cordell WH, Larson TA, Lingeman JE, et al.: Indomethacin suppositories vs intravenously titrated morphine for the treatment of ureteral colic, *Ann Emerg Med* 1994;23:(in press)

22. Goldman G: Biliary colic treatment and acute cholecystitis prevention by prostaglandin inhibitor, *Dig Dis Sci* 34:809-811, 1989.

23. Paris PM, Stewart RD: Analgesia and sedation, In Rosen P, editor: *Emergency medicine: Concepts and clinical practice*, ed 3, St Louis 1992:201-229, Mosby–Year Book.

24. Goldfarb B: Prehospital pain management: Providing physical and psychological care. *Prehospital Care Reports* 2:73-80, 1992.

25. Jacobs TJ: *Patient communication*, Englewoods Cliffs, NJ, 1991, Brady.

6

Altered Level of Consciousness

The patient presenting to the prehospital care provider with an altered level of consciousness is one of the most common encounters in EMS. Many of these conditions may cause significant morbidity, and it is essential that proper care be initiated in the field, often before a diagnosis is available. In most instances, this treatment must be instituted in conjunction with attempts to determine the cause for altered level of consciousness. In addition, the care of these patients must include avoiding possible complications, such as C-spine injury and aspiration. The challenge is to rapidly identify and treat those problems that are reversible in the field and to prevent added morbidity from occurring to patients who have lost their protective reflexes.

Differential Diagnosis

The differential diagnosis for the patient with an altered level of consciousness is extremely long and complex, with many of the causes falling out of the scope of practice for the prehospital care provider. Emphasis, however, should be placed on those conditions that may be effectively treated in the field. A simple and useful mnemonic for the potential causes is AEIOU TIPPS (Box 6-1).

Discussion

The focus of a prehospital care protocol for the patient with altered level of consciousness is to treat those common or easily reversible conditions and to use general supportive measures to protect the patient from harm due to the loss of protective reflexes (such as the gag reflex). These BLS measures should be instituted before any attempt is made to gather a complete history or perform a detailed physical examination.

The first task is to determine the degree of the altered level of consciousness. Unfortunately, a variety of inexact terms are commonly used to describe an individual's level of consciousness. Terms such as stuporous, comatose, semi-comatose, obtunded,

ERIC DAVIS, MD, FACEP

Box 6-1 Mnemonic for Causes of Altered Level of Consciousness

A- Airway - hypoxia and postanoxic encephalopathy
E- Endocrine and metabolic
I- Insulin - hypoglycemia
O- Overdose
U- Uremia and Hepatic encephalopathy
T- Trauma, Tumor
I- Infection - meningitis, encephalitis, brain abscess
P- Primary Neurological - seizures, tumors, strokes
P- Psychological
S- Shock

Table 6-1 Glasgow Coma Scale

Eye Opening	Spontaneous	4 points
	Responds to Speech	3 points
	Responds to Pain	2 points
	No response	1 point
Verbal Response	Oriented × 4 (time, place, person, situation)	5 points
	Confused	4 points
	Inappropriate words	3 points
	Incomprehensible sounds	2 points
	No response	1 point
Motor Response	Obeys commands	6 points
	Localizes pain	5 points
	Withdraws (from pain)	4 points
	Flexion (pain)	3 points
	Extension (pain)	2 points
	No movement	1 point

Total GCS Scores:
14-15 points = 5
11-13 points = 4
8-10 points = 3
5-7 points = 2
3-4 points = 1
A score of <9 indicates severe neurological impairment.

confused, and delirious are all used at times by prehospital care providers. In general, it is best for levels of consciousness to be described on the basis of the response the patient makes to a given stimulus. Field providers should describe the exact reaction of a patient to stimuli, such as loud verbal or painful stimuli. Prehospital care providers should all be trained and familiar with use of the Glasgow Coma Scale (Table 6-1).

A study done with paramedics scoring videotaped patients with altered levels of consciousness confirmed that paramedics can give scores that correlate well with those of ED physicians.[1]

Simultaneously with this determination of unresponsiveness, one must assess and maintain an adequate airway. If the patient is not breathing, respirations should be assisted by whatever means are appropriate (bag-valve-mask, intubation). In the patient with respirations, an oropharyngeal airway may be inserted. When a gag reflex is present, the problem can probably be managed by simple head-tilt maneuvers and supplemental oxygen, but if no gag reflex is present, the patient would probably benefit from an attempt at endotracheal intubation. Should the patient become violent or it become impossible to easily intubate the patient, then the better part of valor is to provide meticulous attention to the airway with use of oropharyngeal airway and bag-valve-mask and suction as necessary. In cases where opioid overdose is suspected, then ventilation can be supported with a bag-valve-mask awaiting the reversal of narcosis with an opiate antagonist. IM naloxone can be expected to work within 3 minutes.[2]

Trauma must always be a consideration in these patients, and appropriate protection of the cervical spine must be undertaken throughout. High flow oxygen should be applied to all patients, and if no contraindication exists, the lateral decubitus position offers additional protection of the airway.

Once the airway is secured, the next step is to monitor the patient's pulse, preferably by use of a portable monitor and blood pressure, and to frequently check vital signs. A common mistake in these patients is to miss shock or an arrhythmia, which can obviously have serious consequences. With satisfactory evaluation of those functions necessary to support life, the prehospital care provider and command physician are able to proceed to the next phase of field care: the diagnosis and treatment of potentially reversible conditions.

The next order in most protocols calls for the establishment of IV access while at the same time drawing blood. The blood obtained may then be tested for a serum glucose level, with exogenous glucose administration based on the result. While the level at which glucose is given to the patient may vary from system to system, most use a level of 80 mg/dl when accompanied by symptoms and below as hypoglycemia. This method of testing is preferable to the blind administration of exogenous glucose to all patients with an altered level of consciousness. Studies have shown that only 25% of those patients falling into this category are hypoglycemic, and the commonly held assumption that an ampule of D-50 "won't hurt anyone" has come under attack. This exogenous administration may result in multiple problems, including skin necrosis (after inadvertent extravasation or subcutaneous infiltration), variable elevations in the serum glucose level, hyperosmolality, hyperkalemia (in certain diabetic patients with hyporenemic hypoaldosteronism), and potentially a poorer neurological outcome in patients with focal or global ischemia.[3-10] It is this last point that is of the most concern since this population is common in EMS and the effect is potentially serious. The observations have been derived from both animal and human studies using both stroke and cardiac arrest. While the exact mechanism has not been absolutely defined, it may be due to an increase in acidosis secondary to the delivery of the metabolic substrate glucose in those areas where blood flow is below that necessary to preserve neuronal viability.[11,12] This then impedes recovery once normal blood flow is restored. While not all studies have supported this hypothesis,[13] the current consensus is that the administration of exogenous glucose may be harmful in many patients, an opinion brought forth convincingly in an article by Browning et al.[14] The measurement of serum glucose level in the field has traditionally been accomplished through the use of reagent test strips (Chemstrip, Dextrostix), which have been found to yield accurate results in some studies but to be less effective in others, with a small but significant number of false positives and false negatives.[15-19] Problems may occur with the interpretation of the color change by prehospital personnel, as well as inaccuracy of the strips, particularly if the strips are old, were stored in unsealed containers, or were exposed to extremes of temperature.[20,21] New glucose measuring devices have recently been introduced that give a digital readout of the serum glucose level from a single drop of the patient's blood and could prove to have use in the prehospital setting.[22] The advantage with this method would be that no interpretation of results is necessary. Non-invasive transcutaneous glucose measurement may soon be available.

After administration of glucose to the hypoglycemic patient, an improvement in mental status is usually seen within 5 minutes. The average increase in serum glucose level following one amp of D-50 is approximately 150.[2] After an improvement in mental status, many patients will refuse further medical care, a practice which has been shown to be generally safe if certain criteria are met.[23] The proposed criteria for safe treatment and non-transport are—

1. History of diabetes mellitus.

2. Pre-treatment blood glucose level <80 mg/dl.

3. Post-treatment blood glucose level >80 mg/dl.

4. Return of normal mental status within 10 minutes of D-50 administration.

5. Absence of complicating factors (chest pain, arrhythmias, dyspnea, seizures, alcohol intoxication, chronic renal failure requiring dialysis, or focal neurological signs/symptoms).[23]

If patients are treated and not transported, it is important for the patient's physician to be contacted to regulate insulin dose or make other dietary changes as necessary. The prehospital care provider or a reliable family member should ensure that the patient's physician is contacted.

It is not an uncommon occurrence for paramedics to have a difficult time establishing IV access in patients with hypoglycemia. In these cases the use of IM glucagon has been shown to be safe and effective.[24] Patients without glycogen stores will not respond well to glucagon, but this is a distinct minority of patients. The mean time to response to glucagon is approximately 6-9 minutes with an increase in glucose level of 100 mg/dl.[24] An amp of D-50 works more quickly and on average increases the glucose level by approximately 150 mg/dl.[24,25]

Care must be taught to EMS providers regarding the use of oral glucose solutions in patients with an altered level of consciousness, since aspiration may occur.[25]

The next step in the protocol is to administer an opiate antagonist, which currently is naloxone (Narcan™). Recent studies have shown the number of patients benefiting from this step to be low (7.8%), and it was found to be safe with very few serious side effects, the most common being precipitation of withdrawal.[26] Some authors have argued for a more selective use of naloxone based upon more selective criteria (respiratory rate <12, miosis, circumstantial evidence of opioid abuse) than just altered level of consciousness. These criteria have not been prospectively studied however. There have been several case reports of side effects, such as hypertension, pulmonary edema, and dysrhythmia production after use of naloxone, but these are all in patients who are having reversal of opioid anesthesia and not in patients without an opioid on board.[27-29] Therefore to use naloxone relatively freely in the field is relatively safe but may add more cost than using more selective criteria. There is no currently available method to test for opioids in the field. This step may be initiated earlier in the sequence if suspicion of opioid overdose is high. There is theoretical risk, however, to those patients who are reversed and then refuse further medical treatment (including transport), since they may lapse back into a coma due to the shorter effective period of naloxone as compared to some opioids. Some advocate a low dose administration (0.4 mg IM or IV), which may reverse the respiration depression but may not reverse the patient to the point of refusing transport. This is a perplexing problem, and the true magnitude of risk has not been studied. Experience in systems that have been fully reversing opioid overdose and allowing transport refusals would suggest the actual risk is quite small.[30] A long-acting (4-6 hour) opioid antagonist, nalmefene, has been released and may help to eliminate this problem. Early results would suggest that nalmefene reverses opioid induced coma but that its onset of reversing the respiratory depression may be slower than naloxone.[2] It may turn out that the safest treatment is the combination of naloxone and nalmefene, allowing both quick reversal of respiratory depression and prolonged action.

In all cases, it is extremely important that the prehospital care provider observe and record any response by the patient to the administered medication. This will greatly aid the emergency department personnel in their treatment.

The final portion of the basic sample protocol is to have the field personnel obtain as much information about the patient from the scene as the situation permits. The approach to this phase should be undertaken in as systematic a way as possible to ensure that no information is omitted. Because the patient cannot give an adequate history, alternative sources, such as bystanders and the physical surroundings, must be used. Have the EMS personnel question people familiar with the patient about the patient's health, the rapidity of the onset of the symptoms, any complaints voiced or signs demonstrated by the patient, or any seizure activity. Places where medications are commonly located (such as bathrooms, medicine cabinets, bedrooms, nightstands, and kitchens) should be searched to provide clues concerning underlying illnesses or possible ingestion. A medic alert bracelet or necklace should be sought. Finally, empty pill containers, liquor bottles, syringes, and other drug paraphernalia should be noted and if possible brought to the emergency department.

If a drug overdose or poisoning is suspected, the field personnel should attempt to gather further pertinent information. The route of exposure should be determined. In the majority of cases, this will be by ingestion, and it should be determined what was ingested (including if it was a mixed ingestion), when it occurred, the amount consumed (especially the maximum possible), and any action taken by the patient or bystanders, including the administration of any "antidotes". This will greatly aid later treatment decisions.

The secondary survey should also be directed toward determining the origin for the alteration of consciousness. Respiratory patterns should be noted, as well as any odor on the patient's breath (acetone=DKA, bitter almonds=cyanide, ETOH). Focal neurological signs suggesting stroke or increased intracranial pressure should be noted and recorded as a baseline for possible progression. Specifically the pupils (dilated bilaterally=cerebral hypoxia, barbiturate overdose; pinpoint=opioid overdose) should be observed. The tongue may be checked for bleeding, which may indicate seizure activity, or swelling, indicating anaphylactic shock, which is an unlikely cause unless there is coexistent hypotension. The head should be carefully examined for signs of trauma. The extremities should be observed for flaccidity (stroke, cervical spine injury), track marks (opioid abuse), posturing (increased intracranial pressure, brain damage), and healed slash marks (previous suicide attempt). The skin may be used to determine temperature (increased=infection or heat illness, decreased=exposure, dehydration, alcohol or barbiturate overdose), and for rashes (infection or allergic reaction). Pay careful attention to respirations with rate, pattern, and depth all noted. In each case the positive findings should be relayed to the command physician.

A final point to be addressed is when medical command should be contacted. This in large part is determined by the individual system depending on the assessment abilities of the paramedics, number of calls handled by command, patient population, preference of EMS medical director, local or state statutes, etc. Generally, it is recommended that medical command should be contacted after glucose determination is made and naloxone administered. This enables the command physician to individualize treatment (as in supplemental doses of naloxone or D-50) or to alter the normal mode of therapy (e.g., sodium bicarbonate in suspected tricyclic antidepressant overdose).

Pitfalls

There is probably no patient category with more potential pitfalls than those presenting with an altered level of consciousness. The large differential, combined with the lack of direct pertinent information due to the inability of the patient to give a history, contribute to a large potential for error.

The first potential pitfall with these patients is that they could be misplaced in the altered level of consciousness protocol. The various forms of shock will obviously cause a decrease in the level of consciousness yet must be treated completely differently. Another common mistake is to misinterpret a normal heart rate as evidence that the patient is not hypovolemic. Patients may be on a medication that prevents an increased heart rate (i.e., a beta blocker). Recent research suggests that a relative bradycardia is common with acute blood loss. Also remember that hypoxia or hypercapnia cause agitation or obtundation, and careful attention must be given to maintaining an adequate airway and providing supplemental oxygen. Aspiration is one of the most significant complications of inadequately protecting the airway in these patients.

The next problematic group are those patients that are diagnosed as being "just drunk". The sheer numbers of these commonly abusive patients, combined with the inherent dislike of caring for them, leads to an attitude of indifference by many field personnel. One must keep in mind that the intoxicated/alcoholic patient is at risk for an increased number of secondary problems.

Possible Problems in Alcoholics

- Liver disease
  a) hepatic encephalopathy
  b) coagulation disorder
  c) hypoglycemia
- Electrolyte abnormalities
- Hypoxia
- Trauma
- Sepsis
- Hypothermia
- Seizures

Trauma, particularly of the head and neck, is always a possibility, and everyone should be aware of the increased risk of subdural hematoma. In all patients with an altered level of consciousness, occult trauma must be a major consideration. Immobilization should be the rule. Mixed drug overdoses are also common, and the administration of an opioid antagonist is a good idea. The alcoholic is also prone to a myriad of medical problems, including hypoglycemia. Those patients with liver disease may not have adequate glycogen stores. In addition, the clouded mentation may cause an error with medication such as insulin. Other complications of alcohol, such as hypothermia, should also be considered.

The patient who has a seizure is another potential source of problems. It is tempting to assume that these patients have an underlying seizure disorder, but one must bear in mind that seizures are also caused by hypoxia, hypoglycemia, trauma, intracranial hemorrhage, stroke, and drug overdoses. The patient that has had a seizure is also more prone to head and neck trauma.

Failure to give an appropriate amount of an opioid antagonist is another pitfall. The synthetic and semisynthetic opioids may require large doses of naloxone for reversal. In a similar light, the hypoglycemic patient may not respond immediately if the hypoglycemia has been of prolonged duration.

Perhaps the most common pitfall is related to the terminology used by prehospital care providers communicating to the command physician. Many terms, such as stuporous, obtunded, semi-conscious, and arousable, are used in an imprecise way. It is not uncommon to hear a description such as "alert but not responsive." It is probably best to describe the level of consciousness in a stimulus response manner, as is done in the Glascow coma scale. The patient's response to verbal and painful stimuli should be relayed in specific terms.

Summary

The command physician must always approach the prehospital management of the patient with altered level of consciousness with a great deal of care and in a systematic fashion. Treatment of these patients must be accomplished simultaneously with maneuvers designed to protect and evaluate the patient. Attention must be given to support the patient's vital functions and to reverse those disorders that are able to be treated in the field. All of this should be accomplished through the guidance of the medical command physician.

SAMPLE CASES

CASE #1

"Medic Command, this is Medic One. We are inbound with a 20-30 minute ETA with an approximately 35-year-old male found by police lying in the street. The police called us and we arrived to find him obtunded and disheveled. He is obviously a street person. He smells strongly of ETOH, and we discovered an empty wine bottle beside him. There isn't anybody around to give us any history on the guy. We placed him on a stretcher and are getting ready to initiate transport. His vital signs are as follows: BP 110 over palp, pulse 120, and respirations 12. The patient is currently asleep and snoring. We are unable to obtain a further physical exam because his coat and clothes are reeking of urine, feces, and vomit. The police have requested we bring him into the E.D. for medical clearance for jail. We just wanted to notify you and wonder if you have any further orders."

How would you proceed?

This is a common type of case and presents difficulties for any number of reasons. One of the more distasteful aspects of the job that is performed by the prehospital care provider is dealing with this sort of patient. The majority of these cases will turn out to be "just drunk", but occasionally one will have an alternative reason or reasons for their altered level of consciousness. Sound medical evaluation and treatment should apply in all cases. First, the patient should have been immobilized. This tenet applies to most "just drunk" patients but particularly to one found in the street, since he may have been a victim of trauma. The patient's airway is the next concern. All altered level of consciousness patients should be placed on oxygen, preferably high flow (6-10 L/M), and the report of snoring should alert the command physician to a potential problem with airway patency. An oral airway should be inserted to check for a gag reflex and keep the airway open. A decision to intubate may be at least partially based on the patient's response to this maneuver.

The vital signs obtained are good but they are only a start. If the situation permits, the patient should be undressed, a distasteful but necessary procedure. The wet clothes may be causing the patient to become hypothermic (no one is sure how long he was down), and a good physical exam is important. It will also make it easier to initiate an IV line. Once the IV is established and blood drawn, a serum glucose level should be checked. As previously stated, this population is prone to hypoglycemia due to decreased glycogen

storage ability in the alcoholic liver. This holds true even if the patient is not diabetic. Naloxone should also be administered, since mixed drug overdose is common.

A more thorough physical exam should also be performed. The patient should be carefully checked for signs of trauma, particularly about the head and neck. The pupils should be observed for both configuration and response to light. The lungs must be examined and auscultated to help determine the adequacy of ventilation and the abdomen inspected for rigidity and other signs of an acute abdomen. The extremities may give clues as far as symmetry of movement, as well as track marks. When this evaluation is complete, one should have at least a tentative list of possible etiologies.

The medicolegal aspects of the "clearance for jail" topic and problems with releasing any patient with an altered level of consciousness to the police are important and fraught with potential hazardous consequences. This topic will be covered in greater detail in Chapter 19.

CASE #2

"General Hospital, this is Unit One. We are inbound with a 26-year-old female found by her mother unconscious in her bed. Apparently the family had been trying to get a hold of her all day and went over this evening. She apparently has taken an unknown quantity of the following medications: valium, S-I-N-E-Q-U-A-N, and has obvious ETOH on board. There are empty pill bottles by her bedside, dated 3 days ago. Family states she has been depressed lately. Vital signs are as follows: BP - 120/palp, pulse 130 and thready, respirations 18. Patient does not respond well to verbal stimuli but is arousable to pain. We have her on O$_2$ and are preparing to give her ipecac and have an ETA of 15 minutes. Do you have any further orders?"

How would you proceed?

This is another common scenario. Syrup of ipecac is generally considered to be a ALS-level drug. However, it is easy to see the problems that may arise and that may be avoided with on-line control. Syrup of ipecac should not be given to a patient with an altered level of consciousness, primarily due to problems with protecting the airway. This patient clearly does not warrant ipecac both because of her level of consciousness and also because the time of ingestion is unknown. Ipecac use may delay the administration of activated charcoal. The short transport time may also weigh against ipecac. The prehospital care providers also failed to demonstrate the patency and function of the airway. An oral airway may be inserted to check for a gag reflex, and based on this along with further information obtained by patient examination may warrant an order by medical command for intubation. The drugs involved in this case may cause respiratory compromise.

An IV line should also have been attempted. It is probably warranted in all patients with an altered level of consciousness for blood draw, glucose level check, and administration of naloxone. It is certainly justified in a patient with the above ingestion (especially tricyclic antidepressant) and who is tachycardiac. An IV line is a good precaution, since these patients may decompensate rapidly.

A final point is that medic command may individualize treatment according to the situation. The current treatment of choice for a tricyclic overdose, and one that could be instituted in the field, is bicarbonate administration. This administration should only be accomplished through contact with the medical command physician. Also, the benzodiazepine antagonist flumazenil could be used in selected patients. The importance of being able to add to the treatment of the prehospital patient cannot be overemphasized.

CASE #3

"Medic command this is Rescue 1. We are in the board room of a large company seeing the vice president who is a 42-year-old female who was complaining of a severe headache all morning and while giving a presentation suddenly lost consciousness. She responds to deep pain by withdrawing her arms to her chest. Her vital signs are a blood pressure of 220 over 108, pulse of 92, and a respiratory rate of 24."

How would you proceed?

This patient should have an IV line established and have her glucose checked. Since there is no reason to suspect an opioid overdose, naloxone can be withheld. The scenario suggests an intracranial catastrophe, and the patient should have her airway supported as necessary and be transported to a center that has neurosurgical capabilities if possible. The paramedics will frequently ask for antihypertensive medications in cases such as this. In this particular case the blood pressure is probably elevated as a protective mechanism to help maintain cerebral perfusion. It would potentially be dangerous to lower the blood pressure in this patient. As in all patients with an altered level of consciousness, careful monitoring and support are essential.

SAMPLE STANDING ORDERS / PROTOCOLS
ALTERED LEVEL OF CONSCIOUSNESS

GOALS

The overall goal in a patient who has a serious altered level of consciousness is PROTECTION. Protective reflexes such as cough and gag are lost; aspiration is an ever-present danger in these patients, and, if it occurs, can be lethal.

The specific goals of protection may be stated as being—

1. To protect the patient from physical harm.
2. To protect the patient's brain from injury due to lack of oxygen or glucose.
3. To protect the patient from aspiration.
4. To reverse several underlying causes of coma that may be present, such as hypoglycemia or opiate depression.
5. To gather information for hospital personnel.

INDICATION

Alteration in normal mental status, ranging from confusion or unusual behavior to unresponsiveness to deep pain.

EXCLUSIONS

1. Head injury or other trauma.
2. Shock or serious cardiac arrhythmia.
   If any of above present, go immediately to proper protocol.

NOTE

Although alcohol is a common cause of altered level of consciousness, it is not commonly a cause of frank coma—that is, total unresponsiveness to pain. In these protocols, NO JUDGMENT IN THE FIELD IS TO BE MADE OF THE IMPORTANCE OF ALCOHOL IN THE GENESIS OF THE PRESENTING SIGNS AND SYMPTOMS. For practical purposes and for the sake of the patient, no one is "just drunk".

PROTOCOL

1. ASSESS LEVEL OF CONSCIOUSNESS and maintain AIRWAY as indicated—left decubitus position with head down helps prevent aspiration. INTUBATE and SUCTION as necessary.
2. OXYGEN 4L NC or 10-15 L mask as needed to maintain pulse ox > 94%.
3. SALINE LOCK IV. Attempt to draw red top tube of blood when starting IV.
4. CHECK CHEMSTRIP READING— IF BELOW 80 mg/dl, give 50 cc of 50% glucose iv push. If no IV access, give glucagon 1 mg IM.
5. CHECK FOR NARCOSIS (respiratory depression, constricted pupils, or drug paraphernalia near patient). If any of these present, titrate NALOXONE 0.4-2 MG IV or IM carefully to avoid combativeness. (May give before #4 if situation is suspicious for opioid overdose.)
6. If no response, continue TO VENTILATE, INTUBATE, AND TRANSPORT. Repeat and record vitals and neuro exam frequently.
7. Consult Command Physician.

References

1. Menegazzi JJ, Davis EA, Sucov AN, et al.: Reliability of the Glasgow coma scale when used by emergency physicians and paramedics, *J Trauma* 34(1):46-48, 1993.
2. Davis EA, Menegazzi JJ, Sucov A: Safety and effectiveness of nalmefene vs. naloxone in opioid and mixed drug overdose in the prehospital care setting, *Prehosp Dis Med* 9(3[2]):S60, 1994.
3. Adler P: Serum glucose changes after administration of 50% dextrose solution: pre- and in-hospital calculations, *Am J Emerg Med* 4(6):504-506, 1986.
4. Goldfarb S, Cox M, Singer I, et al.: Acute hyperkalemia induced by hyperglycemia: hormonal mechanisms, *Ann Int Med* 84(4):426-432, 1976.
5. Pulsinelli W, Levy D, Sigsbee B, et al.: Increased damage after ischemic stroke in patients with hyperglycemia with or without established diabetes mellitus, *Am J Med* 74:540-544, 1983.
6. Longstreth W, Invi T: High blood glucose level on hospital admission and poor neurologic recovery after cardiac arrest, *Ann Neuro* 15(1):59-63, 1984.
7. Longstreth W, Diehr P, Invi T: Prediction of awakening after out-of-hospital cardiac arrest, *N Engl J Med* 308(23):1378-1382, 1983.
8. Siemkowicz E: Hyperglycemia in the reperfusion period hampers recovery from cerebral ischemia, *Acta Neurol Scand* 64(3):207-216, 1981.

9. D'Alecy L, Lundy E, Barton K, et al.: Dextrose containing intravenous fluid impairs outcome and increases death after eight minutes of cardiac arrest and resuscitation in dogs, *Surgery* 100(3):505-511, 1986.

10. de Courten-Myers G, Myers R, Schoofield L: Hyperglycemia enlarges infant size in cerebrovascular occlusion in cats, *Stroke* 19(5):623-630, 1988.

11. Rehncrona S: Brain acidosis, *Ann Emerg Med* 14(8):770-776, 1985.

12. Marsh W, Anderson R, Sundt T: Effect of hyperglycemia on brain pH levels in areas of focal incomplete ischemia in monkeys, *J Neurosurg* 65:693-696, 1986.

13. Matchar DB, Divine GW, Heyman A, et al.: The influence of hyperglycemia on outcome of cerebral infarction, *Ann Int Med* 117:449-456, 1992.

14. Browning R, Olson D, Steven H, et al.: 50% dextrose: antidote or toxin? *Ann Emerg Med* 19(6):683-687, 1990.

15. Maisels M, Lee C: Chemstrip glucose test strips: correlation with true glucose values less than 80mg/dl, *Crit Care Med* 11(4):293-295, 1983.

16. Hogya PT, Yealy DM, Paris PM, et al.: The rapid prehospital estimation of blood glucose using Chemstrip bG, *Prehosp Dis Med* 4:109-113, 1989.

17. Lavery RF, Allegra JR, Cody RP, et al.: A prospective evaluation of glucose reagent teststrips in the prehospital setting, *Am J Emerg Med* 9:304-308, 1991.

18. Jones JL, Ray G, Gough JE, et al.: Determination of prehospital blood glucose: a prospective controlled study, *J Emerg Med* 10:679-682, 1992.

19. Chernow B, Diaz M, Orvess D: Bedside blood glucose determinations in critical care medicine: a comparative analysis of two techniques, *Crit Care Med* 10(7):463-465, 1982.

20. Crist D, Murray B, Jones J: Performance and storage of blood glucose reagent strips (abs), *Prehosp Dis Med* 9[2]:S59, 1994.

21. Herr RD, Metz, Richards M: Chemstrip reliability declines with ambulance storage, *Prehosp Dis Med* 4:64, 1989.

22. Chiasson J, Morrisset R, Hamet P: Precision and costs of techniques for self-monitoring glucose levels, *Can Med Assoc* 130:38-43, 1984.

23. Thompson RH, Wolford RW: Development and evaluation of criteria allowing paramedics to treat and release patients presenting with hypoglycemia: a retrospective study, *Prehosp Dis Med* 6:309-313, 1991.

24. Vukmir RD, Paris PM, Yealy DM: Glucagon: prehospital therapy for hypoglycemia, *Ann Emerg Med* 20:375-379, 1991.

25. Collier A, Steedman DJ, Patrick AW, et al.: Treatment of severe hypoglycemia in an accident and emergency department, *Diabetes Care* 6:712-715, 1987.

26. Hoffman J, Schriger D, Luo J: The empiric use of naloxone in patients with altered mental status: a reappraisal, *Ann Emerg Med* 20(3):246-252, 1991.

27. Azar I, Turndorf H: Severe hypertension and multiple atrial premature contractions following naloxone administration, *Anesth Analg* 58:524-525, 1979.

28. Prough DS: Acute pulmonary edema in healthy teenagers following conservative doses of intravenous naloxone, *Anesthesiology* 60:485-487, 1984.

29. Pallasch TJ, Gill TJ: Naloxone: associated morbidity and mortality, *Oral Surg Oral Med Oral Path* 92:602-603, 1981.

30. Paris PM, Personal experience, City of Pittsburgh EMS.

31. Mossesso V, Paris PM, Stewart RD, et al.: City of Pittsburgh ALS Protocols (adaptation), 1996.

7

Shortness of Breath

Shortness of breath (SOB), medically termed dyspnea, is one of the most frequently encountered complaints in the prehospital setting. The patient with dyspnea presents one of the most challenging management problems for both the prehospital care provider and medical command physician. Early interventions can frequently lead to dramatic patient improvement prior to arrival at the hospital. Unfortunately, there has been very little research on the prehospital management of patients with dyspnea.

Assessment of the patient with respiratory distress can be difficult even for an experienced physician in the emergency department with the assistance of tests not available to the prehospital care provider, such as chest x-rays and EKG. In the field the challenge for the command physician is to rely entirely on the history and physical findings as relayed by the paramedic to form a working diagnosis and initiate prehospital therapy. The paramedic must literally be the eyes and ears of the command physician. The physician must be cognizant that the perceptions of the prehospital clinician may be influenced by commonly disseminated misperceptions regarding the relationship of selected signs and symptoms and ultimate diagnosis. Until very recently, there have been almost no objective measures of the severity of respiratory distress in the field.

The risk-to-benefit ratio must be weighed for each intervention contemplated for use in the prehospital setting. Treatments that are indicated for certain conditions are contraindicated in other conditions. Some of the treatments for specific illnesses may harm the patient if the prehospital diagnosis is incorrect. The interventions that may be used in a given prehospital setting depend on level of training and skill of the paramedics, as well as the extent of direct medical control.

Differential Diagnosis

When presented with a case of respiratory distress, the medical command physician must form an initial differential diagnosis of possible etiologies. Of these, life-threatening conditions must be rapidly identified and appropriately treated. For most paramedics, the major differential diagnosis of a patient with SOB is bronchospasm versus congestive heart failure (CHF). They often have protocols that are broken down into those two entities, but they rarely think of other common, potentially life-threatening illnesses, such as pul-

THOMAS D. FOWLKES, MD

monary embolus or pneumonia. Box 7-1 is a partial list of the differential diagnosis of the patient with dyspnea.

Box 7-1	Non-Traumatic Etiologies of Dyspnea

- Bronchospasm: Asthma, Emphysema, Bronchitis, COPD
- Cardiogenic pulmonary edema - CHF
- Non-cardiogenic pulmonary edema - ARDS
- Spontaneous pneumothorax
- Pneumonia
- Pulmonary embolus
- Physiological hyperventilation (e.g., metabolic acidosis)
- Psychogenic
- Upper airway obstruction
- Pleural effusion
- Neuromuscular disease
- Anaphylaxis

Objective Measures

Given the unreliability of physical findings in patients with dyspnea and the variability in paramedics' skill in interpreting these subjective findings, objective measurements may greatly enhance our ability to focus our evaluation and treatment. In the future, objective measures of airway obstruction, oxygenation, and ventilation will be used to assess the severity of respiratory distress and help to differentiate the etiology. Pulse oximetry is rapidly becoming the standard of care for ALS systems. It provides an easily used and non-invasive means of reliably detecting hypoxemia in the field.[1,2] Prehospital studies have shown that a significant number of cases of hypoxemia detected by pulse oximetry were not suspected on clinical grounds. At present, cost is the primary impediment to its widespread use in the field. Capnography is already established as a reliable means of confirming endotracheal tube placement and in the future may be useful in the field to assess the adequacy of ventilation. Measurements of peak expiratory flow rates (PEFR) provide an objective measurement of airflow obstruction. An emergency department study suggested that the PEFR could be used to differentiate CHF from COPD, but a recent field study done to confirm this initial report failed to show benefit for using this modality to make this diagnostic differentiation.[3,4] Although theoretically PEFR could be used to objectively measure the degree of airway obstruction, one small field study showed

that it was difficult to obtain accurate readings.[5] In the emergency department, use of the PEFR has become the legal standard of care to grade the severity of airway obstruction in asthma and to guide therapy.[6]

Without the use of technology such as above the command physician should be very attuned to asking how many word dyspnea a patient has. When a patient has less than 4-5 word dyspnea the condition should be considered severe and needing aggressive interventions.

Discussion

As with all fields of medicine, the basic premise of prehospital care must be: "First, do no harm." The goal of the medical control physician should be to treat those life-threatening conditions that are treatable in the field without worsening other potentially serious medical conditions if the prehospital diagnosis is incorrect.

There has been very little research on the prehospital treatment of patients with respiratory distress. MacLeod et al. evaluated 118 patients presenting with SOB in an urban EMS system with on-line physician supervision and found that when the ED diagnosis was bronchospasm or CHF, the prehospital diagnosis was correct 86% and 82% of the time respectively.[7] For these two conditions, appropriate treatment was given in 98% and 92% respectively. In 24 patients with other ED diagnoses, prehospital diagnosis matched ED diagnosis in only 33% of cases, but acceptable treatment was given in 79%. This study shows that paramedics are able to appropriately evaluate and treat the common conditions of bronchospasm and CHF with on-line physician supervision. For other diseases, paramedics are less accurate in their assessment but appropriate treatment (primarily supportive) is usually given. It must be emphasized that these findings cannot be generalized to other EMS systems without close on-line physician involvement.

Bronchospasm (COPD/Asthma)

Often the diagnosis of bronchospasm is strongly suggested by the past history and the patient's medications and confirmed by typical findings on physical examination. It is helpful to ascertain the severity of prior episodes, especially the need for previous intubation or steroids and O_2 dependence.

Paramedic training has traditionally overemphasized the possible precipitation of respiratory arrest in CO_2

retainers by use of high flow O_2. Clearly one of the most lethal problems in COPD patients is hypoxia and an important goal of prehospital treatment should be to correct hypoxemia. Paramedics are extremely reluctant to use more than nasal canulas for the bronchospastic patient. Venturi masks provide precise O_2 concentration between 24%-50%, and it is not unreasonable to begin O_2 therapy with these or low-flow O_2 via nasal canula. However, if the patient shows signs of hypoxemia or is even suspected of being hypoxemic, higher flow O_2 should be used as necessary to correct the hypoxemia. The likelihood of precipitating respiratory arrest is very small and can be dealt with by paramedics trained in advanced airway management. Even if unable to intubate, the paramedic can adequately ventilate the patient with a bag-valve-mask. In the future, the use of pulse oximetry in the field should greatly enhance the ability of paramedics to recognize and treat hypoxemia.

Inhaled B_2-agonists have emerged as the first-line treatment of bronchospasm both in the ED and in the field. Inhaled B_2-agonists have been shown to be a safe and effective treatment for reactive airway disease in the field. Paramedics can be trained to reliably distinguish patients who will benefit from B_2-agonists by the history, physical examination, and medications. In addition, few side effects from inhaled selective B_2-agonists are seen.[8]

B-agonists may be given parenterally or inhaled via metered dose inhaler (MDI) or nebulized aerosol. Previously subcutaneous epinephrine or terbutaline have been used extensively for bronchospasm, however the inhaled route has replaced this as the first choice because fewer side effects are seen and the drug is more directly delivered to the site of action. Subcutaneous B-agonists may still be used as adjunctive treatment in severe bronchospasm in a young asthmatic or as treatment of anaphylaxis but should be used as a last resort in the older COPD/asthma patient with possible coronary artery disease.

Nebulized aerosol and MDI delivery of B-agonists have been shown to be equally effective when used appropriately; however, good hand-breath coordination is required.[9] This may not be possible for patients in severe respiratory distress.[10] Therefore, nebulized aerosol is recommended for prehospital use. The recommended dose for aerosol treatments is albuterol 2.5 mg or metaproterenol 5% solution .3 cc in 2.5 cc saline. For severe bronchospasm, this dose may be repeated or may be used continuously during the transport. For small children, one half the adult dose would be appropriate. Nebulized aerosols can also be successfully used through an endotracheal tube or can be applied to a tracheostomy site. For prehospital use the nebulized aerosol treatment should be powered by oxygen from a portable O_2 supply.

Intravenous aminophylline, once a common prehospital modality, now has few field indications. It has largely been replaced by the more efficacious B_2-agonists. In addition, aminophylline's low therapeutic index and the need for drug level monitoring, along with serious doubts about its beneficial effects in the acute management of bronchospasm, have resulted in much less use of aminophylline in emergency departments and the prehospital setting.

Recently there has been great interest in the use of magnesium sulfate in the treatment of severe acute asthma.[11] This offers some promise as a safe helpful adjunct in the field treatment of severe asthma.

One of the most difficult situations a paramedic can face is a patient with bronchospasm and severe hypoxia who is combative and agitated and not allowing therapeutic interventions to be initiated. One agent that may offer theoretical benefit in this difficult situation is ketamine. Ketamine is a dissociative anesthetic that also causes bronchodilation. Despite a report of five cases in the emergency department setting and anecdotal evidence of field benefit, there are no published field trials of this agent as of yet.[12]

It is important to remember that dyspnea in a patient with COPD may be secondary to CHF, pneumonia, pneumothorax, pulmonary embolus, or arrhythmias and treatment must keep these other possible disorders in mind. Bronchospasm may play a role in CHF; thus patients with CHF may benefit from, as well as not be harmed by, B_2-agonists. The medical command physician should err in favor of B_2-agonists when the exact diagnosis is in doubt.

Congestive Heart Failure (CHF)

The working diagnosis of acute pulmonary edema is most clear when there is no previous history of COPD/asthma and there is prior history of CHF, coronary artery disease, or hypertension. A recent retrospective study shows a reduction in mortality for those patients with a discharge diagnosis of CHF who received prehospital treatment with nitroglycerin, Furosemide, or morphine compared with those patients who received only oxygen. However, there was also an apparent increase in mortality in those patients who were "mistreated" with the above medications but who ultimately had a diagnosis other than CHF.[13]

There is some evidence to suggest that nitrates are the preferred first-line treatment in the prehospital treatment of pulmonary edema. In a prehospital study by Hoffman of presumed pulmonary edema, patients who received nitroglycerin and furosemide fared better than patients who received morphine and furosemide.[14] These results should be interpreted cautiously, however, since there were several methodological problems with the study. An important finding of this study was that 23% of the patients were ultimately given a diagnosis other than pulmonary edema.

The beneficial effects of nitroglycerin in pulmonary edema are well described.[15] The primary side effect of nitroglycerin is hypotension, which can be a problem in the patient who is already relatively hypotensive or dehydrated.[16] Often the hypotension, which may be accompanied by bradycardia, is transient and resolves spontaneously or with symptomatic therapy.[17] Hypertensive patients with pulmonary edema should be treated aggressively. Initially 2 sublingual 0.4 mg nitroglycerin should be given and then 1-2 every 3-5 minutes as long as the systolic blood pressure is maintained above 120. For patients with significant hypertension and pulmonary edema, much higher doses of nitroglycerin may be of benefit.

Morphine can be used as a second-line treatment, but one must keep in mind its risks and benefits. Although all of morphine's actions in CHF are not well understood, it clearly reduces myocardial oxygen consumption by decreasing both preload and afterload. There is some research to suggest that it also may increase coronary artery blood flow.[18] Another advantage is the decrease in anxiety that may facilitate increased cooperation with the efforts of the prehospital care provider. Morphine however can decrease the respiratory drive, especially if the underlying condition is not CHF, although this concern is probably overstated. It may also cause hypotension, which may not respond to opioid antagonists, but frequently responds to fluid administration.

Another second-line agent in the prehospital treatment of CHF is IV furosemide. There has been much debate regarding furosemide's action as a venodilator, but clearly it has a role in the treatment of CHF as a diuretic. Therefore in patients with severe CHF, especially if already on furosemide, prehospital treatment with approximately twice the oral dose will at the very least minimize the delay in diuretic therapy and may improve outcome.

The newest modality that is now being studied for prehospital treatment of pulmonary edema is CPAP (continuous positive airway pressure). In the hospital, this modality is gaining support as a means to quickly improve pulmonary edema, decreasing the need for endotracheal intubation.[19] Portable battery-operated CPAP equipment using a nasal mask is currently being investigated in a field trial and preliminary results suggest that it is a reasonable and effective field intervention.[21]

Upper Airway Obstruction

While upper airway obstruction in adults is not common, it is obviously an immediately life-threatening emergency and must be considered in patients with acute respiratory distress. Foreign body aspiration is the most frequent cause, especially in children. The diagnosis may be suggested by a history of onset while eating and the presence of inspiratory distress or stridor, as opposed to expiratory distress with bronchospasm. Recently, there has been more recognition of retropharyngeal infections, including epiglottitis, as a cause of airway obstruction in adults. In addition, angioedema secondary to ACE inhibitors is becoming much more common.

It is critical to rapidly identify the choking victim and relieve the obstruction with the Heimlich maneuver or direct laryngoscopy and Magill forceps. If these maneuvers are not successful and the patient cannot be ventilated, field cricothyrotomy or jet ventilation may be lifesaving. Jet ventilation can be taught to paramedics but is usually not included in the standard paramedic curriculum. Special equipment, including a direct connection to a 50 psi O_2 source, is required. It must be remembered that standard 15 lpm O_2 or a BVM connected to a trans-tracheal catheter will not provide adequate ventilation.

Pneumonia

Pneumonia is especially common in patients with COPD, alcoholism, or immunosuppression and in elderly or institutionalized patients. The diagnosis may be suggested by cough, sputum production, fever/chills, or a friction rub. Pneumonia is infrequently considered by paramedics in the field. The rales that commonly are heard with pneumonia are often equated with CHF by paramedics, and their presence alone often prompts a request for furosemide, etc. Field treatment is primarily supportive with oxygen to treat hypoxemia, although bronchodilators may help alleviate dyspnea caused by reactive airways. If the patient has a fever and is clinically dehydrated, mild fluid resuscitation would be indicated.

Pulmonary Embolus (PE)

Pulmonary embolus is a relatively common life-threatening condition that is under-considered in the field. Again, prehospital treatment is primarily supportive, but the advent of thrombolytic treatment requires the command physician to consider this diagnosis and ensure expeditious transport. The most common symptoms of a pulmonary embolus are chest pain and shortness of breath, but atypical presentations are as much the rule as the exception. Treatment for CHF, especially furosemide and nitroglycerin, can potentially have adverse effects for the hemodynamically unstable patient with a pulmonary embolus.

Pneumothorax

Spontaneous pneumothorax is an uncommon cause of dyspnea. Pleuritic chest pain is often a prominent component, but the history and physical findings are notoriously unreliable. Fortunately, only 1%-2% of spontaneous pneumothoraces go on to tension pneumothoraces. It must be remembered that tension pneumothorax is a clinical, not a radiographic, diagnosis. Paramedic curricula include the signs of tension pneumothorax, but paramedics may or may not be trained in needle decompression. Paramedic protocols should include specific indications for needle decompression (i.e., unilateral diminished breath sounds with tracheal deviation and hypotension or cyanosis). This intervention is dangerous if the diagnosis is incorrect but lifesaving if there is a tension pneumothorax.

Standing Orders / Protocols

Respiratory Distress

The development of protocols for treating the adult non-trauma patient with respiratory distress is difficult at best. It is impractical to have one protocol for all cases of respiratory distress. It is important to construct protocols for the different categories of underlying problems that require different treatments in the field (upper airway obstruction, bronchospasm, acute pulmonary edema, and anaphylaxis). Integral to these protocols is an outline of the

relevant history and physical findings that guide the paramedic to the appropriate protocol. Each protocol should include specific indications and exclusions for its use.

In addition, guidelines for determining the severity of respiratory distress should be included. Early physician contact should be mandated or strongly encouraged for cases of severe dyspnea. Cases of severe respiratory distress may especially benefit from early intubation.

The appendix to this chapter contains a sample series of protocols for dealing with respiratory distress in an urban ALS system that requires direct medical control and has the capability for on-scene physician intervention in selected cases.[22] The dashed lines indicate interventions that may be initiated prior to contact with medical control. Note that under certain conditions the paramedics are also referred to other protocols.

Pitfalls

Perhaps the most common pitfall is that many paramedics place too much reliance on a given sign to make a diagnosis and to the etiology of dyspnea. Physical findings are often unreliable despite the experience of the examiner and do not necessarily correlate with the severity of respiratory distress.

This problem is compounded since a paramedic's differential diagnosis for SOB is often only CHF versus COPD. There is a common misunderstanding that rales equal CHF and wheezing equals COPD. Paramedics are most often not accurate in their assessment of JVD and pedal edema. Table 7-1 shows the large overlap in the physical findings that occurs in conditions causing dyspnea, particularly CHF and COPD.

The field team may make a decision about what they think the underlying diagnosis is and allow that to bias or slant the report given to the physician. For example, it would not be unusual for a paramedic to examine a

Table 7-1 COPD vs. CHF

	Rales	Wheeze	JVD	Pedal edema
COPD	+	+++	++	+
CHF	+++	+	+++	++

Key: +   May be present
      ++   Often present
      +++   Usually present and prominent

patient and find wheezing and attribute it to COPD as opposed to recognizing the possibility of "cardiac asthma". On the other hand, wheezing may be absent with severe airflow obstruction.

The risks and benefits must be weighed before ordering treatment based on the paramedic's assessment. Especially keep in mind the possible risks if the working diagnosis is incorrect. The safety of various interventions for these two conditions is estimated in Table 7-2.

The medical control physician should take into account the skills of the providers, the transport time, and the severity of the respiratory distress in determining which interventions will be performed in the field. In general, on-scene time for the severely dyspneic patient should be limited to approximately 10 minutes, unless endotracheal intubation must be performed at the scene.

Psychogenic hyperventilation is a dangerous diagnosis to make by radio. Many serious conditions, such as pulmonary emboli, hypoxia, sepsis, and metabolic acidosis, can be indistinguishable from psychogenic hyperventilation. Reassurance and O_2 are acceptable treatment for each of these conditions. Pulse oximetry would be very helpful in ruling out hypoxemia as a cause of hyperventilation. **Having patients re-breathe into a paper bag should not be done, since it is clearly inappropriate treatment for the other, more serious possibilities.**

One of the pitfalls that may occur with asthma is for the paramedic to underestimate the severity of an asthma attack. A patient may not initially look severe or may initially be thought to be improving, only to have the sudden onset of extremely severe dyspnea, agitation, and eventual respiratory arrest.

Summary

Dyspnea is a common but unfortunately difficult complaint to diagnose and treat in the field. Paramedics generally are limited in their ability to provide accurate physical findings. Often paramedics' understanding of dyspnea is simply to equate rales with CHF and wheezing with COPD/asthma. The medical command physician should also rely heavily on the patient's history and home medications to formulate a working diagnosis and to guide safe field treatment.

Supportive treatment (e.g., oxygen, airway management, prophylactic IV, monitor) and expeditious transport to the emergency department is always indicated. When the etiology is clear (e.g., CHF with hypertension), aggressive treatment should be begun in the field to attempt to avoid further deterioration and to improve morbidity and mortality. However, the medical command physician should always keep foremost in his mind: "Do no harm!"

Table 7-2   Treatment of CHF vs. COPD

	O_2	Lasix	B-agonist	NTG	MS	Aminophylline
COPD	+++	+−	+++	+−	−	+−
CHF	+++	++	+	+++	++	+−

Key to table:

−	*Potentially harmful*
+−	*Risks exist, limited if any benefit*
+	*Limited risk, uncertain if any benefit*
++	*Useful but not without some side effects or risk*
+++	*Safe, minimal risk*

S A M P L E   C A S E S

CASE # 1

A 74-year-old male with a history of 4 previous MI's and "an enlarged heart" is seen by the paramedics after worsening SOB for the last 2 days. The patient has been unable to lie down to sleep at night and is unable to walk to the bathroom without severe dyspnea. He denies chest pain. Meds include digoxin, furosemide, and nitroglycerin, but wife states he has been out of his meds for 4 days. Paramedics report patient sitting upright on couch in severe respiratory distress, able to speak only one to two words at a time. P-110 RR-32 BP-196/110, heart-regular, sinus tach on monitor; lungs-rales throughout; abdomen unremarkable; skindiaphoretic; 2+ pedal edema.

How would you proceed?

This case depicts classic CHF and will likely be recognized as such by both the paramedics and the medical command physician. The challenge in this case is to provide aggressive enough treatment to turn this patient around and hopefully avoid intubation. Since the diagnosis is relatively certain and the blood pressure is elevated, aggressive use of sublingual nitroglycerin will provide the most benefit. Also since the patient has previously been on furosemide and has not had any for several days, furosemide 40-80 mg IV (or twice his usual dose) would be appropriate. The severity of this case also warrants the judicious use of small, frequent doses of morphine sulfate, keeping in mind the caveats discussed above.

If the patient does not respond to initial treatments or his mental status deteriorates, the patient may require intubation and assisted ventilation. This is a potential candidate for awake, sitting nasal intubation if the medics are appropriately trained. The success of nasotracheal intubation by paramedics depends on adequate training and opportunity for practicing this skill. In addition, the availability of a CO_2 detection technique or some other reliable method to confirm endotracheal tube placement is highly desirable. This case would also be a candidate for CPAP or BiPAP if available (see previous discussion).

CASE # 2

Paramedics are at a local nursing home where they were called for a 76-year-old female with SOB for approximately the last 4 hours. The patient also complains of right-sided chest pain that is worse with inspiration. Patient has a history of 2 CVA's and is completely bedridden due to left hemiparesis. No other significant past history. P-116 RR-28 BP-104/68, A&OX3, moderate respiratory distress; skin-warm/dry, no cyanosis; heart-regular, tachycardia; monitor-sinus tachycardia; lungs-rales in the bases; abdomen-soft, non-tender.

How would you proceed?

In this scenario the diagnosis is unclear and the patient does not fit nicely into any of the specific protocols. The most likely diagnoses are pneumonia and pulmonary embolus, although certainly CHF or metabolic acidosis are possible. Given the patient's mental status and degree of respiratory distress, immediate intubation is not indicated. To avoid further complicating the picture or precipitating hemodynamic compromise, basic supportive measures (high-flow O_2, IV of NS or LR, monitor) and expeditious transport should be adequate for this patient. Since this patient may have a pulmonary embolus and the blood pressure is only 104/68, a fluid challenge would be reasonable. Furosemide is potentially dangerous since the patient's volume status is not known.

CASE # 3

You are consulted by paramedics who are at the home of a 60-year-old female who has had worsening SOB and intermittent chest pain for the last 3 days. The patient currently does not have pain but is sitting upright in a dining room chair wearing home O_2 at 2 lpm and is only able to speak short phrases. She has a past history of "emphysema," requiring several hospitalizations and home O_2. Patient also had an MI 6 months ago. Meds include Albuterol and Atrovent inhalers, Theodur, Lasix, Isordil, and Captopril. She is awake but slightly drowsy in moderate-to-severe respiratory distress. P-80 RR-36 BP-144/96; skin-slight cyanosis of nailbeds; heart-irregular, monitor-Afib at 80; lungs- breath sounds decreased at bases, wheezes in upper fields bilaterally; abdomen-soft, non-tender.

How would you proceed?

Directing field treatment in such cases is particularly difficult for the medical command physician.

(continued)

(continued)

Without actually examining the patient yourself and getting a chest x-ray, it is very difficult to determine whether this exacerbation is primarily due to COPD, CHF, or, as is more likely, a combination of the two. In such cases, supportive measures are paramount, with intubation as required by the clinical condition. Beyond this, specific treatments should only be used if they are unlikely to cause deterioration in the patient's condition if the working diagnosis is incorrect and if they are likely to have a beneficial effect. See Table 7-2. B-agonist treatment would likely be useful in this case since there is at least some degree of bronchospasm and if the etiology is found to be primarily cardiac there would be limited risk.

S A M P L E   P R O T O C O L S
RESPIRATORY DISTRESS (NON-TRAUMA)

This set of protocols is designed to provide guidelines for the management of those patients who present with a subjective sensation of shortness of breath (DYSPNEA), a rapid respiratory rate (TACHYPNEA), airway obstruction, or a combination of the above.

In clinical field practice, dyspnea can be classified as follows:

MILD—can speak normally;
MODERATE—can speak short sentences;
SEVERE—can speak a few words or none at all.

Application of a specific protocol will depend upon the presence or absence of certain elements of history and certain signs and symptoms. They are:

HISTORY
- Onset—sudden or gradual
- Cardiac disease
- Lung disease
- Onset while eating
- Home oxygen use
- Similar problem previously
- Prior allergies/anaphylaxis
- Current medications

PHYSICAL
- Cyanosis
- Inability to phonate (a measure of cord obstruction)
- Inability to speak words, sentences (a measure of severity of dyspnea)
- Respiratory rate
- Use of accessory muscles
- Tracheal indrawing/supraclavicular retraction
- Stridor/audible wheezing
- Breath sounds—clear, equal, wheezing, crackles
- Hyperresonant chest on one side
- Barrel chest (increase in A-P diameter)
- Clear/absent heart sounds
- Neck veins/peripheral edema
- Pursed-lip breathing—indicates problem is chronic
- Ratio of inspiration to expiration

Based on the brief initial history and physical in the field, the patient may be treated with one of three protocols:

Protocol 1: UPPER AIRWAY OBSTRUCTION
Protocol 2: BRONCHOSPASM (Wheezing)
Protocol 3: ACUTE PULMONARY EDEMA

PROTOCOL #1: UPPER AIRWAY OBSTRUCTION

INDICATIONS

1. Patients with respiratory distress suspected of foreign body upper airway obstruction. Suspect if: sudden onset while eating or other object in mouth, inability to phonate, patient holding neck (universal distress signal), stridor.
2. Patients in cardiac arrest that occured while eating

PROTOCOL

A. Patient Conscious:

1. Determine adequacy of air exchange. Signs of *poor* air exchange are—
   - Weak, ineffective cough
   - High-pitched noise while inhaling (stridor)
   - Inability to phonate
   - Cyanosis
   - Decreasing mental status or increasing agitation
   - Pulse ox reading < 92%
2. If adequate air exchange present—
   - Encourage continued coughing
   - Oxygen
   - Transport rapidly in position of comfort
   - Monitor adequacy of air exchange, mental status, vitals, pulse ox, EKG
   - Contact Medical Command
3. IF ADEQUATE AIR EXCHANGE **NOT** PRESENT—
   - Perform Heimlich maneuver repeatedly until obstruction relieved or patient becomes unconscious (see Part B of protocol below)
   - Oxygen

B. Patient Unconscious

1. Attempt to ventilate patient with BVM or demand valve.
2. If unable to ventilate, perform Heimlich maneuver on supine patient until laryngoscope available.
3. Visualize the upper airway with LARYNGOSCOPE.
4. REMOVE OBSTRUCTION WITH MAGILL FORCEPS or SUCTION.
5. If no obstruction visualized, re-attempt to ventilate.
6. If patient remains unconscious, intubate per ETI protocol.
7. If unable to ventilate due to unrelieved obstruction and unable to intubate, perform needle cricothyroid puncture (per procedural protocol).
8. After providing adequate ventilation, assess pulse, blood pressure, pulse ox, and EKG.
9. Contact Medical Command and transport promptly.

PROTOCOL #2: BRONCHOSPASM (WHEEZING)

NOTE

Bronchospasm—the reversible constriction (spasm) of the smooth muscle of the small airways (bronchioles)—is a manifestation of several diseases. The most common are asthma, bronchitis, and emphysema (COPD). However, CHF, pulmonary embolism, and pneumonia may also present with wheezing.

INDICATIONS

1. Respiratory distress with wheezing or prolonged expiratory phase on ascultation.
2. Respiratory distress with history of asthma or COPD and no other apparent cause of dyspnea.

(continued)

(continued)

CONTRAINDICATIONS

Acute CHF/Pulmonary edema—use Protocol #3.

PROTOCOL

1. Assist ventilation/intubate based on mental status, adequacy of air exchange, vitals, pulse oximetry.
   *NOTE: Intubation does not relieve (and may in fact worsen) bronchospasm. This should only be done when patient clearly needs ventilatory assistance or airway protection.
2. OXYGEN—as needed to maintain pulse ox reading > 93%.
3. ALBUTEROL 2.5 mg nebulized with oxygen at 6 L/min.
4. Contact Medical Command.
5. Monitor mental status, air exchange, vitals, pulse ox, and EKG en-route to hospital.

6. Repeated albuterol treatments.
7. Epinephrine 0.3 cc of 1:1000 sol. SC for patients unable to cooperate with albuterol treatment or in severe distress.

PROTOCOL #3: ACUTE PULMONARY EDEMA / CONGESTIVE HEART FAILURE

INDICATIONS

1. Respiratory distress with history/exam suggestive of heart failure, such as chest pain, diaphoresis, crackles in lungs, pink frothy sputum, peripheral edema, or past history of CHF, MI, or heart disease.
2. Respiratory distress associated with SBP >180 or DBP >120.

EXCLUSIONS

1. Cardiac dysrhythmia—go to appropriate protocol (Cardiac dysrhythmias).
2. Shock (poor perfusion or SBP <100)—go to appropriate protocol (Cardiogenic shock).

PROTOCOL

1. ASSIST VENTILATION/INTUBATE if mental status decreased or inadequate air exchange.
2. SIT PATIENT UP—as straight as possible, legs dangling over bed or stretches (if possible).
3. OXYGEN—15 L/min by face mask if tolerated, 6 L/min by N/C if not.
4. ASSESS vital signs, pulse ox, lung sounds, pedal edema, ECG rhythm.
5. NITROGLYCERIN—0.8 mg sublingual (2 sprays or 2 tablets) every 3-5 minutes if SBP is greater than 140 mmHg.
6. Saline lock IV.
7. Contact Medical Command and initiate patient transfer.
8. Monitor level of consciousness, vitals, pulse ox, air exchange, and EKG en-route to hospital.
   NOTE: Ultimate therapy for CHF is intubation. This is usually unnecessary with aggressive medical care but should be done if patient develops decreased LOC, hypotension, or worsening dyspnea.

9. Increased or decreased dosage of NTG based on patient's blood pressure and respiratory distress.
   NOTE: Nitroglycerin is the primary intervention for treatment of CHF; it should be used aggressively as long as blood pressure permits.
10. If patient has chronic CHF or peripheral edema, FUROSEMIDE 40-100 mg IV push.
    (Standard IV dose for patient on Lasix is same as his/her usual oral dose.)
11. If patient remains hypertensive and in severe respiratory distress, MORPHINE SULPHATE 2-5 mg IV bolus over 2 minutes. May repeat this dose based on patient response.
    *Observe carefully for respiratory depression after giving morphine, and be prepared to intubate.
12. If wheezing persists after initial dose of NTG, albuterol 2.5 mg nebulized may be given.

References

1. McGuire TJ, Pointer JE: Evaluation of a pulse oximeter in the prehospital setting, *Ann Emerg Med* 17:1058-1062, 1989.

2. Sughey K, Hess D, Eitel D, et al.: An evaluation of pulse oximetry in prehospital care, *Ann Emerg Med* 20:887-891, 1991.

3. McNamara RM, Cionni DJ: Utility of peak expiratory flow rate in the differentiation of acute dyspnea, *Chest* 101:129-132, 1992.

4. Kelly JM, Delbridge TR, Sullivan MP, et al.: Assessment of the usefulness of peak expiratory flow rate to differentiate out-of-hospital CHF and COPD patients, *Prehosp Dis Med* 9(supp 3): S56, 1994.

5. Heller MB, Melton JB, Paris PM, et al.: Data collection by paramedics for prehospital research (abstract), *Ann Emerg Med* 17:414, 1988.

6. Rubsamen DS: The doctor, the asthmatic patient, and the law (editorial), *Ann Allergy* 71:493-494, 1993.

7. MacLeod BA, et al.: The accuracy of prehospital diagnosis in patients with dyspnea (abstract), *Ann Emerg Med* 19:459, 1990.

8. Eitel DR, et al.: Prehospital administration of inhaled metaproterenol, *Ann Emerg Med* 19:1412-1417, 1990.

9. Hawkins J, et al.: Metered-dose aerosolized bronchodilators in prehospital care: a feasibility study, *J Emerg Med* 4:273-277, 1986.

10. Cabanes LR, et al.: Bronchial hyperresponsiveness to methacholine in patients with impaired left ventricular function, *N Engl J Med* 320:1317-1322, 1989.

11. Kuitert LM, Kletchko SL: Intravenous magnesium sulfate in acute, life-threatening asthma, *Ann Emerg Med* 20:1243-1245, 1991.

12. L'Hommedieu CS, Arens JJ: The use of Ketamine for the emergency intubation of patients with status asthmaticus, *Ann Emerg Med* 16:568-571, 1987.

13. Wuerz RC, Meador SA: Effect of prehospital medications on mortality and length of stay in congestive heart failure, *Ann Emerg Med* 21:669-674, 1992.

14. Hoffman JR, Reynolds S: Comparison of nitroglycerin, morphine, and furosemide in treatment of presumed pre-hospital pulmonary edema, *Chest* 92:586-593, 1987.

15. Bussman WD, Schapp D: Effects of sub-lingual nitroglycerin in emergency treatment of severe pulmonary edema, *Am J Cardiol* 41:931-934, 1978.

16. Wasserberger J, Balasubramaniam S: Complications in prehospital use of nitroglycerin, *Ann Emerg Med* 11:116, 1982.

17. Wuerz R, Swope G, Meador S, et al.: Safety of prehospital nitroglycerin, *Ann Emerg Med* 23:31-36, 1994.

18. Leaman DM, Nellis SH, Zelis F, et al.: Effects of morphine sulfate on human coronary blood flow, *Am J Cardiol* 41:324-326, 1978.

19. Bernsten AD, Holt AW, Vedig AE, et al.: Treatment of severe cardiogenic pulmonary edema with continuous positive airway pressure delivered by face mask, *N Engl J Med* 325:1825-1830, 1991.

20. Sullivan MP, Kisdaddon RT, Menegazzi J, et al.: The use of continuous positive airway pressure (CPAP) for the treatment of acute cardiogenic pulmonary edema in the prehospital setting. City of Pgh Division of EMS.

21. Yealy DM, Plewa MC, Stewart RD: An evaluation of cannulae and oxygen sources for pediatric jet ventilation, *Amer J Emerg Med* 9(1):20-23, 1991.

22. Mosesso V, Stewart RD, Paris PM, et al.: City of Pittsburgh ALS Protocols (Adaptation), 1996.

8

Chest Pain

In the early 1960s, prehospital care of patients consisted of only transport. In 1967, Pantridge and Geddes reported on a new mobile ICU that successfully resuscitated 10 of 10 prehospital cardiac arrest victims, who were initially seen for chest pain.[1] Half of these patients were long-term survivors. With more modern ALS, increased technology has been brought into the field. In the case of cardiac ischemia, nearly all therapies that can be done in the ED (e.g., airway management, arrhythmia control, thrombolytics, etc.), can be initiated in the field. Paramedic reports have become very sophisticated, giving detailed descriptions of the pain and associated symptoms, helping the command physician to differentiate ischemic from nonischemic chest pain. The goal of emergency cardiac care has always been preservation of myocardial tissue, prevention of sudden death, and resuscitation from cardiac arrest when it does occur. Rest, oxygenation, and prevention of hypotension prevent further damage but do little to regain lost tissue. The advent of thrombolysis and angioplasty has greatly changed the prehospital approach for the patient with chest pain.

Perhaps the most important element that must be considered in the field treatment of chest pain is TIME. Time to definitive intervention (thrombolytics or angioplasty) now is more critical than ever in the treatment of coronary occlusion. Time to reestablishing perfusion to ischemic myocardium must decrease if precious myocardium is to be saved. Mortality can also be greatly reduced with the early administration of thrombolytics. In one large multicenter trial, there was a 47% reduction in mortality if thrombolytics were administered within 1 hour of symptoms.[2] Command physicians must readdress priorities for the care of cardiac patients with time as a crucial factor to be considered in the risk/benefit ratio of any field intervention or use of time.

There are three major components in the timeline from onset of symptoms of myocardial ischemia to definitive care:

1. Onset of symptoms to seeking medical care
2. Prehospital care
3. Delay from hospital arrival until thrombolytic administration or angioplasty.

SANDRA M. SCHNEIDER, MD, FACEP

The longest delay occurs in the first phase, where most individuals wait for several hours before seeking medical care.[3] Many public information campaigns are now underway to encourage patients with chest pain to seek care earlier and to do so by contacting their local EMS system and not driving or having their family or friends drive them to the hospital.[4]

Chest pain is a common prehospital complaint (with an incidence of 100-200 calls/100,000 population), but only 12%-30% of patients with chest pain have acute myocardial infarctions.[3-5] Using standard cardiac care for all patients with chest pain is not only expensive and time consuming but may have detrimental effects in selected patients. Nitroglycerin may compromise patients with non-cardiac chest pain, such as pulmonary embolism. Prophylactic lidocaine may cause side effects. In our zeal to provide "the best" in cardiac care, we must be selective and conservative in its application to the larger group of patients who do not have cardiac disease.

Differential Diagnosis

ACLS and BCLS training, and even the media, have all stressed cardiac disease as the "killer". Is it any wonder that paramedics (and some physicians) classify all chest pain as either cardiac and noncardiac (i.e., not important disease)? There is a very large differential diagnosis of the symptom of chest pain. Many etiologies of non-ischemic chest pain are life threatening and need to be considered. Paramedics often receive little training on conditions such as dissecting aortic aneurysm and pulmonary emboli. Box 8-1 lists the more common or important causes of chest pain.

Despite all the attention cardiac disease receives, most chest pain patients will have another, non-cardiac cause for their discomfort. Some of the most important causes (i.e., may lead to rapid death) include dissecting aortic aneurysm, pulmonary embolism, pericarditis, and tension pneumothorax. In addition, some patients will have chest trauma (pneumothorax or hemothorax, flail chest, etc.) not covered in this chapter.

Suspected Ischemia

Cardiac pain is commonly, but not always, substernal, heavy (crushing) discomfort with radiation to the neck or arms. Accompanying diaphoresis or vomiting are important signs suggestive of a life-threatening condition. Healthy, young women under the age of 40 are unlikely to have ischemic disease unless they are diabetic, have had pelvic surgery, or use cocaine. The risk of ischemic disease for males becomes significant after the age of 30 or even younger for diabetics.

Subtle details of the history can be extremely helpful to create an accurate suspicion of the correct diagnosis. Paramedics should be taught to obtain and report the important descriptors of chest pain that are sometimes remembered by use of the mnemonic PQRST (Box 8-2).

Unfortunately, not all patients with ischemic disease present with "typical" substernal chest discomfort. Many patients have atypical presentations—isolated arm or jaw pain, epigastric discomfort, or the absence of pain. This is particularly true in the elderly (> 75 years old) where chest discomfort occurs less than half the time.[6] Diabetics also commonly have "silent MIs." The elderly and diabetics commonly present with shortness of breath (SOB),

Box 8-1   Causes of Chest Pain

- Myocardial ischemia
- Pulmonary embolus
- Aortic dissection
- Esophagitis
- Chest wall pain
- Pneumonia
- Pleuritis
- Pericarditis
- Neuropathic
- Thoracic outlet syndrome
- Pneumothorax
- Psychogenic

Box 8-2   Historical Aspects of Chest Pain

P- What **provoked** the pain or what was the patient doing when the pain started?
Q- What is the **quality** of pain; is it burning, aching, squeezing, stabbing?
R- Is there any **radiation** of the pain; does it go to neck, jaw, back, or arms?
S- How **severe** is the pain? On a scale of 1-10, with 10 being the worst pain of one's life, what is the pain currently and what was it earlier?
T- What are the **temporal** aspects of the pain? How long has it been present? Has it occurred before and when?

weakness, or just a subtle mental status change. The sudden onset of pulmonary edema in a patient without peripheral edema should strongly suggest acute cardiac ischemia.

Some patients have typical symptoms, but their denial is so strong that the history is vague and misleading. This is particularly true of "Type A," executive personalities and certain ethnic groups. Repeated questioning and a healthy degree of suspicion help to identify these patients.

Cocaine Use

The acute or chronic use of cocaine may cause coronary artery vasoconstriction and acute ischemia. In addition, it causes myofibril necrosis in bands throughout the myocardium serving as a focus for ventricular (and atrial) arrhythmias. Drug use, specifically "crack" use, makes a patient a high risk for coronary ischemia. Very frequently, patients are reluctant to relay this information and since they may be very young, paramedics may not seriously consider the possibility of myocardial ischemia.

Bronchospasm

Patients with bronchospasm may complain of chest tightness. Wheezing may be inaudible if bronchospasm is severe. The bronchospasm that is associated with a complaint of chest tightness may be due to pulmonary disease or congestive heart failure (CHF). In a patient with CHF, the chest pressure sensation must be considered due to myocardial ischemia until the patient is fully evaluated in the ED. In patients with only a history of asthma who may be younger, it is commonly appropriate to consider complaints of chest tightness to be due to the bronchospasm itself until the patient is evaluated. An elaborate discussion of the differential diagnosis and treatment of dyspnea in the field is presented in Chapter 7. Other less common gastrointestinal causes of chest pain include inflammatory diseases of the stomach, duodenum, and pancreas.

Gastrointestinal Disease

Disorders of the gastrointestinal tract (esophageal reflux and spasm) are a common cause of a variety of symptoms including burning, substernal pain, or tightness. Nitrates often relieve the pain of esophageal spasm. Antacids can relieve the burning (reflux) but can also relieve the pain of myocardial infarction in some patients. A trial of nitrates in the field may ease chest pain, but relief should not be interpreted as proving the etiology of the pain was myocardial ischemia.

Pleuritic Chest Pain

Any irritation of the pleural surface causes pleuritic chest pain. When the onset is sudden, the cause may be serious, most notably, pulmonary embolism or pneumothorax. Even when the onset is more insidious, potentially life-threatening causes should be considered, e.g., pericarditis. Often the cause is a benign viral disorder (pleurodynia) or may remain obscure (musculoskeletal).

Perhaps the most important cause of pleuritic chest pain and one of the most difficult to diagnose is pulmonary embolism (PE). Often considered the great imitator, PEs can mimic cardiac disease, cause severe pleuritic pain, or present with acute dyspnea without any chest discomfort, often labeled "hyperventilation." Patients are frequently anxious, which fools the prehospital care provider into assuming the etiology of the patient's complaints is due to anxiety and the patient is simply hyperventilating.

Patients who are immobile, on estrogens (oral contraceptives), have leg pain/swelling, or recent pelvic surgery are at a much higher risk for a PE. There are estimated to be over 650,000 PE cases each year, many occurring in patients with no obvious risk factors.[7]

The sudden onset of dyspnea, cyanosis, and pleuritic pain is classic, but the pain can be heavy and squeezing. Vasodilators, such as nitrates and opiates, reduce preload and cause severe hypotension in patients with a PE.

If the patient is hemodynamically compromised and the diagnosis of PE is strongly suspected, the receiving hospital may consider preparing a thrombolytic agent for expeditious administration.

Dissecting Aortic Aneurysm

Dissecting aortic aneurysms occur in patients with a history of hypertension and patients with Marfan's syndrome. The pain is classically felt as a tearing into the back, but many other presentations may occur. Comparison of upper extremity blood pressures is occasionally useful but impractical for the field. Dissecting aortic aneurysms are rarely diagnosed in the field and are often missed in the ED. Even if aortic dissection is strongly suspected, most EMS systems do not carry the common drugs used to control blood pressure and cardiac contractility in this entity.

Pericarditis

The pain of pericarditis often mimics that of pleuritic pain that is relieved to some extent by sitting up or leaning forward. Pericardial rubs are infrequently heard in the ED and can be very transient. It is unlikely they could be detected in the field. Pericarditis occurs in patients with renal failure, within the few weeks after coronary bypass, and in otherwise healthy individuals.

Pneumothorax

The development of a spontaneous pneumothorax may cause pleuritic chest pain. Loss of breath sounds on the affected side and jugular venous distention may not be detected in the field. On rare occasion, such patients may go on to develop a tension pneumothorax associated with more severe dyspnea and hypotension. Always consider this diagnosis in trauma and asthmatic/COPD patients, especially if they are in cardiac arrest. Some patients will have bilateral tension pneumothoraces.

Pneumonia

Pneumonia can present as pleuritic chest pain and fever, but immunosuppressed patients (including those with AIDS) may be afebrile and complain only of chest heaviness and dyspnea. Rales and other auscultatory findings of an infiltrate are often not appreciated in the field. Prehospital care consists of oxygen, and in elderly or very ill patients, IV and ECG monitor.

Musculoskeletal Pain

The most common etiology of chest pain is musculoskeletal or "undetermined cause". Though these patients rarely die of their disease, their anxiety and health-care costs rival those with cardiac etiology. Often paramedics (and physicians) later dismiss valid complaints when voiced by a patient who had repeatedly "cried wolf." Reproducible chest wall tenderness can occur with true cardiac ischemia and should not be used to totally dismiss cardiac ischemia, particularly in the field. However, most patients with chest wall pain require little care other than transport. Musculoskeletal pain is a diagnosis that should not be made in the field.

Discussion

"Safe" Transport

Despite the availability of sophisticated prehospital care systems, many patients with chest pain continue to delay coming to the ED. Massive public education efforts designed to heighten awareness of cardiac symptoms and their importance have had little impact on patients'

denial of potential danger and delays in seeking prompt treatment.[8] Even when patients decide to seek treatment, they may use their own automobile, often on the advice of their physicians. Continued public education, often through popular television shows (not "educational") and national access to 9-1-1 will hopefully improve this situation. Clearly more education is needed, beginning with health-care professionals.

All patients should receive supplemental oxygen that theoretically improves oxygen delivery to the myocardium. Oxygen therapy may be titrated with the use of pulse oximetry to monitor the arterial content of oxygen noninvasively. It is a rapid, inexpensive, and non-invasive clue to oxygen needs, but its results must be interpreted with caution. There is a tendency to think that any result greater than 90% is good, when results in the low 90s may correlate with a Po_2 level in the 50s. Pulse oximetry may not be accurate in patients with severe hypotension, peripheral vasoconstriction, dark nail polish, or dyshemoglobinopathies.

Patients should receive increased amounts of oxygen until their O_2 saturation is $> 95\%$ (unless the patient also has significant lung disease). The patient with severe COPD should be watched for the development of confusion or somnolence, an indication of CO_2 retention. Any patient with continued low saturations that are believed to be accurate despite maximal supplemental oxygen should be considered for possible intubation and rapid transport.

Pain Relief

Regardless of the etiology of chest pain, pain relief should be attempted, provided it does not endanger the patient's hemodynamic status. The relief of pain reduces anxiety and decreases the catecholamine effect that decreases myocardial oxygen consumption. This is particularly beneficial in preserving the myocardium, but it also improves overall patient comfort.

There are three major analgesics used to provide acute pain relief in the field: opioids, nitroglycerin, and nitrous oxide.

Opioids are very helpful since they provide both analgesia and anxiolysis. Morphine, the most commonly used opioid for chest pain, decreases systemic and peripheral vascular resistance and decreases the cardiovascular response to stress. Morphine is also believed to have the potentially beneficial action of decreasing coronary artery resistance.[9] Hypotension is an idiosyncratic reaction to morphine that may occur more often when the rate of administration exceeds 5 mg morphine per minute or when given to elderly or vasoconstricted patients. This hypotension is often associated with a slowing of the pulse. The hypotension is almost always self-limited and responds to administration of fluids.

Nitroglycerin decreases myocardial oxygen demand and may also increase collateral blood flow. It may also be effective in patients with esophageal spasm. When using nitroglycerin, it is desirable to have an IV initiated as soon as possible to treat hypotension or bradycardia that may occasionally occur as a result of the nitroglycerin.

Nitrous oxide has less hemodynamic effects but does relieve apprehension and some pain. It may be used in the field when opioids and nitroglycerin are contraindicated by hypotension or drug allergy. Nitrous oxide should not be combined with opioids, since the combination may result in a significant decrease in cardiac output.[10]

Perhaps the most commonly ignored form of providing comfort to patients in pain is proper use of communication techniques. These can be particularly helpful in patients having ischemic chest pain, since the patients may have many fears associated with the implications of the pain.[11]

Dysrhythmia Suppressants

Patients with acute cardiac ischemia and occasionally other causes of chest pain are at risk of ventricular dysrhythmias. Hypoxemia is an important, *correctable* cause of dysrhythmias.

Lidocaine was previously recommended for ventricular fibrillation prophylaxis in all patients suspected of acute myocardial ischemia. In two recent reviews, prophylactic lidocaine failed to improve survival and both authors report a slight increase in deaths in the patient group receiving prophylactic lidocaine (an unexplained phenomena).[12,13] The American Heart Association no longer recommends routine prophylaxis with lidocaine.[14] Current recommendations are to use lidocaine in the treatment of symptomatic ventricular dysrhythmias and in patients following termination of ventricular tachycardia or ventricular fibrillation. Many patients have PVCs chronically without symptoms and without long-term consequences. Some patients will be aware of their frequent benign PVCs. Paramedics commonly ask for lidocaine in any patient with PVCs, and it is important to explain the rationale for withholding the drug.

Side effects of lidocaine may be common, occurring in 39%-64% of cases in some series.[15] These adverse effects include hypotension, seizures, and CNS depression. Life-threatening events, such as asystole, occurred in 5 of the 285 patients in one study.[14] Doses of lidocaine need to be decreased and the drug needs to be used cautiously in patients already on an oral congener of lidocaine, such as tocainide.[16]

The dysrhythmic suppressant level of lidocaine is 1.5 to 6 mcg/ml. Several dosage schemes are available to maintain blood levels in this range. The following is an example of one that has been suggested by the American Heart Association:[14]

Infusion Method:

In non-cardiac arrest an initial bolus of 1-1.5 mg/kg followed by a maintenance infusion at a rate of 30-50 mcg/kg/min (2-4 mg/min) is required to achieve therapeutic levels of lidocaine rapidly. To prevent subtherapeutic lidocaine levels after the initial bolus, a second bolus of 0.5 mg/kg is recommended after 10 minutes. If ventricular ectopy persists, additional bolus injections of 0.5-0.75 mg/kg can be given every 5-10 minutes to a total dose of 3 mg/kg. The maintenance infusion should be titrated according to clinical needs and plasma lidocaine concentrations.[14]

Lidocaine is rapidly distributed through the body (initial plasma half life is 10 minutes). An infusion may not keep plasma levels therapeutic in the initial phase, therefore a second bolus is necessary. The maintenance dose (bolus or infusion) of lidocaine should be decreased in patients with decreased hepatic flow, such as in congestive heart failure, shock, or acute myocardial infarction. Elderly patients have a decrease in their volume of distribution and therefore require a decrease in their infusion dosage.

Continuous infusions are difficult to accurately control in the field. Therefore a bolus method is used by many systems.

Bolus Method:

1-1.5 mg/kg mg IV given every 5-10 min to maximum dose of 225 mg (3 mg/kg). In patients with congestive heart failure or liver disease, doses after the initial loading dose should be halved.

Thrombolysis

In the past, little attention was placed on field times of patients with acute cardiac complaints. An IV line, oxygen, and monitoring were established with some haste, but the patient may not have been transported until analgesics and communication with the base station were completed. With the availability of thrombolysis, field times must be kept to an *absolute minimum*. This means rapid institution of cardiac monitoring, oxygen, IV, and in many cases pain relief given during transport. Few patients with chest pain actually have an acute myocardial infarction, and fewer still are candidates for thrombolytic therapy. ST segment elevation on the prehospital rhythm ECG is not sensitive or specific enough to determine the need for thrombolysis when used as the sole criteria for myocardial infarction. On-line medical command and paramedics using 12-lead ECG telemetry can accurately identify patients appropriate for thrombolysis.[17,18] In Salt Lake City, this has saved 20-25 minutes from ED arrival to thrombolysis, without increasing on-scene or transport time.[19]

Since time to thrombolysis is critical, prehospital administration of thrombolytics is appealing. Several European studies have demonstrated safe use of these drugs in the field, generally using physician-staffed ambulances. Time saved by prehospital thrombolysis varies but averages about 1 hour in some European and U.S. studies.[20] In the largest prehospital thrombolytic trial, "The Myocardial Infarction Triage and Intervention Trial" (MITI), the group treated in the field had a 1.2% mortality versus 8.7% for the group treated in the hospital.[21] A recent study done in Milwaukee showed that paramedics were capable of properly identifying appropriate candidates for thrombolytics and administering the agents in the field.[22] In this study, the time from paramedic arrival to administration of drug averaged 40 minutes versus the control group, which was treated at the hospital an average of 70 minutes after paramedic arrival. While this 30-minute savings has significant clinical advantage, it may be possible in many systems with relatively short transport times to achieve the 40-minute treatment time and still have the thrombolytic administered in the hospital. Certainly for systems with prolonged transport times, field administration becomes more attractive. Field administration of thrombolysis may not be feasible for most prehospital systems. Even for systems where thrombolytics are not administered in the field, paramedics may perform a valuable function by screening for con-

traindications to thrombolytic therapy, saving precious time once the patient is at the hospital.

Atypical Chest Pain

Perhaps the most confusing patients are those with some components of cardiac pain and some symptoms of gastrointestinal pain (for example, the patient with a little burning, a little belching, and a mild SOB). These individuals are difficult enough to diagnose in the ED. Patients at risk of cardiac disease—previous history of MI, over age 40 (50 in women), heavy smokers, hypertensives—should be presumed to have cardiac disease even if the story is atypical. These patients should receive oxygen, an IV line, and monitoring until their symptoms are better analyzed in the ED. Avoid labeling these high-risk patients as "crocks", since very often they will later develop true cardiac disease.

Silent MI

Beware of patients, particularly the elderly or those with diabetes or hypertension, who present with acute SOB, fatigue, or acute pulmonary edema. These symptoms may indicate a silent myocardial infarction. Patients with a silent myocardial infarction are five times as likely to have life-threatening complications and three times as likely to die than patients with atypical chest pain.[23] One of the new technologies that may play an important role in detecting silent and nonsilent ischemia in the field is the use of portable 12-lead continuous ST segment monitoring. In an early study of the field use of this technology, several patients had machine documented transient ischemic changes in the ST segments that would not have been detected in the ED.[24]

Elderly Patients

Less than 40% of patients over the age of 85 describe chest discomfort or pain with acute myocardial infarction.[2] Common presenting symptoms in this age group include acute confusion, weakness, SOB, and acute pulmonary edema.

The elderly often have liver dysfunction, which may interfere with lidocaine metabolism; infusion rates need to be reduced by approximately 50%. The elderly are also more susceptible to the sedative, hypotensive, and respiratory suppression effects of opioids.

Hypotension

The acute cardiac ischemia patient with hypotension (including those precipitated by opioid or nitroglycerin therapy) is a difficult management problem. Though analgesics seem indicated for pain relief, they may cause hemodynamic compromise. In some patients the decrease in preload and afterload may actually cause the cardiac output to increase. Patients with a borderline low blood pressure, such as 90 to 100 mm/Hg systolic, may be treated with very small doses of morphine sulfate (1-2 mg IV) titrated to the desired effect. Patients who become hypotensive (excluding those in CHF) may respond to a fluid challenge or Trendelenburg position. Patients with significant hypotension in the field should be rapidly transported. Nitrous oxide can provide anxiety relief generally without hypotension, although pain relief may be variable. Nitrous oxide should not be combined with opioid use, since the combination may decrease cardiac output.

Hyperventilation

Patients hyperventilate for a variety of reasons, including anxiety, pain, pulmonary embolism, and aspirin toxicity.

In the past, it was popular to treat many of these patients with a paper bag (to elevate their PCO_2 level). The hypoxemia caused by rebreathing expired air can cause disaster if the "hysterical" patient really has a pulmonary embolism. Rebreathing masks should be used with *extreme* caution and only if a pulse oximeter is available. Paper bags should be totally avoided in the field.

Summary

Chest pain is one of the most commonly treated complaints by EMS providers. There are many new developments that require a revision of traditional treatment patterns. Technology now allows us to actually reestablish the circulation to ischemic and infarcting myocardium in cases of coronary occlusion. The EMS system must play a larger role than ever in the chain of survival not only for cardiac arrest but for cardiac ischemia. As technology advances however we must always be cognizant of one of the most important factors in the treatment of patients with chest pain with life-threatening conditions—TIME.

SAMPLE CASES

CASE #1

"Medic command, this is medic one."

"Medic command, over."

"We are currently at a local bank seeing the vice president who is 50 years old. The patient states there is nothing wrong with him; his co-workers overreacted. He states he began having indigestion about an hour after eating. The indigestion was partially relieved by belching, although some chest discomfort continues. The patient has some mild nausea and SOB. He has never had similar pain before. The patient is on an anti-hypertensive, brand unknown, and he smokes two packs a day. On physical examination, his blood pressure is 140/100, pulse 110 and regular, respirations are 28 and unlabored. The patient is cool, clammy and his clothes are soaked with sweat. His chest is clear to auscultation. The monitor shows a normal sinus rhythm with a ventricular bigeminy pattern. The PVCs appear to be unifocal. There appears to be some ST depression on the monitor. We have an ETA of 10-15 minutes. How would you like to proceed?"

DISCUSSION

This is a typical patient at high risk for an acute myocardial infarction. The patient has many risk factors and relatively classic pain, although he may be subjectively denying his symptoms. Short field time is appropriate since he may be a candidate for thrombolysis. If available, transmission of a 12-lead EKG may mobilize personnel for rapid administration of thrombolysis. Recognize that the ST depression on the monitor is not diagnostic. The paramedics may be able to screen for contraindications to thrombolytics. While the American Heart Association no longer recommends lidocaine prophylaxis, they do state that patients who are having an acute myocardial infarction and who display symptomatic ventricular irritability may benefit from lidocaine therapy.[25] Since the field setting is less controlled than a coronary care unit, many clinicians still choose to treat "warning dysrhythmias" in the field in patients who are likely to be having an acute myocardial infarction.

SAMPLE ORDERS

1. Oxygen 2 L/min by nasal canula.
2. IV NS at KVO rate.
3. Apply a cardiac monitor.
4. Administer one nitroglycerin tablet or buccal spray every 5 minutes, as long as blood pressure remains above 100 systolic or until chest discomfort is eliminated.
5. Transport *expeditiously* in a supine position (or with the head slightly elevated).
6. Frequent check of vital signs.
7. Lidocaine 75 mg IV over 1-2 minutes. Repeat bolus every 5-10 minutes to a maximum of 225 mg.

CASE #2

"We are at the home of an 85-year-old female who called with a complaint of being sick. The patient is extremely vague about her history. When she got up this morning, she was feeling well. Shortly after eating breakfast, she began to feel weak and lightheaded. She broke out in a sweat, and it was more difficult for her to breathe while she walked around. She denies any pain. The patient has a past medical history of cardiac disease. She had a myocardial infarction approximately 1 year ago with similar symptoms. The patient is currently on Tocainide, Lasix, Digoxin, Ecotrin, Synthroid, Procardia, Peri-Colace, Halcion, Periactin, Timoptic, and Allopurinol. The patient is lying in bed, somewhat diaphoretic. Vital signs—blood pressure 90/60, respirations are 28 and mildly labored, pulse is 80. Chest has rales at the bases. There is 2+ pitting edema of the ankles. Monitor is showing a normal sinus rhythm. ETA is 5 minutes. How would you like to proceed?"

DISCUSSION

This elderly patient poses several problems. She does not present with chest pain, but rather a variety of vague symptoms, which together should suggest ischemic cardiac disease (particularly since the same symptoms occurred with the previous myocardial infarction). The patient is on Tocainide (a lidocaine-like oral antiarrhythmic), which may complicate lidocaine therapy. Lidocaine therapy added to therapeutic Tocainide levels may cause seizures and other toxicities.[16] A reduced dose of lidocaine (bolus or infusion) would be used—or the drug avoided if possible. Also the lidocaine infusion dosage would need to be further reduced because of her geriatric metabolism and her CHF with hepatic insufficiency. Since the patient is currently without dysrhythmias, prophylactic lidocaine is best withheld. The patient is hypotensive and requires a reduced dose of analgesics. If her respiratory distress were severe (and rales heard), diuretics could be given but might worsen her hypotension.

SAMPLE ORDERS

1. Oxygen.
3. Cardiac monitor.
2. IV NS KVO.
4. Consider very small doses of morphine (1-2 mg) IV.

CASE #3

"We are seeing a 28-year-old female complaining of severe substernal chest pain and SOB. Her symptoms began approximately 1 hour ago while she was playing tennis and the pain is still present despite rest. She describes it as a heavy pressure radiating into her jaw and down her arm. She also complains of SOB.

"The patient has previously been well. She is on no medications. She admits to using cocaine regularly and did some crack this morning just before getting the pain. Also, be advised, she may be pregnant.

"On physical exam, she is cold and clammy, BP 150/100, pulse 120, regular respiration 25. Chest is clear. Monitor shows a sinus tachycardia with occasional PVCs. ETA is 10 minutes.

"How would you like to proceed?"

DISCUSSION

This patient would normally be in a low-risk group (menstruating female) but her use of cocaine puts her at high risk for cardiac damage. She should be treated as a possible myocardial infarction.

SAMPLE ORDERS

1. Cardiac monitor.
2. IV D5W KVO.
3. Oxygen, 10 L by face mask.
4. Pain relief (morphine or nitrates) en-route to hospital.

CASE #4

"We are seeing a 19-year-old female complaining of intermittent, sharp, stabbing chest pain. Patient states the pain has been coming and going for the past month but seems worse today. Each pain lasts less only seconds. The patient denies SOB, nausea, and lightheadedness. She states her grandfather died last month of a heart attack. She is on no medications and denies drug use. The pain is not increased with deep breath or motion.

"On exam the patient is clearly anxious. BP 130/70, pulse 100, respirations 20. Chest is clear. Monitor shows a normal sinus rhythm.

"How would you like to proceed?"

DISCUSSION

This patient is at low risk for ischemic chest pain. She can be transported with BLS services only. She has no known exposure to cocaine, is young, and should have estrogen protection. Her pain is extremely brief (cardiac pain generally lasts for > 5 min). She has no associated symptoms—SOB, diaphoresis. She also has no symptoms consistent with pulmonary embolus or pericarditis.

SAMPLE ORDERS

1. Transport.
2. Oxygen is optional.

References

1. Pantridge JF, Geddes JS: A mobile intensive care unit in the management of myocardial infarction, *Lancet* 2: 271-273, 1967.

2. Gruppo Italiano per lo studio della streptochinasi nell'infarcto miocardico (GISSI). Effectiveness of intravenous thrombolytic treatment in acute myocardial infarction, *Lancet* i:397-402, 1986.

3. Christenson JM, Aufderheide TP: Pre-hospital management of acute myocardial infarction, *Acad Emerg Med* 1:140-143, 1994.

4. LaRossa JH, Horan MJ, Passamani ER, editors: *Proceedings of the National Heart, Lung, and Blood Institute symposium on rapid identification and treatment of acute myocardial infarction,* U.S. Department of Health and Human Services, 1991.

5. City of Pittsburgh EMS Data, 1990.

6. Bayer AJ, Chadha JS, Farag R, et al.: Changing presentation of myocardial infarction with increasing old age, *J Am Geriatr Soc* 34:263-266, 1986.

7. Frieman DG, Suyemoto J, Wessler S: Frequency of pulmonary thromboembolism in man, *N Engl J Med* 272:1270-1274, 1965.

8. Ho MT, Eisenberg MS, Litwin PE, et al.: Delay between onset of chest pain and seeking medical care: the effect of public education, *Ann Emerg Med* 18:727-731, 1989.

9. Sethna DH, Moffit EA, Gray FJ, et al.: Cardiovascular effects of morphine in patients with coronary artery disease, *Anesth Analg* 61:109-114, 1982.

10. McDermmott RW, Stanley TH: The cardiovascular effects of low concentrations of nitrous oxide during morphine anesthesia, *Anesthesiology* 41:89-91, 1974.

11. Jacobs DT: Patient communication: *for first responders and EMS personnel,* Englewood Cliffs, NJ, 1991, Brady.

12. Collins R, Peto R: Effects of prophylactic lidocaine in suspected acute myocardial infarction: an overview of results from the randomized controlled trials, *JAMA* 268:1910-1916, 1988.

13. Hine LK, Laird N, Hewitt P, et al.: Meta-analytic evidence against prophylactic use of lidocaine in acute myocardial infarction, *Arch Intern Med* 149:2694-2698, 1989.

14. Cummins RO, editor: *Textbook of advanced cardiac life support,* American Heart Association, 1994, p. 7-7.

15. Rademaker AW, Kellen J, Tam YK, et al.: Character of adverse effects of prophylactic lidocaine in the coronary care unit, *Clin Pharmacol Ther* 40:71-80, 1986.

16. Schuster MR, Paris PM, Kaplan RM, et al.: Effect on the seizure threshold in dogs of tocainide/lidocaine administration, *Ann Emerg Med* 16:749-751, 1987.

17. Otto LA, Aufderheide TP: Evaluation of ST segment elevation criteria for the prehospital electrocardiographic diagnosis of acute myocardial infarction, *Ann Emerg Med* 23:17-24, 1994.

18. Cummins RO, Eisenberg MS: From pain to reperfusion: what role for the prehospital 12-lead EKG? *Ann Emerg Med* 19:1343-1346, 1990.

19. Karagounis L, Ipsen SK, Jessop MR, et al.: Impact of field transmitted electrocardiography on time to in-hospital thrombolytic therapy in acute myocardial infarction, *Am J Cardiol* 66:786-791, 1990.

20. Weaver WD, Cerqueira M, Hallstrom AP, et al.: Prehospital-initiated vs hospital-initiated thrombolytic therapy: the myocardial infarction triage and intervention trial, *JAMA* 270:1211-1216, 1993.

21. The European Myocardial Infarction Project Group: Prehospital thrombolytic therapy in patients with suspected myocardial infarction, *N Engl J Med* 329:383-389, 1993.

22. Aufderheide TA, Keelan MH, Lawrence SW, et al.: The Milwaukee pre-hospital chest pain project: a randomized trial of pre-hospital versus hospital based thrombolytic therapy for acute myocardial infarction patients (abstract), *Acad Emerg Med* 1:A8, 1994.

23. Fesmire FM, Wears RL: The utility of the presence or absence of chest pain in patients with suspected acute myocardial infarction, *Am J Emerg Med* 7:372-377, 1989.

24. O'Toole KS, Paris PM, Menegazzi JJ, et al.: Evaluation of continuous twelve-lead ST segment monitoring by paramedics (abstract), *Acad Emerg Med* 1:A58, 1994.

25. Billi JE, Cummins RO, editors: *Instructors manual for advanced cardiac life support,* American Heart Association, 1994:C6-17.

SAMPLE STANDING ORDERS / PROTOCOLS
CHEST PAIN

GOALS

1. The prevention of and resuscitation from sudden death.
2. Prompt transport to hospital for administration of thrombolytic agent.
3. The reduction of myocardial ischemia.
4. The relief of pain and anxiety.

INDICATIONS

This protocol is to be applied to any of the following patients:

1. Those over age 25 complaining of non-pleuritic pain in the anterior chest, described as pressing, tight, dull, constricting, band-like, or heavy.
2. Those over age 25 with non-pleuritic chest pain, or epigastric, neck, jaw, or arm pain associated with nausea, vomiting, apprehension, pallor, sweating, or dyspnea.

PROTOCOL

1. INITIAL CONTACT—reassure, place supine or semi-Fowlers position, explain procedures.
2. OXYGEN—via nasal canula 4-6 L/min or face mask 10-15 L/min as needed to maintain pulse ox > 94%.
3. Take HISTORY OF PAIN: P, Q, R, S, and T. (Provocation, Quality, Radiation, Severity, Timing)
4. Place EKG MONITOR
   - Continue below if sinus rhythm with rate 60-140. IF NOT, go to arrhythmia protocols.
5. EXAM and VITALS
   **If blood pressure less than 100 mmHg systolic, CONTACT MEDICAL COMMAND physician BEFORE proceeding with protocol.

6. NITROGLYCERIN 0.4 mg by intraoral spray (or sublingual tablet).
   *NOTE: B/P MUST be above 100 systolic.
7. IV saline lock. IF systolic BP < 100, LR or NS Maxidrip with fluid challenge quantity to be determined.
8. BEGIN TRANSPORT as soon as possible to allow early administration of thrombolytic. MONITOR VITALS and EKG closely while en-route.
9. Contact Medical Command as early as possible.
10. NTG—0.4 mg every 3-5 minutes for continued chest pain.
    - Recheck BP prior to each administration to ensure > 100.
    - If BP decreases to < 100 or BP decreases with signs of poor perfusion, elevate legs and give IVF LR 250 cc boluses as needed.
11. MORPHINE SULFATE 2-3 mg IV if chest pain is moderate to severe and unrelieved by 3 doses of NTG SL. This dose may be repeated as needed and as tolerated.
12. Lidocaine 1 mg/kg IVP for multifocal PVCs, PVCs > 6/min, couplets or R-on-T. (Reserved for patients thought to be having an acute myocardial infarction, this is a bit more liberal than current AHA guidelines.)
    - Initial bolus should be followed by 0.5 mg/kg Q10 min up to 3 mg/kg (maximum of 4 additional doses), EXCEPT in patients with decreased perfusion (CHF or shock), liver disease, or over age 70, who should receive follow-up doses of 0.25 mg/kg up to a total of 2 mg/kg (maximum of 4 additional doses).

9

Dysrhythmias

EMS physicians often use the same approach in the field and the hospital to provide or guide patient care even though the goals in each area differ. Prehospital care of patients with dysrhythmias focuses on treating all life-threatening or imminently life-threatening rhythm changes over a short period (minutes). In the ED and hospital, a longer period (hours to days) is available to achieve these goals, plus identify other nonlethal rhythms and deliver definitive long-term treatment. It is this confusion over the basic goals of dysrhythmia management in these two settings that can complicate medical command.

This chapter discusses a pragmatic method of providing medical direction for nonarrest dysrhythmias. The most important field observations and actions will be highlighted to help simplify the approach when giving verbal commands or creating written protocols. We assume the presence of basic electrocardiograph (ECG) interpretation skills. A decidedly "low tech" approach to the problems will be used, emphasizing simple tools including a brief history, physical exam, and standard 4-electrode field ECG monitor. Similarly, the interventions suggested will be streamlined to those that are effective and easily given in the prehospital setting. In general, the approach offered is consistent with the AHA ACLS guidelines, although areas where simplification or an alternative are offered will be highlighted.

The Basic Principles of Medical Command for Dysrhythmias

Three basic sources of information are available during the assessment of field dysrhythmias: patient history, physical examination, and the ECG. Rarely will any one of these suffice in choosing a treatment option; rather, the combination of these three data sources can help streamline care.[1-2]

Four steps can be used to manage patients with dysrhythmias in the field. Often, treatment decisions can be started before completing all steps, allowing an economy of effort. We will review these steps, highlighting areas where sufficient information is available to justify action or observation.

DONALD M. YEALY, MD, FACEP   CARL W. GOSSETT, MD, FACEP

Step One: Are There Symptoms and How Do They Relate to the Rhythm?

Two groups of patients present with dysrhythmias: asymptomatic patients or those with incidental rhythm changes and patients with symptomatic rhythm changes. Incidental dysrhythmias may relate to the symptoms but are the result (not the cause) of another problem and do not worsen immediate outcome. Patients with an incidental dysrhythmia or who are asymptomatic rarely require field rhythm-directed treatment.

Those with incidental dysrhythmias require treatment of any underlying acute condition (e.g., analgesia for pain or oxygen for hypoxemia). For example, a 67-year-old male patient with a history of "extra heart beats" transported for an isolated ankle injury displays a sinus tachycardia (from pain) and occasional premature ventricular complexes but no other symptoms or abnormalities on physical exam. He requires splinting and analgesia, not antidysrhythmics. This should not be confused with dysrhythmias accompanying symptoms, such as frequent or complex ventricular extrasystoles associated with ischemic chest pain.

Step Two: Identify Stable and Unstable Patients

Since asymptomatic or incidental dysrhythmias usually require no direct treatment, we can shift the prehospital focus to those dysrhythmias associated with symptoms. Although many patients display symptoms attributable to the change from a "normal" rhythm, most tolerate these well. Two broad categories can be created to classify patients based on the severity of symptoms: stable and unstable. Unstable patients are likely to suffer harm or deteriorate; the providers and EMS physician must identify these patients and rapidly intervene. The best method of identifying unstable patients is to seek signs of inadequate end-organ perfusion that are a result of the rhythm disturbance.[2] A few short historical questions and physical exam steps can accomplish this in minutes.

The following *must* be sought in the initial phases of patient evaluation:

- Hypotension—arbitrarily defined as a systolic blood pressure below 90 mmHg.
- Chest pain, shortness of breath (SOB), or rales (signifying inadequate myocardial perfusion)

- Altered consciousness, from mild agitation or somnolence to obtundation or coma (signifying CNS hypoperfusion)

Delayed capillary refill and lowered skin temperature are often sought to identify poor perfusion; however, the subjective nature of these observations and multiple other causes limit their utility in the field.

Assessing instability is not an "all or none" phenomenon but a continuum. The presence of either a severe or . one sign/symptom of hypoperfusion is diagnostic of an unstable rhythm; a single mildly abnormal finding suggests instability. The blood pressure is the simplest method of assessing circulatory adequacy, but it alone may be insufficient in accurately classifying patients. A patient with a blood pressure of 90 mmHg systolic, rales, and a depressed sensorium is clearly unstable; if awake and with no rales, chest pain, or other symptoms, he or she occupies a "borderline" position. Similarly, agitation suggests mild CNS hypoperfusion, while coma is associated with more profound derangement.

In the absence of clear evidence of instability, each patient can receive a more complete evaluation, although the total prehospital time should not be unduly prolonged. Stable and borderline patients are usually treated with pharmacological agents. Unstable patients need rapid therapy, usually with electrical interventions, such as countershock or external pacing. Symptomatic but stable or borderline unstable patients can be initially treated with pharmacological agents, with other electrical devices nearby in the case of deterioration. The more deranged any isolated sign or symptom of instability that is present (e.g., coma versus mild anxiety) should push the provider toward more aggressive treatment.

Step Three: Classify the ECG Findings

After assessing stability, the field providers need to categorize the ECG. Again, it is tempting to use a traditional approach, separating dysrhythmias into dozens of categories. In the field evaluation, a simpler scheme can be used based on the assessment of stability and three ECG features: QRS complex rate, regularity, and duration.

ECG interpretation is performed in two ways: by command physicians receiving transmitted tracings or by the field teams. Transmitted ECG tracings are hampered primarily by technical problems (which occasionally can cloud salient features) or limitations in the reader's skills (which are best addressed by on-going education when needed). Field providers can learn the basics of ECG interpretation, and most paramedics can classify the common and lethal rhythms with good accuracy. However, misclassification of QRS duration and rate may occur in up to 20%-30% of tachycardias.[3] Protocols and on-line command decisions must assume that the potential for misclassification exists and take actions to minimize the adverse outcomes that can result. Our strategies, which follow, apply to both field and transmitted ECG interpretation. In all steps, ECG interpretation must be done from a printed strip and not "guesstimated" from the monitor to lessen misclassification.

Rate

Initially, the rate should be classified as fast (>120/minute), slow (<60/minute), or normal/near normal (60-120/minute) based on the frequency of QRS complexes over 6 seconds (two large "hash marks" on the ECG strip) multiplied by ten. After the estimation of rate, sinus P waves should be sought in those patients with normal or fast rates. These P waves should always precede the QRS complexes with a consistent appearance and relationship (i.e., distance from the QRS complexes).

As a simple rule, all nonsinus fast rhythms in unstable patients deserve immediate countershock with 100 Joules (J). Often, lower energy levels can convert specific rhythms (SVT or atrial flutter), but little benefit is gained by attempting to make fine distinctions in these unstable patients. Although changes in heart rate that fall into the "normal" range can cause symptoms, these are usually of little importance in field management.

Slow dysrhythmias require no further classification after assessing stability. All other details (e.g., P wave characteristics, Type I or II second degree block, junctional versus ventricular escape, etc...) are of little value in the prehospital management of patients. Slow stable dysrhythmias need no intervention besides monitoring for deterioration. Slow dysrhythmias in unstable patients should be treated with external pacing or atropine (0.5-1.0 mg IV in adults up to 2-3 mg total). Transcutaneous pacing is best done as early as possible to maximize clinical capture and restoration of normal or near normal perfusion.[4-5]

Previously, isoproterenol (2 mg in 250-500 cc of crystalloid titrated to heart rate and symptoms) was suggested for atropine-resistant bradycardias. With the availability of external pacemakers in the field and the poor clinical effectiveness of isoproterenol, this treatment is not currently recommended. In adults, epinephrine and dopamine infusion should be used only when heart rate has been normalized or if other measures fail.

Some command physicians may request field providers to measure the QRS duration in symptomatic bradycardia. Theoretically, a QRS of >0.12 seconds (three small boxes on the ECG strip) may represent ventricular escape and worsen with atropine.[1] In practice, clinical harm is rarely seen and easily treated with transcutaneous pacing, allowing this step to be omitted.

Regularity and Duration

In contrast to bradycardias, if the ventricular rate is fast, the regularity and duration of the QRS complexes should be assessed. Regularity is divided into two categories: mostly or completely regular and chaotic (or "irregularly irregular" without any pattern). Chaotic rhythms are usually due to atrial fibrillation, irrespective of the appearance of the baseline or QRS duration. Other less common causes include multifocal atrial tachycardia and frequent extrasystoles (either atrial, ventricular, or junctional).

To ease the process of measuring duration, ask the field teams to run an ECG strip. From this, they or the command physician (if transmitted) can measure in "small boxes" how wide the QRS duration is and look for irregularity. Each small box represents 0.04 seconds at normal paper speed. This approach will limit mathematical or conversion errors. Evaluating printed strips helps with detecting irregularity, which may be difficult to appreciate on a monitor if the ventricular rate is > 150/minute. In these cases, close tracking on a 6-second ECG strip may help detect chaos and identify atrial fibrillation.

Those rhythms with a QRS duration of less than three boxes (0.12 seconds) are termed *narrow complex* dysrhythmias. Conversely, any rhythm with a QRS duration of greater than three boxes is considered a *wide complex* dysrhythmia. Nearly all narrow complex rhythms originate from atrial or nodal (i.e., supraventricular) sources. Wide complex rhythms can originate from a ventricular source or a supraventricular source. In the latter situation, some abnormality in ventricular conduction is responsible for the prolonged QRS duration. In the field, attempts to separate the myriad causes of wide complex tachydysrhythmias rarely alters therapy, which is based on the clinical stability of the patient, basic history, and the simple ECG characteristics previously defined.

Unstable Tachydysrhythmias

Aside from sinus tachycardia, all other unstable patients with a wide complex tachydysrhythmia (WCT) or a narrow complex tachydysrhythmia (NCT) deserve countershock(s), irrespective of the exact source (ventricular or supraventricular). The initial energy level used to treat tachycardias is based on the QRS pattern. If the QRS pattern is regular (or nearly regular) in any unstable patient with a tachydysrhythmia, 100 J should be used, followed by increasing energy up to 360 J if unsuccessful. As noted previously, some rhythms may require less energy but attempts to carefully titrate this lifesaving therapy in unstable patients is of little pragmatic benefit.

In those subjects with an unstable nonsinus WCT, lidocaine should be given after successful countershock. The initial dose of lidocaine is 1-1.5 mg/kg, followed by 0.5-0.75 mg/kg every 5-10 minutes (up to 3 mg/kg) and a continuous drip at 2-4 mg/min.[1-2] This will reduce the risk of recurrent ventricular tachycardia after conversion and cause no harm in supraventricular rhythms. Conversely, no follow-up drugs are needed in the field after cardioverting an NCT.

If the QRS complexes are chaotic, the most common diagnosis is atrial fibrillation. When chaos and a QRS duration of >three boxes appear together, atrial fibrillation with altered conduction is the diagnosis. All *fast chaotic* rhythms in unstable patients should be cardioverted with 50 J initially and titrated up as needed. No post-countershock medications are needed.

One practical point: if regularity versus irregularity cannot be established during assessment of a patient with an *unstable* WCT or NCT, 100 J is a good starting energy level for countershock. Similarly, if simplicity of treatment protocols is sought, 100 J is reasonable for all unstable nonsinus tachycardias, since the extra energy delivered to the rapid atrial fibrillation patient is unlikely to cause harm or worsen discomfort compared to 50 J.

Step Four: Focused Actions to Evaluate Stable but Symptomatic and "Borderline" Patients

Up to this point, little specific history and only a few basic physical exam and ECG reading skills have been required. This is intentional, so as not to "clutter" the field evaluation of those who need it the most (the unstable patient) or do not need it at all (the asymptomatic patient). The remaining patients are those with symptoms, albeit none clearly identifying instability. Here, a few questions and actions can help to deliver the appropriate prehospital care.

History

An abridged past medical history alone can influence field therapy; the field teams should focus on cardiac-related problems in stable patients. For example, patients who present with a new onset WCT with a history of previous myocardial infarction are much more likely to have ventricular tachycardia than a supraventricular rhythm with abnormal conduction. Similarly, those with a history of a previous dysrhythmia who present with similar symptoms again are likely to have recurrence rather than a new dysrhythmia. Neither of these clinical rules is infallible, but these data can help guide therapy. Other points are also helpful; for example, a patient with a history of poorly controlled hypertension presenting with a blood pressure of 98/50 mmHg suggests a dramatic change, prompting more aggressive treatment.

History can influence the dosing of field agents. Patients with liver or heart failure, and those age 65 and older, should receive lower lidocaine infusion rates. An inquiry about allergies may help avert a catastrophic iatrogenic complication.

The current medications can provide a clue to any previous conditions or guide field drug therapy. For example, the use of digoxin or a calcium channel blocker for "palpitations" would suggest an underlying supraventricular dysrhythmia (e.g., atrial fibrillation or paroxysmal SVT). Those subjects on mexiletine or tocainamide (both lidocaine congeners) should receive lower lidocaine doses to avert additive toxicity.[6]

Physical Exam

In addition to a search for signs of instability, some manipulations can help when assessing and managing tachycardias. Specifically, actions that alter AV node conduction (termed "vagal maneuvers") can help terminate or uncover a specific dysrhythmia. In the patient under 50 years old, carotid body massage can be attempted; this procedure is often restricted or prohibited in the field because of poorly documented concerns about embolization. The Valsalva maneuver can be used with massage (where allowed) in young patients or as the sole maneuver in those over 50 years old. Other maneuvers, including ocular and rectal massage, ice packs or cold-water dunking, and rapid inflation of PASG, are of dubious value and are not routinely recommended.

Stable Narrow Complex Tachydysrhythmias

In patients who are symptomatic but stable or with one singular "borderline" symptom of instability (e.g., dizzy or anxious with a blood pressure of 92 mmHg systolic), certain actions are indicated. Patients with a regular NCT between 120 and 140/minute are likely to have a sinus tachycardia and require no antidysrhythmic treatment. Stable patients with a *regular* NCT at a rate of 140/minute or greater should have vagal maneuvers performed in an attempt to terminate the rhythm. Sometimes, this uncovers sinus P waves, clarifying the etiology. When sinus P waves are seen, treatment is directed at the cause, not the rhythm.

Those with minor symptoms (e.g., isolated subjective dizziness or "palpitations") do not require field treatment beyond vagal maneuvers. For those with more prominent symptoms during a *regular* NCT at 140/minute or greater, give adenosine (6-12 mg as a rapid IV bolus followed with a flush).[1,3,7] The smaller initial dose (6 mg) is effective about 60% of the time, and it should be repeated within 2 minutes up at the higher doses at least twice more before discarding this agent in those refractory to the first dose.

Adenosine is effective in 85%-90% of patients with a regular NCT. Even in those who 'fail,' adenosine may uncover hidden sinus or flutter waves, clarifying the diagnosis. The drug has a duration of effect of 20 seconds or less, and recurrence of an NCT may occur in 10%-58% of cases. It is common for patients to complain of transient chest pain, flushing, or dyspnea during adenosine treatment. Some patients may experience bradycardia or asystole after adenosine; usually, this lasts seconds but may require temporary external pacing if prolonged. Contrary to popular belief, adenosine can occasionally terminate ventricular tachycardia[8], although the majority of patients are unaffected.

Verapamil (2.5-5 mg IV initially followed by 5-10 mg in 15-30 minutes if unsuccessful) will terminate 85%-90% regular NCT.[9] However, verapamil can cause hypotension and CHF; because of these disadvantages, we prefer adenosine in the field. Whenever giving verapamil in the field, it must be absolutely clear that the QRS duration is less than three boxes (0.12 seconds). This will help avoid the hemodynamic collapse seen with this drug in ventricular tachycardia or atrial fibrillation with an accessory pathway. If hypotension occurs after IV verapamil in the absence of bradycardia, it is treated with saline infusions, IV calcium salts (5-10 cc of a 10% $CaCl_2$ solution), or catecholamines (dopamine or epinephrine).

Current research suggests that even with close monitoring, WCT are erroneously classified as narrow in up to 20% of cases. Because of this, many command physicians prefer to avoid verapamil and use adenosine in the field for all NCT.

For those patients with a chaotic NCT, atrial fibrillation is the likely rhythm; if mildly symptomatic, no field treatment is required. An example of this is an elderly patient with an irregular NCT at a rate of 130/minute complaining of weakness; although rapid atrial fibrillation can contribute to the symptoms, no field treatment is needed in the absence of other clear signs or symptoms of decompensation. Those with instability deserve immediate countershock with 50-100 J. If transport is prolonged and either borderline symptoms or a rate of 140-180/min, verapamil (2.5-5 mg IV) is an option. Diltiazem (0.25 mg/kg IV) will control the ventricular rate in 85%-90% cases of rapid atrial fibrillation with lower incidence of hypotension compared to verapamil but has not been studied in the prehospital setting.

One pitfall in the treatment of stable NCT must be highlighted: when the rate is >250/minute, the risk of decompensation rises and the ability to detect irregularity is limited.[2] Because of this, all adults with a heart rate >250/minute should be cardioverted with 100 J, even if apparently stable.

Stable Wide Complex Tachydysrhythmias

As noted earlier, WCT can be due to VT or SVT with abnormal conduction. Until proven, field providers should assume all new WCT are due to VT. Hospital data recently suggest that about two thirds of patients with a new WCT have VT; with a history of previous myocardial infarction, this frequency of VT increases to 90%. Although it is possible to assemble evidence to detect supraventricular rhythms from a detailed exam and 12-lead ECG, these data are not easily obtainable in the field. Thus, actions in managing WCT should either treat or cause no harm in VT.

All unstable patients with a WCT should be cardioverted with 100 J. When stable or borderline, a few simple measures can help stratify patients. It is always an option to observe this group, intervening only if conditions worsen.

If P waves precede each QRS complex during a stable WCT at a rate of 140/minute or less, a supraventricular source (especially sinus or atrial tachycardia) is likely, although VT is a remote possibility. Treatment focuses on correcting any potential causes (e.g., pain, hypovolemia, hypoxemia) and observation. Irregular QRS complexes suggest atrial fibrillation or multifocal atrial tachycardia; neither requires field rhythm directed therapy in stable patients, although other actions (e.g., oxygen, bronchodilators) may be needed.

When no clear PQRS relationship exists, differentiating between SVT and VT is difficult during a WCT. These key features help determine a clinical course of action:

■ Patients with new onset WCT and a history of previous myocardial infarction or VT very likely will have VT.

■ VT will not often slow during vagal maneuvers; therefore, slowing of a WCT during these efforts suggests SVT. The absence of change does *not* diagnose VT.

■ Most VT does not respond to adenosine, where SVT slows or terminates. Conversely, lidocaine has little effect on most SVT and will terminate 75%-85% of VT.

■ VT is usually regular and rarely seen at a rate of >220/minute. Any chaotic WCT should be considered atrial fibrillation with abnormal conduction. When a chaotic WCT at a rate of >220/minute occurs, atrial fibrillation with the Wolff-Parkinson-White syndrome is likely to be present; this rhythm is prone to deterioration.

From these clinical observations, the following scheme can be used in approaching stable patients with a WCT.

■ All stable patients with a *regular WCT at a rate of 120-220/minute* should receive vagal maneuvers. Those who slow should receive adenosine (6-12 mg IV). If no slowing with vagal maneuvers occurs, one of three paths should be taken:

■ Young (age <50 years), previously healthy patients with a stable *regular WCT* that slows with vagal maneuvers should receive adenosine. If this fails, lidocaine (1.0-1.5 mg/kg up to 3 mg/kg) should be given. If lidocaine converts the rhythm, a continuous drip at 2-4 mg/kg and repeat boluses at 5-10 minutes of 0.5 mg/kg should be given during transport to prevent recurrence (with lower infusion rates used in those over the age of 65 years, with a history of CHF or liver disease).

■ Patients with a history of a previous myocardial infarction, VT, or over the age of 50 years presenting with a stable regular WCT should be treated with lidocaine as outlined above.

■ Because of the risk of deterioration, any patient with a WCT at a rate of >250/minute deserves countershock with 100 J, irrespective of symptoms.

■ Patients with a chaotic WCT usually have atrial fibrillation with altered conduction; if stable with a heart rate of <200/min, they should receive close observation and rapid transport. If the rate elevates to 220/minute or higher, immediate countershock with 100 J is indicated.

Other agents are available but have a limited role in the field. Procainamide (50-100 mg IV every 1-2 minutes up to a maximum of 17 mg/kg or until side effects occur) treats both VT and SVT. Bretylium (5 mg/kg IV) terminates some cases of refractory VT and ventricular fibrillation. The difficulty administering procainamide and close monitoring needed during administration of both (especially for hypotension), limit the usefulness of these in most field situations.

Pitfalls

Rhythm Strips versus Monitor Interpretation

Besides clearly abnormal rhythms (e.g., obvious ventricular tachycardia or severe bradycardia), ECG interpretation should be taken from a tracing and not "guesstimated" from the monitor screen. It is tempting to avoid obtaining strips, but misclassifications may result from a "screen look". These strips are valuable in the ED evaluation, documenting conditions before and after field treatment, which helps unravel the causes in certain dysrhythmias. Also, at least two leads should be sampled.

Synchronization and Sedation During Countershock

When possible, it is preferable to deliver any countershock synchronized with the intrinsic QRS complexes. Synchronization helps avoid depolarization during the vulnerable phases of repolarization, theoretically decreasing the risk of post-countershock ventricular fibrillation. During most dysrhythmias, this is not a problem; the defibrillator unit senses the underlying QRS pattern and delivers the shock at the appropriate time. When the rhythm is extremely fast, irregular, or the QRS complexes are markedly abnormal (i.e., very wide or small), sensing is difficult. In these cases, an unsynchronized countershock is appropriate. Electrophysiological data do not support

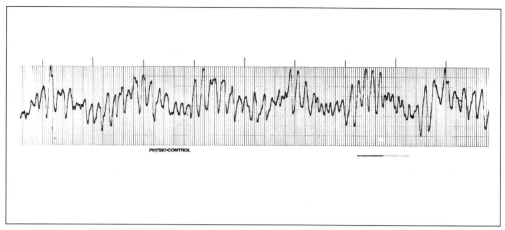

Figure 9-1. The classic 1-lead ECG appearance (lead II here) of TdP from a 57-year-old woman with sudden death. Note the shifting of the QRS complex axis and appearance. This patient failed multiple countershocks, transcutaneous pacing, and lidocaine therapy but was resuscitated after magnesium was administered.

the notion that this will increase the likelihood of ventricular fibrillation (VF). If post-countershock VF occurs, repeat countershock is usually successful in restoring an organized rhythm.

Sedation with a benzodiazepine (midazolam or diazepam) before countershock may improve patient comfort. However, unstable patients should not have electrical therapy delayed while awaiting clinical sedation.

The Problem of PVCs

When to treat premature ventricular complexes (PVCs) in the field can be a source of confusion. If the PVCs are asymptomatic or trivial, there is no proven benefit from treatment. PVCs associated with more pronounced symptoms should receive an antidysrhythmic, usually lidocaine. Although oft-cited lists of ominous ECG "warning" signs exist (e.g., multiform, > 6 minutes, couplets, R-on-T, or runs of PVCs), treatment of these and other asymptomatic PVCs does not usually confer any benefit.

The prophylactic use of lidocaine for all patients with chest pain to reduce the risk of VF is no longer recommended. Instead, therapy should be based on the effect of the PVCs on symptoms or if the aforementioned higher risk patterns are seen.

Pediatric Dysrhythmias

When evaluating pediatric tachycardias, one crucial difference compared with adults must be stressed: children under the age of 5 years can sustain a sinus tachycardia at much higher rates (up to 200-225/minute) in response to physiological stresses. Because of this, a search for hypovolemia, hypercapnia, and hypoxemia is mandatory in stable children with NCT before drug therapy is used. A volume challenge with 10-20 cc/kg of saline may also be useful before other therapies.

Although some guidelines distinguish between energy levels when performing synchronized versus unsynchronized countershock, the utility of this is dubious. To keep treatments simple but effective, unstable children should receive countershock with 2 J/kg. Otherwise, antidysrhythmic principles are similar to those outlined earlier, with agents given in the appropriate mg/kg doses.

Pediatric nonarrest bradycardias are also usually secondary to another cause, often respiratory distress. When symptomatic, these rhythms are treated primarily with epinephrine and airway maneuvers and rarely need transcutaneous pacing or atropine (0.02 mg/kg/dose).

Torsades de Pointes

This rare dysrhythmia classically presents with paroxysms of syncope and polymorphic ("twisting") wide QRS complexes, each lasting 20-30 seconds (Figure 9-1). Torsades de pointes (TdP) in adults is usually "pause dependent," flourishing when the intrinsic heart rate drops below 80-100/minute. A variety of antidysrhythmic (especially class IA and IC agents), antihistamine, antimicrobial, and psychoactive drugs, along with metabolic disorders, pre-cipitate TdP. Field treatment consists of countershock when unstable and transcutaneous overdrive pacing or iso-proterenol (titrated to a heart rate > 120/minute). Mag-nesium sulfate, 2 grams as a rapid IV bolus, is also suggested for those who fail countershock.

A more practical problem with TdP is the search for it—specifically, patients with VT or VF often display some changes in QRS complex appearance. Field providers may mistake these variations for the classic (but rare) QRS twisting. If recurrent polymorphic VT occurs in a patient with one or more of the above risks, treatment should be started. Otherwise, orders and protocols should focus on the treatment of common VT.

Summary

Prehospital dysrhythmia evaluation must be tailored to the time restraints, physical limitations, and outcome needs that are specific to the field setting. Decision trees should be simple and effective, focusing on treating patients, not rhythms. Medical command and protocols must iden-tify and treat all unstable patients; those subjects without symptoms or with trivial symptoms do not require rhythm-directed therapies. For the remaining symptomatic but sta-ble patients, a few key steps should be taken to help manage each case.

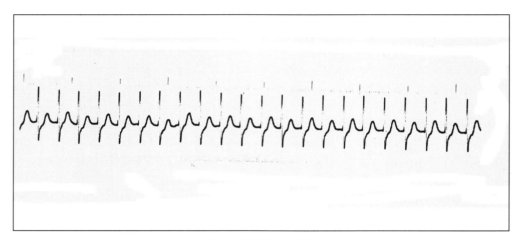

Figure 9-2. Case #2.

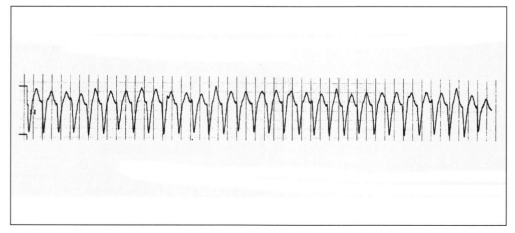

Figure 9-3. Case #3.

SAMPLE CASES

CASE #1

A 52-year-old white male presents with weakness and dyspnea. He is somnolent with rales in all lung fields. His blood pressure is 60 mmHg palpable, and his heart rate is 40/minute, confirmed on the ECG monitor. What further assessment and treatment are needed?

DISCUSSION

This is an unstable patient with bradycardia. A rhythm strip should be obtained and immediate transcutaneous pacing initiated to elevate the heart rate to >60/min and resolve symptoms. If not available, atropine should be administered.

CASE #2

A 22-year-old female with a history of "rapid heart beats" complains of palpitations. She is not taking any medications currently, and she denies any other symptoms. Her blood pressure is 102/66 mmHg with a heart rate of 180/minute and regular; the lung exam is clear. How should she be managed?

DISCUSSION

This is a stable tachycardia; further evaluation should include an ECG strip to determine QRS regularity and duration. Figure 9-2 identifies her rhythm to be a regular NCT (less than three boxes wide). Vagal maneu-

vers should be performed. If these fail, either close observation and transport or adenosine 6-12 mg IV can be chosen. Verapamil (5 mg IV) would also be reasonable for this stable patient.

CASE #3

A 72-year-old 70 kg male with a previous myocardial infarction and "skipped heart beats" presents with dizziness. His medications include procainamide, diltiazem, and nitroglycerin. His initial vital signs are: blood pressure 92/40 mmHg; heart rate 200/minute and regular; respirations 18/minute. His lung fields are clear, he denies chest pain, and he is awake and oriented. How should he be managed?

DISCUSSION

This is a "borderline" unstable patient, with one finding (mild hypotension) suggesting poor perfusion; an ECG strip must be obtained. In this case, a regular WCT (QRS > three boxes wide, Figure 9-3) at a rate of 200/minute is seen. From his history and ECG, VT is likely. The best course is to give lidocaine (1.5 mg/kg IV—100 mg in this patient—and repeat up to 3 mg/kg total); if this fails or deterioration is noted, cardioversion with 100 J is indicated. If lidocaine is successful, a continuous drip and follow-up bolus should be given. If worsening hypotension or any other sign of hypoperfusion develops, immediate countershock is indicated.

References

1. American Heart Association: *Textbook of advanced cardiac life support,* Dallas, 1994.

2. Yealy DM, Stapcyznski JS: Dysrhythmias. In Rosen P, et al., (editors): *Emergency medicine: concepts and clinical practice,* ed 3, St Louis, 1992, Mosby.

3. McCabe J, Menegazzi JJ, Adhar G, et al.: Intravenous adenosine in the prehospital treatment of supraventricular tachycardia, *Ann Emerg Med* 21:358-361, 1992.

4. Hedges JR, Syverud SA, Dalsey WC, et al.: Prehospital trial of emergency transcutaneous pacing, *Circulation* 76:1337-1340, 1987.

5. Paris PM, Stewart RD, Kaplan RM, et al.: Transcutaneous pacing for bradyasystolic cardiac arrest in prehospital care, *Ann Emerg Med* 14:320-323, 1985.

6. Shuster MR, Paris PM, Kaplan RM, et al.: Effect on seizure threshold in dogs of tocainide/lidocaine administration, *Ann Emerg Med* 16:749-751, 1987.

7. Wrenn K: Management strategies in wide QRS complex tachycardia, *Am J Emerg Med* 9:592-597, 1991.

8. Wilber DJ, Baerman J, Olshansky B, et al.: Adenosine-sensitive ventricular tachycardia: clinical characteristics and response to catheter ablation, *Circulation* 87:126-134, 1993.

9. O'Toole KS, Heller MB, Menegazzi JJ, et al.: Intravenous verapamil in the treatment of paroxysmal supraventricular tachycardia, *Ann Emerg Med* 19:279-285, 1990.

Cardiac Arrest

For those involved in EMS, cardiac arrest represents the pinnacle of challenges. The cardiac arrest brings to bear, right here and now, the very essence of who we are and what we do as EMS providers. The cardiac arrest thrusts upon us the challenge of life and death that is undertaken in a more deliberate manner throughout our entire career. Some may say that cardiac arrest is a straightforward diagnosis and its treatment delineated by well-defined protocols. Nonetheless, this condition symbolizes the struggle for life that medicine is all about. These cases not only test our medical knowledge and clinical skills in an unforgiving, time-pressured manner, but they invoke strong physiological and emotional forces both in caregivers and in bystanders. Newer field personnel experience an unmatched surge of adrenaline, while old-timers may view such calls as hopeless and routine. Both responses may hinder the prehospital care provider from functioning as efficiently and expeditiously as possible in a situation in which time is our biggest enemy.

The provision of the highest quality care in such instances requires that the entire system be in a constant state of readiness. Call takers must be trained to recognize potential cardiac arrest calls and promptly dispatch appropriate units including the closest emergency responder. Equipment must be properly stocked and in working condition. Personnel must be well-trained and empowered with appropriate resources and the authority to immediately initiate lifesaving interventions. Finally, a medical command physician who understands the prehospital cardiac arrest scenario, knows the medics' capabilities and resources, and is able to provide expert and level-headed guidance must be continuously available. It is the medical director's responsibility to ensure that all of these components of the system are in place.

This chapter will discuss the important issues involved in providing high-quality medical control (both off-line and on-line) for prehospital care of the patient in cardiac arrest.

Off-Line Command

To be effective at reducing mortality from prehospital cardiac arrest, the EMS system must be well prepared and in a constant state of readiness. In the following section, we will briefly discuss a few areas that should be of particular concern to both the med-

VINCE N. MOSESSO, JR, MD, FACEP

Box 10-1 The Chain of Survival

Early Access → Early → Early → Early
to EMS CPR Defibrillation ACLS

ical directors and system administrators. Attention to these areas is necessary to enable medical command physicians and field personnel to provide the highest possible care to the patient in cardiac arrest.

Rapid Response

The most important determinant of survival from sudden cardiac death is the rapidity with which treatment is provided, as symbolized by the AHAs Chain of Survival (Box 10-1).[1,2] Current research indicates that the most important intervention to affect survival rates is defibrillation. While 70%-80% of patients in ventricular fibrillation can be successfully converted to a perfusing rhythm if countershocked within 3 minutes of the onset of ventricular fibrillation, this success rate deteriorates rapidly with every passing moment.[3] Studies in Seattle have demonstrated a significant benefit from CPR if initiated within 5 minutes of collapse and if followed by ACLS care within 10 minutes.[4] Larsen has reported on the survival effect of time to initiation of various interventions and developed the following equation:

Survival rate = 67%-(2.3% per minute to CPR)-(1.1% per minute to defibrillation)-(2.1% per minute to ACLS).[5]

This 10- to 12-minute window of opportunity can easily (and generally does) get squandered unnecessarily. A series of events must all occur in swift succession for EMS providers to even have a chance at successful resuscitation. These events include—

- recognition of arrest (by public)
- notification of public safety answering point (PSAP)
- dispatch of response unit
- initiation of response
- arrival at scene
- arrival at bedside
- delivery of therapy

Since delay in achieving any of the above tasks correlates directly with increased mortality, it is the medical director's and administration's responsibility to work on improving these components of the system.

For example, the medical director should be aware exactly what the dispatch time is in the system, as well as the other components, such as response time and average time from arrival at bedside to delivery of electrical therapy.

An excellent example of the importance of strong medical control can be found in the city of Houston. In Houston, annual survival from ventricular fibrillation improved from 0% to 21% over a 5-year period after the hiring of a medical director who became actively involved in training personnel in cardiac arrest management and implemented immediate bedside defibrillation on standing orders.[6] Stewart has described the importance of strong and authoritative medical control and writes that "without dedicated medical leadership, the EMS system of a community flirts with mediocrity."[7]

Training

Cardiac arrest is a condition that demands timeliness and accuracy of proper interventions. It is ruthlessly unforgiving to delays in administering proper therapy. Therefore, all field personnel must be extremely well-versed in recognizing and instituting initial treatment for this condition. Field crews must be able to work synchronously with each other so that multiple critical interventions can be performed as rapidly as possible. We suggest that field crews be run through practice scenarios so that system-wide protocols that reflect the most efficient use of personnel can be instituted and so that individual crews become proficient at working together. These practical scenarios also allow medical directors and administrative personnel to evaluate current protocols, policies, and equipment and to implement modifications that facilitate a more rapid and efficient provision of care.

Personnel must be able to use various specialty pieces of equipment with the utmost proficiency in this setting. Therefore, it may be beneficial for periodic review of the use of equipment such as monitor-defibrillators, external pacers, pulse oximeters, CO_2 detectors, mechanical CPR devices and of skills such as endotracheal intubation and intraosseous infusion. Even in busy systems, there is often a significant proportion of personnel who do not perform these various skills or use specific equipment for months at a time.

Protocols/Standing Orders

Protocols provide a system-wide standard so that field personnel and command physicians understand and are facile in the system's approach to various conditions. Standing orders are those steps of individual protocols that field personnel are permitted to perform without on-line medical command. Cardiac arrest is one of the indisputable conditions when prehospital care providers should operate initially on standing orders and not delay critical interventions to contact the command physician. The extent of these standing orders will be system and condition specific, but should at a minimum include ECG rhythm determination, immediate defibrillation for ventricular fibrillation and pulseless ventricular tachycardia, and definitive airway management. Additional reasonable standing orders include IV access and administration of first-line ACLS drugs, such as epinephrine. The protocols and standing orders used in the City of Pittsburgh EMS are provided as an Appendix to this chapter.

Continuous Quality Improvement

While a comprehensive and effective quality improvement program is in essence a continual reappraisal of the entire system, in this section we will point out only a few items that deal specifically with cardiac arrest. Perhaps the most important issue is timeliness of service. In the treatment of cardiac arrest, time reduces directly to survival. The faster a system can access a patient, provide electric countershock, and manage the airway correlates directly with that system's success rate in regards to resuscitation. Therefore, a high priority should be given to evaluating important time intervals previously alluded to, including call received to unit dispatched and to unit arrival, patient access time after unit arrival on scene, and call received to first defibrillation. Decreasing delay by the public in activating the EMS system is of obvious importance but beyond the scope of this text. The quality improvement program should also review proper protocol implementation, skills performance such as intubation, ECG interpretation, and IV initiation, and the timeliness of these procedures as well.

The recently published Utstein style for reporting of cardiac arrest data attempts to provide some common denominators for comparing resuscitation rates between various systems.[8] Systems may want to use this format to compare their performance with that of other systems.

On-Line Command

While it is critical that field personnel provide initial care through standing orders so that interventions are performed as rapidly as possible, it is just as important that on-line medical command be involved after this initial period. We strongly discourage use of intermediaries between the command provider (whether it be a physician or a specially trained nurse) and the field crew; this provides unnecessary delay and promotes miscommunication. These problems become magnified in critical conditions like cardiac arrest.

The command physician must know the system intimately, including a thorough understanding of patient care protocols, a working knowledge of what medications field personnel have available and how they are supplied, and what types of equipment, such as external pacemakers, CO_2 detectors, pulse oximeters, automatic ventilators, mechanical CPR devices, and IO infusion devices, are available. It is also helpful if the command physician and paramedic are familiar with each other and have worked together previously.

Perhaps the most important attribute that the command physician can bring to the situation is a calm demeanor and clear thinking. Field personnel are caught in an uncontrolled setting that is often quite raucous and complicated by anxiety-ridden bystanders and family members. Field personnel also have many psychomotor skills to perform and can become thoroughly occupied by practical necessities at the scene. The following case illustrates this point. The patient, who collapsed at a family gathering, was wedged between the bathtub and the commode, covered with stool, and being tugged at by numerous panicked relatives. Simply taking care of the logistics of maneuvering the patient into a position so that defibrillation and airway management could be properly performed, getting bystanders out of the way, and paying some attention to becoming unnecessarily soiled was itself quite a challenge for the EMS crew. The command physician's ability to elicit a past medical history of renal failure, a missed dialysis session, and the recognition of a wide QRS bradycardia suggested the presence of severe hyperkalemia. The administration of sodium bicarbonate and calcium chloride led to the patient's subsequent resuscitation.

The command physician should take advantage of his or her distance from the scene and should use the resultant solitude to gather all the important data available and to evaluate the situation as a whole. He or she should ensure that basics of care are done, including prompt defibrillation of ventricular fibrillation, proper airway management, absolute confirmation of endotracheal tube placement, and the basic steps of the appropriate protocol. He or she should then determine if special interventions are indicated and decide when transport to the hospital should be initiated versus cessation of resuscitative efforts at the scene.

A significant challenge is to accomplish all of this with conservative radio use. This is perhaps the biggest trap for the novice or inexperienced command physician. Directives must be as brief and concise as possible while still being very precise and understandable. Avoid soliciting information that will not change your instructions to the field team or the preparation of the receiving facility. There is much data of interest or even of use in the ED that will not influence prehospital treatment. Extreme diligence in use of radio time will avoid unnecessary distraction of field personnel.

Pitfalls

While a majority of cardiac arrests are due to myocardial ischemia or primary ventricular fibrillation and require standard ACLS care, the command physician must be the watchdog for those situations when a specific intervention may be appropriate and could lead to the successful resuscitation of a patient who otherwise would die. The most common and important of these situations are listed in the AHAs ACLS algorithms for pulseless electrical activity (PEA) and asystole. The astute command physician will pick up clues to these conditions and prompt prehospital care providers to investigate further and treat accordingly. These interventions are often outside the scope of protocols or rarely performed. A few specific example cases follow.

Perhaps the most obvious atypical cardiac arrest is that associated with major trauma, which in some cases may be occult. Command physicians should ensure that field personnel initiate rapid transport of these patients; initial defibrillation and airway management are probably the only two interventions that should be done on scene. If crews are properly trained, needle decompression of suspected tension pneumothorax should be done immediately as well; venous access and volume infusion should be accomplished en-route to the hospital.

Another condition paramedics may not think of is the presence of hyperkalemia, as in the example discussed earlier. While this is probably a fairly unusual cause of cardiac arrest, it is an entity that the command physician should know when to consider, since it can be treated in the field with calcium and bicarbonate infusions. A case of severe hyperkalemia leading to cardiac arrest, including 26 continuous minutes of asystole, with subsequent complete recovery was recently published. The authors present an excellent discussion of treatment of hyperkalemia in the arrest setting.[9]

Asthmatic patients present a particularly challenging scenario. When these patients arrest they are severely hypoxic and hypercapnic, so initial management should be to ensure oxygenation and ventilation. Field personnel may be particularly distraught in these cases (patient often young, arrests in front of medics), and the command physician must confidently guide field personnel to achieve adequate airway patency and ventilation, preferably by intubation, in a patient who may have trismus or laryngeal spasm. Command physicians should recall the high incidence of tension pneumothorax in these patients and consider ordering empirical bilateral chest decompression.[10] This is also one of the few indications for isoproterenol, if it is still in the medics' drug box; another good alternative is ketamine, a dissociative anesthetic with bronchodilator activity. These drugs are obviously in addition to standard epinephrine and atropine.

Another difficult situation is the severely hypothermic patient. Field personnel will usually be alert for this condition in patients with acute exposures in cold weather and cold-water immersions. The astute command physician will consider this diagnosis in patients predisposed to urban (chronic), as well as secondary, hypothermia when it may not be so obvious. Field personnel should be reminded that these patients require prompt transport for rewarming and that the usual ACLS protocols other than initial defibrillation and airway management are not effective.

Occult hypovolemia is another unusual etiology that the command physician's depth of knowledge may assist in detecting. An example is the case of a middle-aged male who collapsed and was found to be in a tachycardic rhythm at a rate of 160 without pulses or other signs of life. Paramedics obtained a history of diabetes and checked blood sugar level with a chemical reagent strip; the glucose level was markedly elevated. The command physician's questioning elicited a history from the patient's wife of increasing urinary frequency and thirst over the past week; therefore, the presence of diabetic ketoacidosis with severe hypovolemia was entertained and the patient was given a large volume of crystalloid fluid with subsequent resuscitation. Other conditions to which the command physician may be able to elicit clues would be previous diagnosis of abdominal aortic aneurysm or gastrointestinal bleeding.

Additional examples of specific conditions in which the training and knowledge of a command physician is of value could be presented. The point, however, is that the command physician must be vigilant for such situations and must avoid assuming that every cardiac arrest is secondary to cardiac ischemia or dysrhythmia; such assumption may not be unexpected of field personnel but should not be the bane of the experienced and astute command physician.

Care After Resuscitation

Paramedic and EMT training places heavy emphasis on initial resuscitative interventions, stressing ACLS protocols. There is much less training in caring for patients after the return of spontaneous circulation. These critical patients whose life is now in the hands of the field crew and their command physician require specifically tailored care. The role of the command physician is to assess each patient individually and to determine the appropriate post-resuscitative therapy for each patient. This, of course, includes ensuring adequacy of ventilation and oxygenation, maintenance of blood pressure with fluids or vasopressors, and any specific therapeutics that may seem appropriate. Use of antidysrhythmic agents, such as lidocaine or bretylium, for ventricular dysrhythmias must be carefully considered, especially in the face of AV block or bradycardia; there may be a role for external pacing in these patients as well. The command physician should insist on frequent updates on patient condition and watch for any trends in deterioration. These should include vital signs, ECG monitoring, pulse oximetry, if available, and reassessment of lung sounds and neurological status.

The command physician should also be prepared to deal with a wide variety of dysrhythmias, since these are common in the post-arrest setting. While many paramedics are very adept at ECG interpretation, their training usually encompasses common and lethal dysrhyth-

mias. Post-arrest rhythms often are complex and do not fit neatly into textbook categories. You may need to elicit descriptions of these rhythms in systems that do not use telemetry to make appropriate therapeutic decisions. Paramedics should be guided to provide specific critical information, such as correlation of P waves to the QRS and the width of the QRS complex, when precise rhythm diagnosis would alter management.

Cessation of Resuscitation Efforts vs. Hospital Transport

An important decision to be made in treating prehospital cardiac arrest is whether to cease resuscitative efforts in the field or to transport to the local ED. This is a complex issue with social and ethical implications beyond pure medical decision-making. A growing body of evidence in the medical literature has found that patients who receive appropriate ACLS, remain in asystole for greater than 20-30 minutes, and are then transported to a hospital are unlikely to be resuscitated.[11] Several EMS experts have endorsed the concept that, after an adequate trial of ACLS, resuscitation should be ceased and there is no medical reason to transport these patients to the hospital.[12-14] This principle is applicable only to the patient with sustained pulselessness from a suspected cardiac etiology and does not apply to patients with drug overdose, hypothermia, trauma, and other special conditions. There has been some concern that ceasing resuscitative efforts at the scene would be poorly accepted by family and friends, but this was found to be false in at least two studies.[15,16] These reports suggest that nontransport is well-accepted and often preferred if proper counseling and explanation are given to family members at the scene. Nonetheless, circumstances at the scene may suggest that transport to the hospital should be done for purely social concerns. The command physician should rely on information relayed by the field crew to make this determination. Field crews should be trained in dealing with survivors of deceased loved ones before such a policy is implemented.

If the decision is made to not pronounce at the scene, care should be taken to avoid unnecessary delay in transporting the patient. The appropriate time to begin transport will be dictated by the specifics of each case, but in general there is probably not much to be gained after the initial interventions of defibrillation and airway management and two or three rounds of ACLS drugs.

Finally, consideration should be given for prompt transport in special situations based on resources available at the receiving facility. For example, immediate cardiopulmonary bypass is being studied at one center for patients with witnessed arrest and short down times.

Summary

Caring for the patient in cardiac arrest is the final battle in the war between life and death for medical personnel. While certain actions may be routine, this condition is clearly the ultimate challenge for the EMS system. The command physician must step forward in his or her role as captain of the system and, more than in any other situation, must provide leadership and guidance to field personnel. While initial care may be provided through protocols, the challenge to the command physician, as well as the field crew, is to effectively battle against the constraints of time and to astutely discover the special circumstances for which specific therapy may lead to the saving of a life. We have outlined the preparation and the actions necessary for command physicians to successfully overcome this challenge.

S A M P L E   C A S E S

In this section, we will present several cases of prehospital cardiac arrests. For each initial presentation, two different scenarios of on-line medical control will unfold. These scenarios illustrate the difference between adequate and superior medical command.

CASE # 1

INITIAL PRESENTATION

Medics are dispatched to a 54-year-old male who is "going in and out of consciousness." Upon medics' arrival, the patient is pulseless, apneic, and in ventricular tachycardia. Medics defibrillate three times in rapid succession without rhythm conversion. They intubate, initiate an IV, and administer epinephrine 1 mg IV. While contacting medical command, they defibrillate again and note temporary conversion to sinus tachycardia without pulses. The patient reverts to ventricular tachycardia.

MEDICAL COMMAND
Scenario A (fair response)

The command physician orders lidocaine 1.5 mg per kg IV push and defibrillation 1 minute after drug administration. These orders are carried out and there is brief conversion to sinus rhythm, but degeneration into ventricular tachycardia quickly recurs. Command physician orders epinephrine 1 mg IV every 5 minutes and orders Bretylium 5 mg per kg IV push followed by defibrillation. Defibrillation is unsuccessful and the command physician orders Bretylium 1 g IV push followed by another defibrillation. The arrest is worked for about 45 minutes and the patient is finally pronounced in asystole.

MEDICAL COMMAND
Scenario B (excellent response)

The command physician orders lidocaine 1.5 mg per kg IV push followed by defibrillation. Again, the patient converts briefly to a sinus rhythm, which then degenerates into ventricular tachycardia. The command physician asks for any available history and the paramedics respond that the patient has a past history of hypertension and was recently discharged from the hospital after admission for new onset atrial fibrillation. They also report that he was started on a new but unknown medication. The command physician then asks for a description of the rhythm. The paramedics review the ECG and describe the rhythm as a wide, complex tachycardia, fairly regular, and with a regularly alternating amplitude. After looking more carefully at the rhythm, medics recognize that it may be Torsades de pointes (TdP). The command physician orders magnesium sulfate 2 g IV push followed by defibrillation. The rhythm converts to sinus but again degenerates into ventricular tachycardia. The command physician orders an additional 2 g of magnesium sulfate IV followed by defibrillation. This time the patient converts to and remains in sinus tachycardia. He regains a pulse and blood pressure and is transported to the ED where his condition stabilizes. At the hospital, it is confirmed that the patient had indeed been started on quinidine for medical therapy of new atrial fibrillation.

Keys to the case:

- Elicit more complete history
- Obtain description, not just name, of ECG rhythm
- Treat identified specific conditions aggressively

CASE # 2

INITIAL PRESENTATION

The air-medical crew responds to the scene of a motor vehicle accident with multiple casualties. Ground EMS initially direct one crew member to the ambulance for a middle-aged female in cardiac arrest. As the crew member begins to evaluate the patient, his partner calls him to assist with another patient, who is still entrapped. Medical command is contacted to give preliminary notification of multiple patients with major trauma.

MEDICAL COMMAND
Scenario A (fair response)

The flight crew reports they have two patients: a middle-aged female in cardiac arrest from blunt trauma whom ground EMS attempted to resuscitate without success, and a potentially critical middle-aged male entrapped for over 20 minutes to whom they are just now gaining access. They report that they will not fly the patient in traumatic arrest per protocol and will provide further information on the male patient as soon as possible. The command physician concurs with this decision and awaits further reports.

MEDICAL COMMAND
Scenario B (excellent response)

The flight crew reports they are seeing a middle-aged female in blunt traumatic arrest on whom ground EMS has been unsuccessfully attempting resuscitation and a middle-aged male who is entrapped and not yet accessed. They report their intention to consider the blunt traumatic arrest patient a DOA due to the low survival rate in this situation and state they will provide further information when they access the entrapped patient. The command physician asks that one member of the crew perform a quick assessment of the patient in traumatic arrest ensuring that—

a. There have been no signs of life since ground EMS arrival.
b. There are no signs of life by flight crew examinations.
c. There is no evidence of an acutely reversible condition, such as tension pneumothorax, airway obstruction, or ventricular fibrillation.
d. The patient has been properly intubated and is being adequately ventilated.

The flight crew reluctantly agrees to perform this assessment and notes that the patient has markedly poor lung compliance upon attempting to ventilate. Breath sounds on the left are diminished. After checking depth of tube insertion, the flight medic performs needle thoracostomy on the left chest, which results in a rush of air and improved compliance. The patient develops weak carotid and femoral pulses. Meanwhile, the other flight crew member reports that the entrapped patient is alert and oriented, has a pulse rate of 100 and a blood pressure of 110 systolic, and has

no significant respiratory distress. Thus, the decision is made to fly the patient who was initially in traumatic arrest to a trauma center, while the patient initially entrapped is transported by ground.

Keys to the case:

■ Directing crew to check critical parameters that may be overlooked due to on-scene distractions
■ Actively listening and interacting with medics even on "preliminary report"

CASE #3

INITIAL PRESENTATION

Paramedics are called to the home of a 44-year-old female who collapsed in front of her family. Family members state that the patient, who is now pulseless and apneic, had been feeling very weak and lethargic since awakening a few hours earlier and was recently discharged from the hospital after a heart operation. Paramedics quickly apply the quick look paddles, note ventricular fibrillation, and defibrillate. The ECG rhythm converts to a supraventricular tachycardia with weak pulses. While contacting medical command, pulses are lost and paramedics intubate the patient.

MEDICAL COMMAND
Scenario A (fair response)

The command physician orders epinephrine 2 mg through the endotracheal tube and administration of IV fluid wide open as soon as venous access is obtained. The medics quickly initiate a large-bore IV and begin fluid administration. The patient's rhythm degenerates into ventricular fibrillation and the command physician orders defibrillation. The rhythm does not convert and the command physician orders lidocaine 1.5 mg per kg IV. There is a brief conversion to a supraventricular tachycardia with questionable pulses. The command physician orders continuation of IV fluid, as well as initiation of a dopamine drip. Upon loss of pulse, the command physician orders epinephrine 1 mg IV push. The patient subsequently goes into ventricular fibrillation and is unable to be resuscitated.

MEDICAL COMMAND
Scenario B (excellent response)

The command physician orders epinephrine 2 mg down the endotracheal tube and administration of IV fluid wide open as soon as venous access is achieved. As IV fluids are begun, the patient again goes into ventricular fibrillation and is defibrillated into a supraven-

(continued)

(continued)

tricular rhythm without pulses. The command physician asks for further information concerning the cardiac surgery, and medics learn from family that the patient was discharged several days ago after open heart surgery for valve replacement. The command physician suspects the presence of post-operative pericardial tamponade. He directs the medics to continue rapid infusion of crystalloid IV fluids and to immediately package the patient for transport to the nearest emergency department. He then contacts the emergency physician at the receiving facility and explains his suspicion. The physician there prepares for periocardiocentesis. Upon arrival of the patient, 60 cc of non-clotting blood is aspirated and the patient regains pulses.

Keys to the case:

- Eliciting more complete history of present illness
- Recognizing potentially reversible cause of pulseless electrical activity (PEA)
- Directing medics to deviate from standard protocol for specific condition
- Communicating proactively with receiving facility

S A M P L E   P R O T O C O L S

CARDIAC ARREST

PROTOCOL: Medical Cardiac Arrest - Initial Care

NOTE
The key to successful resuscitation from sudden cardiac death is to rapidly recognize and treat ventricular fibrillation: **"Don't Wait, Defibrillate."**

INDICATIONS
All patients found unresponsive to "shake and shout" without pulses. (Note that agonal respirations may be present in recently arrested patients.)

EXCLUSIONS
1. Patients fitting DOA Protocol.
2. Arrest associated with major trauma.
3. Arrest associated with hypothermia.
4. Children less than 50 kg—use Pediatric protocols.

PROTOCOL
1. DETERMINE CARDIAC RHYTHM:

A. VF OR VT
Defibrillate 3 times in rapid succession:
- 200, 300, then 360 J
- No pulse check between shocks if no change on monitor and no patient response
- Keep paddles on patient between shocks

B. ASYSTOLE
Check for electrical activity in another lead:
- Defibrillate as above if VF found

C. PULSELESS ELECTRICAL ACTIVITY
Proceed to step #2

2. BEGIN BLS—Maintain airway patency via positioning and suctioning as necessary. Hyperventilate with 100% oxygen. Chest compressions at rate of 100/min.
3. CONTACT MEDICAL COMMAND—report arrest, request MD and other help if needed.

4. REASSESS PULSE, BREATHING, AND ECG RHYTHM:
   A. NO PULSE
      - CPR
      - Intubate (Follow Intubation Protocol)
      - IV LR regular drip with large bore at KVO rate (preferably at/above antecubital fossa or use external jugular)
      - Epinephrine 1:10,000 sol. 2 mg ET or 1 mg IV via first route available
      - Go to appropriate protocol:
         VF/VT
         Asystole or PEA (EMD)
   B. PULSE PRESENT
      - Assess vitals and ECG rhythm
      - Support airway and breathing as needed:
         - Intubate if unresponsive or inadequate ventilation
         - Oxygen 15 L/min face mask if not intubated
      - IV LR regular drip with large bore at KVO rate
      - If HR <60 or >150, go to the appropriate protocol for
         bradycardia or
         tachycardia
      - Contact Medical Command for further orders

PROTOCOL: VENTRICULAR FIBRILLATION/PULSELESS VENTRICULAR TACHYCARDIA

NOTES
1. Protocol assumes VF/VT persists throughout.
2. Reassess pulses after each intervention (except between initial 3 shocks).

PROTOCOL
1. FOLLOW PROTOCOL MEDICAL CARDIAC ARREST-INITIAL CARE:
   A. DEFIBRILLATE 3 times in rapid succession:
      - 200, 300, then 360 J
      - No pulse check between shocks if no charge on monitor and no patient response
      - Keep paddles on patient between shocks
   B. BEGIN BLS—Maintain airway patency via positioning and suctioning as necessary. Hyperventilate with 100% oxygen. Chest compressions at rate of 100/min.
   C. CONTACT MEDICAL COMMAND—report arrest, request MD and other help if needed.
   D. INTUBATE as soon as possible—follow Intubation Protocol.
   E. IV LR regular drip with large bore at KVO rate (preferably at/above antecubital fossa or use external jugular).
   F. EPINEPHRINE 1:10,000 sol. 2 mg ET or 1 mg IV via first route available.
      Repeat EPINEPHRINE every 3 min
2. DEFIBRILLATE 360 J, 30 sec after epinephrine.
3. LIDOCAINE 100 mg IV OR 200 mg ET, CPR for 30 sec, then defibrillate 360 J.
4. LIDOCAINE 100 mg IV OR 200 mg ET, CPR for 30 sec, then defibrillate 360 J.
5. BRETYLIUM 500 mg IV push, CPR for 30 sec, then defibrillate 360 J.
6. REASSESS ET tube position, ECG leads and monitor (proper lead selected), O_2 supply and patient—recheck after every patient movement frequently during resuscitation.
7. MAGNESIUM SULFATE 2 gm IV push, CPR for 30 sec, then defibrillate 360 J.
8. BRETYLIUM 1000 mg IV push, CPR for 30 sec, then defibrillate 360 J.
9. CONTINUE EPINEPHRINE (1 mg IV push or 2 mg ET) every 3 min and drug-shock sequence for persistent VF/VT.
10. Additional orders may include—
   A. SODIUM BICARBONATE 1 mEq/kg IV push then 0.5 mEq/kg every 10 min may be given:
      - Use early in arrest if preexisting metabolic acidosis, hyperkalemia, or tricyclic antidepressant overdose suspected
      - During prolonged resuscitation if ventilation adequate
      - Upon return of pulse after long period of arrest
   B. PROCAINAMIDE 20 mg/min IV up to 17 mg/kg (max=1000 mg) (Carried by EMS Physicians)
   C. Higher doses of EPINEPHRINE

(continued)

(continued)

    D. Additional MAGNESIUM SULFATE

    E. Multiple sequential shocks between drugs.

11. Upon return of pulse with supraventricular rhythm at rate greater than 60/min, patient should receive either lidocaine or bretylium (dose determined by case specifics).

12. If no return of pulse, refer to Protocol: Ceasing Resuscitative Efforts.

13. IV may be converted to Saline Lock before patient transfer.

PROTOCOL: ASYSTOLE AND PULSELESS ELECTRICAL ACTIVITY (PEA) [ELECTRICAL-MECHANICAL DISSOCIATION (EMD)]

INDICATION

All pulseless patients with any ECG rhythm other than VF and VT.

PROTOCOL

1. FOLLOW PROTOCOL: MEDICAL CARDIAC ARREST - INITIAL CARE:

    A. Determine cardiac rhythm:
- If asystole, confirm absence of VF by checking another lead

    B. BEGIN BLS—Maintain airway patency via positioning and suctioning as necessary. Hyperventilate with 100% oxygen. Chest compressions at rate of 100/min.

    C. CONTACT MEDICAL COMMAND—report arrest, request MD and other help if needed.

    D. INTUBATE—follow Intubation Protocol.

    E. IV LR regular drip with large bore at KVO rate (preferably at/above antecubital fossa or use external jugular)

    F. EPINEPHRINE 1:10,000 sol. 1 mg IV OR 2 mg ET via first route available

      **Repeat EPINEPHRINE every 3 min while in arrest.

2. SEARCH FOR POTENTIALLY TREATABLE CAUSES OF ARREST, in the following order:

    A. HYPOXIA:
- If primary event was respiratory, improved ventilation often leads to successful resuscitation
- Ensure excellent ventilation
- Ensure oxygen is flowing to patient
- Ensure tube is in trachea (see Intubation Protocol)

    B. RATE < 50:
- Transcutaneous pacing (Refer to External Pacing Protocol)
- If pacer not immediately available, give atropine 2 mg ET or 1 mg IV; repeat every 3 min. if necessary up to 3 mg
- If increase in rate does not result in palable pulse, consider and treat other potential causes

    C. HYPOVOLEMIA:

    Consider this to be present in *all* patients with clear lung sounds and not in obvious fluid overload state.
- LR 500 cc IV bolus; continue IVF wide open if no response and obvious case of hypovolemia
- Frequently reassess for pulmonary edema
- Command physician may order additional fluid

    D. TENSION PNEUMOTHORAX:

    Assume this to be present in all asthmatics who arrest; suspect after drug snorting and any recent chest trauma or invasive procedure involving the thorax.
- Perform needle decompression of chest (refer to Needle Thoracentesis Protocol); both sides should be done in asthmatics unless reveals presence on one side

    E. HYPERKALEMIA/METABOLIC ACIDOSIS:

    Suspect in patients with renal failure or severe infections.
- Sodium bicarbonate 1 mEq/kg IV push
- Command physician may order calcium or additional bicarbonate

    F. DRUG OVERDOSE/TOXIC EXPOSURE:
- Attempt to determine specific substance and notify command physician for appropriate interventions

G. HYPOTHERMIA:
- Refer to Protocol: Hypothermia Cardiac Arrest
3. REFER TO PROTOCOL: Ceasing Resuscitative Efforts.
4. IV may be converted to Saline Lock before patient transfer.

PROTOCOL: TRAUMATIC CARDIAC ARREST

INDICATIONS

All patients found unresponsive and pulseless after major blunt or penetrating trauma.

EXCLUSIONS

Those patients fitting DOA Protocol. When in doubt about whether to start the protocol, begin and then consult Command physician.

MAXIMUM ON-SCENE TIME: *10 MIN.*

(Unless entrapment, which should be documented on trip sheet.)

PROTOCOL

1. BEGIN BLS—Maintain open airway using jaw thrust *without* head tilt. Suction as necessary. Hyperventilate with 100% oxygen. Chest compressions at rate of 100/min. Maintain cervical spine immobilization.
2. DETERMINE ECG RHYTHM—Defibrillate × 3 if VF or VT.
3. CONTROL *SEVERE* EXTERNAL BLEEDING with constant direct pressure. In case of life-threatening hemorrhage, tourniquet is appropriate only as a last resort.
4. INTUBATE WITH IN-LINE STABILIZATION of cervical spine (per Endotracheal Intubation Protocol). Maximum two attempts at scene. If unable to ventilate patient—notify command physician immediately of this problem. If equipment not ready or other delay in intubation, go to #5 and attempt intubation en-route.
5. IMMOBILIZE quickly with longboard and cervical collar and TRANSFER rapidly to vehicle.
6. EXPEDITE TRANSPORT to nearest Trauma Center. Apply (PASG) for blunt trauma and for penetrating trauma below diaphragm, if enough help available (set up on long board prior to patient); however, *do not delay transport for PASG.*
7. NOTIFY MEDICAL COMMAND of TRAUMATIC ARREST. Medical command will notify Command Physician and Trauma Center.
8. EN-ROUTE:
   A. Reassess airway, ventilation, tube position, and oxygen supply. Continue CPR if no pulses. Intubate if not done at scene. Monitor ECG.
   B. In case of blunt trauma and of penetrating trauma *below* diaphragm, inflate all chambers of PASG until velcro crackles.
   C. Start 2 large bore IVs LR regular drip and run wide open under pressure (use of IV pressure bags recommended).
   D. Provide brief report to Command Physician and Trauma Center.

NOTE

The single most important intervention by far is AIRWAY MANAGEMENT. All efforts must be directed at providing adequate VENTILATION until this is accomplished. (This does not necessarily mean intubation, although this is preferred.)

PROTOCOL: HYPOTHERMIC CARDIAC ARREST

INDICATIONS

Patients unresponsive to "shake and shout" who are pulseless, have no signs of life, and sustain significant cold exposure. This includes elderly and chronically ill patients with prolonged exposure to mild temperatures.

NOTES

1. Patients may appear clinically dead due to severe depression of cardiac and CNS functions but resuscitation with full neurological recovery is possible.

(continued)

(continued)

2. Pulses and respiratory effort may be extremely difficult to detect, so these should be checked for full 30 sec.

PROTOCOL

1. DETERMINE CARDIAC RHYTHM:

A. VF OR VT
Defibrillate 3 times in rapid succession:
- 200, 300, then 360 J
- No pulse check between shocks if no change on monitor and no patient response
- Keep paddles on patient between shocks

B. ASYSTOLE
Check for electrical activity in another lead:
- defibrillate as above if VF found

C. PULSELESS ELECTRICAL ACTIVITY
Proceed to step #2

2. BEGIN BLS—Maintain airway patency via positioning and suctioning as necessary. Hyperventilate with 100% oxygen. Chest compressions at rate of 100/min if no palable pulse *and no other signs of life.*
3. CONTACT MEDICAL COMMAND—report arrest, request MD and other help if needed.
4. REASSESS PULSE, BREATHING, AND ECG RHYTHM:

A. NO PULSE
- CPR
- Intubate (Follow Intubation Protocol)
- IV LR regular drip with large bore at wide open rate (preferably above antecubital fossa or use external jugular)
- *Epinephrine 1:10,000 sol. 2 mg ET or 1 mg IV via first route available

B. PULSE PRESENT
- Assess vital and ECG rhythm
- Intubate if unresponsive or inadequate ventilation (Follow Intubation Protocol)
- Oxygen 15 L/min face mask if not intubated
- IV LR regular drip with large bore at wide open rate up to 1 L

5. PACKAGE PATIENT AND INITIATE IMMEDIATE TRANSPORT.
Consider transport to facility with capability for emergency cardiopulmonary bypass.
6. EN-ROUTE:
A. Continue CPR in no pulse.
B. Continue LR 1 L wide open (warmed if possible).
C. Remove wet clothes and cover with dry blankets as time permits.
D. Increase temperature in vehicle.
E. Avoid rough movements if patient not in VF.
F. Contact command physician for further orders.

*Note: In case of severe hypothermia (<30° C) no drugs should be given. Above 30° C, drugs should be given at longer than standard intervals. Since core temperature cannot be checked in field, we will transport rapidly and command physician can use discretion based on specifics of the case.

PROTOCOL: CEASING RESUSCITATIVE EFFORTS

INDICATIONS

Patients in cardiac arrest for whom cardiac resuscitation has been initiated but has not led to spontaneous circulation.

EXCLUSIONS

1. Hypothermia
2. Trauma arrest
3. Patients who meet DOA criteria per DOA protocols.

PROTOCOL

Resuscitation efforts may be discontinued if *ALL* of the following conditions are met *AND* the Command Physician authorizes the discontinuation.

1. Arrest duration > 30 min.
2. Current rhythm is not VF or VT.
3. No sustained spontaneous circulation (palpable pulse for > 1 min) within the last 10 minutes.
4. No potentially reversible condition identified (e.g., antidepressant overdose).
5. Patient has received adequate trial of ALS interventions as determined by Command Physician.
6. Age >18.
7. No contradictory ethical or legal concerns (eg., public location, family support needs).

NOTE

1. Command Physicians may use discretion to cease resuscitation after less than 30 min if cardiac unresponsiveness determined after trial of ACLS appropriate to clinical situation.
2. Command Physician does *not* need to be on scene to cease resuscitation.
3. It is strongly recommended that a decision be made to either transport or cease resuscitation at scene once resuscitation efforts have persisted for 30 min. Transport may be initiated sooner if logistics permit.

References

1. Roth R, Stewart RD, Rogers K, et al.: Out-of-hospital cardiac arrest: factors associated with survival, *Ann Emerg Med* 13:237-244, 1984.

2. Eisenberg MS, Horwood BT, Cummins RO, et al.: Cardiac arrest and resuscitation: a tale of 29 cities, *Ann Emerg Med* 19:179-186, 1990.

3. Weaver WD, Cobb LA, Hallstrom AP, et al.: Factors influencing survival after out-of-hospital cardiac arrest, *J Am Coll Cardio* 7:752-757, 1986.

4. Cummins RO, Eisenberg MS, Hallstrom AP, et al.: Survival of out-of-hospital cardiac arrest with early initiation of cardiopulmonary resuscitation, *Am J Emerg Med* 3:114-119, 1985.

5. Larsen MP, Eisenberg MS, Cummins RO, et al.: Predicting survival from out of hospital cardiac arrest: a graphic model, *Ann Emerg Med* 22:1652-1658, 1993.

6. Pepe PE, Mattox KL, Duke JH, et al.: Effect of full-time, specialized physician supervision on the success of a large, urban emergency medical services system, *Clin Care Med*; 21:1279-1286, 1993.

7. Stewart RD: Medical direction in emergency medical services: the role of the physician, *Emerg Med Clin NA* (1):119-132, 1987.

8. American Heart Association: Recommended guidelines for uniform reporting of data from out-of-hospital cardiac arrest: the 'Utstein style', *Resuscitation* 22(1):1-26, 1996.

9. Quick G, Bastani B: Prolonged asystolic hyperkalemic cardiac arrest with no neurologic sequelae, *Ann Emerg Med* 24:305-311, 1994.

10. Josephson EB, Goetting MG: Bilateral tube thoracostomies (abstract), *Ann Emerg Med* 18:457, 1989.

11. Kellerman AL, Hackman BB, Somes G: Predicting the outcome of unsuccessful prehospital advanced cardiac life support, *JAMA* 270:1433-1436, 1993.

12. Bonin MJ, Pepe PE, Kimball KT, et al.: Distinct criteria for termination of resuscitation in the out-of-hospital setting, *JAMA* 270:1457-1462, 1993.

13. Kellerman AL: Criteria for dead-on-arrivals, prehospital termination of CPR, and do-not-resuscitate orders, *Ann Emerg Med* 22:47-51, 1993.

14. Gray WA, Capone RJ, Most AS: Unsuccessful emergency medical resuscitation—are continued efforts in the emergency department justified? *N Engl J Med* 325:1393-1398, 1991.

15. Fosnocht DE, Delbridge TR, Garrison HG, et al.: Surviving relatives' acceptance of the decision to terminate resuscitation in the field, *Ann Emerg Med* 22:919, 1993.

16. Schmidt TA, Harrahill MA: Family response to death in the field, *Ann Emerg Med* 22:918, 1993.

11

Hypotension and Shock

Shock can be defined as the widespread reduction in tissue perfusion, which if prolonged, can lead to cellular and organ dysfunction and death. The late stages of shock indicated by marked alteration of vital signs and mental status are easily recognized by prehospital care providers. However, the early stages of shock that present with subtle alterations in mental status and vital signs are easily overlooked or misinterpreted.

Prehospital care providers often equate "normal" vital signs with normal cardiovascular status. The field team may be lulled into a false sense of security if the early signs of shock are overlooked, only to be caught off guard when the patient "crashes" during transport. Early recognition and aggressive treatment of shock may prevent progression to the profound stages of shock and death in potentially salvageable patients.

Unfortunately, the tools available for the diagnosis of shock in the field are very limited. Primarily, the command physician relies on the observations of the field team along with the clinical history. Likewise, the tools for treating shock in the field are limited to fluid infusion, IV vasopressors, PASG, or a combination of these.

Overall, the command physician is to first interpret the patient's clinical condition based on the evaluation provided by the field team and second to devise a treatment plan using the limited resources available in the field. Shock is truly one of the life-threatening emergencies that must be treated early and aggressively in the field to prevent progression and subsequent morbidity and mortality. Time is a critical factor in the prehospital treatment of shock. This chapter will identify several pitfalls associated with the diagnosis and treatment of shock and will help establish an overall thought process for dealing with shock in the field.

Evaluation

The most common problem associated with the evaluation and treatment of shock in the field is its identification. The accuracy of vital signs obtained by prehospital care providers must be kept in mind. Cayten[1] found an error rate of over 20% for EMTs obtaining vital signs in a non-emergent setting compared to a standard set by a nurse research specialist. The tolerance limits set by the researchers were relatively strict, and many of

RONALD N. ROTH, MD, FACEP

the "errors" would have no clinical significance. However, several errors were noted to be quite significant. They suggest that when critical medical decisions will be based on the data gathered in the field, multiple measures should be obtained.

In the noisy field environment, providers often measure blood pressure by palpation rather than auscultation. Blood pressure by palpation provides only an estimate of systolic pressure.

"Normal" vital signs do not necessarily correlate with the presence or absence of shock. For children, the norm of 120/80 mmHg is not applicable (Table 11-1). In addition, adults with previous hypertension may actually be relatively hypotensive with a blood pressure of 120/80 mmHg and may require emergent treatment. Therefore, the patient's age, size, and present and past medical history must be taken into consideration along with the blood pressure. An abnormal blood pressure must be used in conjunction with the signs and symptoms provided by the prehospital care providers. The petite 45 kg 16-year old female with lower abdominal pain and a blood pressure of 88/palpation may have a ruptured ectopic pregnancy or may normally run a blood pressure of 88 systolic. An elderly patient with significant epistaxis may be hypertensive due to catecholamine release and vasoconstriction despite being relatively volume depleted. The presence of signs and symptoms of system-wide reduction in tissue perfusion, such as tachycardia, tachypnea, mental status changes, and cool, clammy skin, would strongly suggest shock. Therefore in the diagnosis and treatment of hypotension in the field, the command physician should look for systemic signs of shock as described in Box 11-1. Previously healthy victims of acute hypo-

volemic shock may maintain relatively normal vital signs with up to 25% blood volume loss.[2] Sympathetic nervous system stimulation with vasoconstriction and increased cardiac contractility can maintain blood pressure in the face of decreasing vascular volume. In some patients with intraabdominal bleeding (abdominal aneurysm, ectopic pregnancy, etc.) the pulse may be relatively bradycardic despite significant blood loss. Obviously, it is beneficial to recognize hypovolemia early before significant alterations in vital signs and organ damage occur.

Orthostatic vital signs are often evaluated in the emergency department. The most sensitive test is lying to standing with a pulse increase of 30 bpm after 1 minute of standing.[3] Symptoms of lightheadedness or dizziness would also be considered a positive test. Orthostatic blood pressure checks are rarely done in the field. Occasionally they are performed unknowingly by the patient who initially refuses treatment while lying down then stands up to leave the scene and suffers a syncopal episode. This demonstration of orthostatic hypotension is often helpful in convincing the patient to allow treatment and transport. In addition, orthostatics may occasionally be helpful in the field, by direct order of the command physician, if the patient's diagnosis is unclear and prolonged treatment or transport is expected, such as in the rural or wilderness setting.

The ATLS course for physicians recommends capillary refill as a clinical test for hypovolemia.[2] However, in a study of blood donors and ED patients with evidence of hypovolemia, Schringer and Baraff[4] found capillary refill not to be a useful test for mild-to-moderate hypovolemia. For a 450 ml blood loss the sensitivity of capillary refill

Age	Average Weight (Kg)	Heart Rate (Min-Max)	Systolic Blood Pressure (Min-Max)
Birth	3.5	90-190	50-70
6 Mos.	7	85-180	65-106
1 Yr.	10	80-150	72-110
3 Yr.	14	80-140	78-114
6 Yr.	20	70-120	80-116
8 Yr.	26	70-110	84-122
12 Yr.	40	60-110	94-136
15 Yr.	50	55-100	100-142

Table 11-1 Normal Vital Signs for Children

Box 11-1 Signs and Symptoms of Shock

Cardiovascular
- Hypotension, tachycardia, arrhythmias

Central Nervous System
- Confusion, agitation
- Alterations in level of consciousness

Respiratory
- Tachypnea, dyspnea

Skin
- Pallor, diaphoresis
- Cyanosis, mottling

in detecting hypovolemia was 11% with a specificity of 89%. This suggests that capillary refill may not be a useful test for evaluating shock in the field.

To aid in the treatment of shock in the field, we often find it helpful to classify the etiologies of shock. Most prehospital care providers are familiar with the pumps, fluids, pipes model of the cardiovascular system with the pump representing the heart, pipes the vascular system, and fluid the components of blood. It is often helpful for the command physician to divide the causes of shock into problems with the pump, the pipes, or the fluid. Table 11-2 divides the causes of shock into four general categories.

The etiologies of shock by category are listed in Box 11-2. Categorizing shock in these four categories not only helps the prehospital care provider but the command physician organize thoughts and develop treatment modalities.

Treatment

Knowing the limited treatment options for the management of hypotension in the field (fluids, vasopressors, PASG) and having the etiologies of shock and hypotension placed in four categories, we can now develop a scheme for treatment. First, treat the primary problem if possible. Often the primary problem is obvious and the initial management is possible. Frequently, the treatment options are very straightforward. The treatment of hypotension in a young, healthy victim of a gunshot wound to the arm is obviously direct pressure to the wound, rapid transport to the hospital with IV fluids, and possibly PASG as an option. The treatment of hypotension in a cardiac patient with a sinus bradycardic rhythm obviously requires atropine and possibly external pacing. The patient suffering from anaphylaxis may require both fluids and vasopressors (epinephrine) to optimally reverse hypotension. Occasionally, the primary problem may be obvious but not treatable in the field, such as cardiac tamponade. Less

often, but most difficult to manage, is the hypotensive patient without an obvious cause of hypotension. The hypotensive cardiac patient not in pulmonary edema and the hypotensive trauma victim without obvious external injuries or internal bleeding provide a challenge for the command physician.

Box 11-2   Etiologies of Shock

Hypovolemia
- External fluid loss
  - Hemorrhage
  - Gastrointestinal losses
  - Renal losses
  - Cutaneous loss
- Internal fluid loss
  - Fractures
  - Intestinal obstruction
  - Hemothorax
  - Hemoperitoneum

Cardiogenic Shock
- Myocardial infarction
- Arrhythmias
- Cardiomyopathy
- Acute valvular incompetence
- Myocardial contusion

Obstructive Shock
- Pulmonary embolus
- Tension pneumothorax
- Cardiac tamponade
- Severe aortic stenosis
- Venacaval obstruction

Distributive Shock
- Drug induced
- Spinal cord injury
- Sepsis
- Anaphylaxis
- Anoxia

Table 11-2 Causes of Shock

Type of Shock	Disorder	Example
Hypovolemic	decreased fluid	hemorrhage, GI loss, burns
Distributive	increased pipe size	spinal cord injury, anaphylaxis, sepsis
Obstruction	pipe obstruction	pulmonary embolus, tension pneumothorax, cardiac tamponade
Cardiogenic	pump problems	MI, dysrhythmia, cardiomyopathy

Treating hypotension and shock caused by hypovolemia would include replacement of fluid volume and possibly the use of PASG. Treating distributive shock involves the combination of pressors to constrict the dilated vasculature and fluids to fill the expanded vascular tree. The PASG may also be useful in distributive shock because of their ability to increase peripheral vascular resistance. The treatment of obstructive shock must be individualized. If possible the obstruction should be removed (i.e., the pneumothorax decompressed). However, when the primary problem cannot be treated successfully in the field (i.e., pulmonary embolus) fluids are often helpful in increasing preload and temporarily overcoming the obstruction. As in obstructive shock, treatment of cardiogenic shock requires individualization. Dysrhythmias causing hypotension including bradycardias and tachycardias will most likely be obvious and should be treated appropriately. Pump failure is as difficult to diagnose and treat in the field as it is in the ED without invasive monitoring. Adult patients without obvious pulmonary edema may receive fluid challenges of approximately 150-300 cc crystalloid (NS or LR) with reevaluation of vital signs after each fluid challenge. An improvement in the patient's condition with fluid challenges suggests that improving preload would be beneficial to the patient's cardiovascular status. A worsening of the patient's condition with a fluid challenge or obvious pulmonary edema on initial evaluation make additional fluid challenges inappropriate. Therefore treatment with pressors, such as Dopamine or Dobutamine, would be more appropriate. Ideally, pressors should be initiated at low doses in the field and then titrated to effect. The command physician must realize that drips are often difficult to manage in the field and must be watched closely.

In a few disconcerting situations the primary etiology for hypotension is not obvious and may not be identifiable by the field team. Looking at the individual etiologies for shock (hypovolemic, distributive, cardiogenic, and obstructive) the bottom line in shock treatment is whether to give fluids. In hypovolemic shock, distributive shock, and obstruction, fluids are an appropriate initial treatment for hypotension. Some cases of cardiogenic shock will respond to fluids. However, fluids should not be given to patients in cardiogenic shock with florid pulmonary edema. In other cases, response to fluid challenges should dictate whether additional fluid challenges should be given or trial of pressors should be used.

Any treatment scheme for treating shock in the field should keep the following factors in mind:

1. Need to establish and maintain the **ABC**s (**A**irway **B**reathing **C**irculation).
2. Need for definitive care.
3. Transport time to the hospital.
4. Resources in the field.
5. Skills of the prehospital care provider in the field.

In the urban setting with a very short transport time, the victim of a penetrating cardiac wound might benefit most from airway maintenance and rapid transport to the hospital without IV access being established in the field.[5] On the other hand, with longer transport times and in the rural setting, the patient with intraabdominal bleeding would most likely benefit from carefully titrated crystalloid volume infusion during the transport time. Fluids should be initiated while the patient is en-route to the hospital, thereby not prolonging scene time and time until definitive care can be obtained. The ideal quantity of fluids to administer is not known (see Controversies). When rapid fluid infusion is required, fluids should be infused with either pressure bags or manual pressure on the IV bag.[6] In addition, the use of large bore trauma tubing and short large bore IV catheters can also maximize volume infusion (Box 11-3).[7]

Occasionally shock will be refractory to initial attempts at resuscitation. This may reflect the need for definitive care in the hospital (i.e., thoracotomy, laparotomy). If after vigorous field treatment of shock the patient remains hypotensive, other etiologies for the hypotension must be considered. Refractory hypotension may be the result of inadequate volume replacement, inadequate oxygenation, cardiac tamponade, tension pneumothorax, acidemia, myocardial infarction, or medications.

Pitfalls

Inability of the field team to recognize the shock state is the initial pitfall associated with the prehospital care for shock in the field. The inaccuracy of vital signs obtained by the field team[1] and the difficulty recognizing poor perfusion and not just hypotension as an indicator of shock may allow patients in shock to go unrecognized.

Box 11-3   Factors Associated with Rapid Fluid Infusion

Catheter
    short length
    large diameter
    proper design

Tubing
    short length
    large diameter

Fluid
    high viscosity
    infused under pressure

Average flow rates in ml/min (tap water)		
Catheter	**Gravity Flow**	**200 mmHg Pressure**
Deseret Angiocath 14 gauge, 2" length	173	405
Deseret Angiocath 16 gauge, 4" length	108	231
USCI Introducer 8 French, 5½" length	243	540
From Mateer et al.[7]		

The benefit of any prehospital procedure must be weighed against any potential risk of the procedure. In general, a major pitfall associated with most prehospital care procedures is the time delay until definitive care can be obtained. It is clear from the work of Pantridge in Belfast[8] that for victims of myocardial infarction, some aspects of definitive care can be delivered in the field (defibrillation and arrhythmia management). However, for trauma victims with internal hemorrhage, definitive care can only be provided in the hospital. Therefore any procedure that delays delivery of definitive care must be critically evaluated.

The role of fluid administration in major trauma cases was evaluated by Smith et al.[5], who looked at 52 cases of prehospital stabilization of multiple trauma victims. He found that time to establish an IV ranged from 8.6-12.6 minutes and over one fourth of the IV attempts were unsuccessful. In all cases, the time for IV insertion exceeded the transport time. An average of only 1 liter of fluid was infused in the most critical patients.

Honigman,[9] on the other hand, looked at 70 patients with penetrating cardiac injuries. Scene time for these patients averaged 10.7 minutes. On-scene time did not correlate with the number of prehospital procedures performed including intubation, PASG application, or IV insertion. In a study evaluating the impact of ALS compared with BLS in trauma, Jacobs et al.[10] reported that ALS-resuscitated patients had higher Champion trauma scores upon arrival to the hospital. In addition, ALS interventions did not delay transport time to the hospital as compared to BLS units. Other investigators have described the feasibility of starting IV access while actually en-route to the hospital. They have coined the term "Zero-time Prehospital IV."[11] These studies suggest that ALS procedures can be performed on scene or during transport without increasing scene time. However, strong medical control and adequate paramedic ALS training are essential.

Excess fluid administration can cause problems in the prehospital setting. Trauma victims with isolated head injuries who receive excess fluids can develop worsened cerebral swelling. In addition, excess fluids may precipitate congestive heart failure (CHF) in susceptible individuals.

Controversies

Recently, several authors have challenged the time-honored practice of attempting to restore a normal blood pressure in a patient with uncontrolled hemorrhage.[12-16] These authors suggest that volume resuscitation prior to controlling hemorrhage may be detrimental. With uncontrolled hemorrhage states, aggressive crystalloid infusion may result in an elevated blood pressure. Several animal studies suggest that attempts at restoring the blood pressure to normal values in uncontrolled hemorrhage may increase hemorrhage volumes, destabilize the early platelet plug, cause profound hemodilution of clotting factors, and ultimately result in higher mortality.[13-14] The "desired" level of hypotension in patients with uncontrolled hemorrhage states in the field has yet to be determined.

Studies by Martin[15] in Houston and Kaweski[12] in San Diego suggest that mortality after trauma is not influenced by prehospital fluid administration. Survival to hospital discharge rates were not significantly different for patients receiving fluids versus patients not receiving fluids in the field. Both studies were performed in systems with relatively short scene and transport times. In addition, the Houston study only evaluated victims of penetrating trauma.

Despite numerous studies, the role of PASG in the pre-hospital care of hypotension remains controversial. Supporters of the prehospital use of PASG state that PASG raises systemic blood pressure, makes vascular access easier, tamponades internal bleeding, and splints fractures.[17-20] PASG detractors suggest that time spent on applying the device delays the time until definitive care can be given with questionable benefits.[21-25] In a prospective, randomized study comparing alternate day PASG use vs. no-PASG, Mattox reported an overall mortality of 31% in the PASG group vs. 25% in the no-PASG group (p=0.05).[25] This study analyzed the results of 784 adult victims of blunt or penetrating trauma with an initial systolic blood pressure of 90 mmHg or less as measured by City of Houston paramedics. The overwhelming majority of the patients in this study were victims of penetrating trauma, and transport times were relatively short (13-14 minutes). For the subgroup of patients with an initial field blood pressure of less than 50 mmHg, survival was actually better in the PASG group (38.2%) vs. no-PASG group (29.2%). However, the difference failed to achieve statistical significance in this subgroup (169 patients).

In a retrospective chart review of 142 trauma victims with blood pressures less than 50 mmHg, Cayten found survival rate from blunt or penetrating trauma significantly higher among PASG (13.6%) vs. no-PASG (9.4%) patients (p=0.055). The improvement in survival occurred despite an average scene time that was 4.7 minutes longer in the PASG group.[26] Cayten concluded that PASG should be considered medically acceptable in patients with profound hypotension pending randomized controlled studies.

Despite the controversy surrounding the use of PASG, many systems continue to use this device. The PASG can be placed on a longboard or stretcher in preparation for the patient. The patient can be placed directly on the open PASG and the device can be applied with minimal delay and inflated en-route.

The reported indications for the application of PASG include—

1. absolute hypovolemia,

2. relative hypovolemia (distributive shock),

3. tamponade of intrabdominal and pelvic bleeding.

The only absolute contraindication for PASG application is pulmonary edema. A relative contraindication for the PASG is third-trimester pregnancy. The abdominal compartment should not be inflated during this stage of pregnancy. Controversy exists as to the benefits or dangers of PASG use with supradiaphragmatic bleeding, suspected increased intracerebral pressure, and during cardiac arrest.

The true controversy about the use of any field procedure is does the procedure truly make a difference in patient outcome?[27] This question, with regards to the PASG and IV fluid therapy, unfortunately, has yet to be answered. For patients with uncontrolled hemorrhage, blood pressure should probably be sustained just high enough to maintain mentation.

Summary

In summary, hypotension is a relative term for patients in the field and must be correlated with the patient's clinical condition including age, size, and present and past medical history. Ideally, we would ask the paramedic to identify signs of systemic decreased tissue perfusion and the presence of shock. Treatment modalities for shock and hypotension are often limited to fluids, pressors, and PASG. Often the primary problem causing hypotension in the field is obvious and can be readily treated. Occasionally the primary problem precipitating the hypotension is obvious but not readily treated in the field.

The most difficult patients to manage are hypotensive patients without an obvious cause for their hypotension. The ultimate question in the treatment of shock in the field is whether to give or withhold fluids. Fluids are an appropriate initial treatment for hypotension caused by hypovolemic shock, distributive shock, and obstruction. Some cases of cardiogenic shock will respond to fluids. However, fluids should not be given to patients in cardiogenic shock with florid pulmonary edema. The response to fluid challenges should dictate the use of additional fluid challenges or determine if vasopressors should be attempted.

Finally, the potential benefit of performing any procedure in the field must be weighed against the potential risk of delaying definitive care.

S A M P L E   C A S E S

CASE # 1

Paramedics report that they are seeing a 65-year-old male with a history of an abdominal aortic aneurysm (AAA), coronary artery disease, and recent prostate surgery with an in-dwelling urinary bladder catheter, who was complaining of abdominal pain and dizziness on standing. The patient is alert and oriented with a BP of 60/palp, pulse of 95, and respirations of 16. Medics note that he is pale and diaphoretic. Their evaluation was remarkable for clear lungs and no evidence of JVD or peripheral edema. The abdomen is slightly distended and tender. Monitor shows sinus rhythm at a rate of 95. The medics are 25 minutes from the nearest hospital and are requesting orders from Medic Command. The patient is taking oral antibiotics and has no allergies.

How would you proceed?

Although the parties involved in this case were rightly concerned about a leaking AAA, other etiologies of hypotension and shock in this patient may include a perforated abdominal viscus, an inferior wall myocardial infarction (MI), gastrointestinal bleeding, or sepsis.

Fluid therapy would be appropriate for hypovolemic, cardiogenic, distributive, or obstructive shock with no signs of fluid overload. Suspecting an abdominal catastrophe, Medic Command should direct field personnel to expedite transport. IV access should be established en-route, at least one large bore (14-16 gauge) catheter. A fluid challenge of 300-500 cc of crystalloid should be rapidly infused under pressure. PASG should be applied and inflated en-route in an attempt to raise systolic blood pressure and to tamponade possible internal bleeding. The patient should be reevaluated frequently, and the operating room and surgical team should be notified by the command physician.

CASE # 2

Medics are requesting orders on a 68-year-old female in acute respiratory distress. She has a past medical history of coronary artery disease and CHF. At the present time she is alert to her name and place only with jugular venous distention (JVD) to her ears in a sitting position. Auscultation of the lungs reveals rales halfway up bilaterally. The medics also note that she has significant peripheral edema. Her vital signs are BP 70/palp, pulse 40, and respirations 36. Her medications include digoxin, furosemide, and potassium. She has no known drug allergies. EKG monitor shows sinus bradycardia rate of 40. The medics have placed the patient on oxygen by face mask and are establishing a line of D_5W.

How would you proceed?

This patient is clearly in shock despite adequate (or excess) fluid status. Her presentation strongly suggests cardiogenic shock with bradycardia as a primary problem. While the airway is being secured, by intubation if necessary, the bradycardia should be addressed as per ACLS protocols. If available, an external pacemaker should be placed on the patient and pacing should be started immediately. Atropine should be administered to increase the intrinsic heart rate. If the patient remained hypotensive despite an increase in her heart rate with the atropine and pacer, a vasopressor infusion, such as dopamine or dobutamine, should be initiated. Note that drug infusions are very difficult to regulate in a moving ambulance. Preferably, the field team should initiate an infusion of dopamine or dobutamine at a concentration and rate ordered by the physician and then titrate the infusion to the patient's response. CHF must be treated aggressively in the field to prevent a poor outcome. Unfortunately, many of the first-line drugs used for CHF in the field (nitroglycerin, furosemide, morphine) can induce hypotension and must be withheld in the field treatment of the hypotensive patient. Fluids and PASG are contraindicated in this patient with cardiogenic shock and pulmonary edema.

CASE # 3

A 65-year-old man with a history of hypertension, coronary artery disease, and MI was working on his roof on a hot, sunny day. He struck a beehive with his hammer and suffered a fall approximately 6 feet from the roof.

Upon arrival of the two-person paramedic crew, the patient was unresponsive, lying on the ground. A primary survey was performed and the airway was secured by endotracheal intubation. During their report to medic command the paramedics noted that the patient was relatively bradycardic, heart rate 65, blood pressure of 60/systolic, and had clear and equal lung sounds. Secondary survey revealed no signs of external or obvious sources of internal bleeding, urticaria, facial swelling, internal or external trauma, or arrhythmias. The medics have the PASG on the stretcher, ready to receive the patient. The paramedics estimate a 20-minute transport time to the nearest trauma center.

How would you proceed?

The etiologies of hypotension in this patient are

possibly endless (Box 11-4). However, the initial evaluation and treatment would be independent of the etiology. The patient showed no signs of fluid overload, therefore interventions to be performed by the paramedics en-route to the hospital should include large-bore IV access and a fluid challenge of at least 150 ccs NS or LR. The PASG could also be inflated during transport. Response to these interventions should dictate further therapy.

The patient in this scenario remained hypotensive despite inflation of the PASG and repeated fluid challenges (200 cc trial infused rapidly under pressure for a total of 1000). A dopamine drip at 20 μg/kg/min was initiated with moderate improvement of the patient's blood pressure and perfusion. However the patient remained unresponsive and without spontaneous movement.

BOX 11-4	Possible Etiologies of Hypotension in Sample Case #3

1. Internal bleeding
2. Spinal cord injury
3. Dehydration
4. Cardiac contusion
5. Cardiac tamponade
6. Myocardial infarction
7. Drugs
8. Tension pneumothorax
9. Anaphylaxis
10. Cardiac dysrhythmias

Evaluation at the trauma center revealed a cervical spine fracture and ECG changes suggestive of an inferior wall MI.

CASE #4

Paramedics have initiated hospital transport of a 25-year-old female who cut both of her wrists in an apparent suicide attempt. Upon arrival of the paramedics at the scene, the patient was awake, but drowsy, with active bleeding from both wrists. The field team estimates a 900 cc blood loss on scene. The bleeding is now controlled with direct pressure, and 2 large-bore IV catheters have been established. The patient's present blood pressure is 60 mmHg systolic. The IV fluids (NS) are running wide open.

How would you proceed?

Clearly, this patient is suffering from hypovolemic shock and requires fluid resuscitation. In this case, the hemorrhage is controlled and fluids should be administered at a wide open rate with pressure applied to the IV fluid bag to increase the flow. Unlike the uncontrolled hemorrhage model, where aggressive fluid administration may lead to increased bleeding, this patient's bleeding is controlled. Therefore, fluid volume should be rapidly replaced.

References

1. Cayten CG, Herrmann N, Cole LW, et al.: Assessing the validity of EMS data, *JACEP* 7:390-396, 1978.

2. American College of Surgeons Committee on Trauma: *Advanced trauma life support (ATLS) course,* Chicago, American College of Surgeons, 1988.

3. Knopp R, Claypool R, Leonard D: Use of the tilt test in measuring acute blood loss, *Ann Emerg Med* 9:72-75, 1980.

4. Schriger DL, Barraff LJ: Capillary refill: is it a useful predictor of hypovolemic states? *Ann Emerg Med* 20:601-605, 1991.

5. Smith P, Bodai BI, Hill AS, et al.: Prehospital stabilization of critically injured patients: a failed concept, *J Trauma* 25:65-70, 1985.

6. White SJ, Hamilton WA, Veronesi JF: A comparison of field techniques used to pressure-infuse intravenous fluids, *Prehosp Disaster Med* 6:129-134, 1991.

7. Mateer JR: Rapid fluid resuscitation with central venous catheters, *Ann Emerg Med* 12:149-152, 1983.

8. Pantridge JF, Geddes JS: A mobile intensive care unit in the management of myocardial infarction, *Lancet* 2:271-273, 1967.

9. Honigman B, Rohweda K, Moov EE, et al.: Prehospital advanced trauma life support for penetrating cardiac wounds, *Abstract Annals* 18:474, 1989.

10. Jacobs LM, Sinclair A, Beiser A, et al.: Prehospital advanced life support: benefits in trauma, *J Trauma* 24:8-13, 1984.

11. O'Gorman M, Trabulsy P, Pilcher DB: Zero-time prehospital IV, *J Trauma* 29:84-86, 1989.

12. Kaweski SM, Sise MJ, Virgilio RW: The effect of prehospital fluids on survival in trauma patients, *J Trauma* 30:1215-1219, 1990.

13. Kowalenko T, Stern S, Dronen S, et al.: Improved outcome with hypotensive resuscitation of uncontrolled hemorrhagic shock in a swine model, *J Trauma* 33:349-353, 1992.

14. Stern S, Dronen S, Birrer P, et al.: Effect of blood pressure on hemorrhagic volume and survival in a near fatal hemorrhage model incorporating a vascular injury, *Ann Emerg Med* 22:155-163, 1993.

15. Martin R, Bickell W, Pepe P, et al.: Prospective evaluation of preoperative fluid resuscitation in hypotensive patients with penetrating truncal injury: a preliminary report, *J Trauma* 33:354-362, 1992.

16. Bickell WH: Are victims of injury sometimes victimized by attempts at fluid resuscitation? (editorial), *Ann Emerg Med* 22:225-226, 1993.

17. Gaffney FA, Thal ER, Taylor WF: Hemodynamic effects of medical antishock trousers, *J Trauma* 21:931-937, 1981.

18. Flint LM, Brown A, Richardson JD, et al.: Definitive control of bleeding for severe pelvic fractures, *Ann Surg* 189:709-716, 1979.

19. Cutler BS, Daggett WM: Application of the "G-Suit" to the control of hemorrhage in massive trauma, *Ann Surg* 173:511-514.

20. McSwain NE Jr: Pneumatic antishock garment: state of the art 1988, *Ann Emerg Med* 17:506-525, 1988.

21. Bickell WH, Pepe PE, et al.: Effect of antishock trousers on the trauma score: a prospective analysis in the urban setting, *Ann Emerg Med* 14:218-222, 1985.

22. Mattox KL, Bickell WH, Pepe PE, et al.: Prospective randomized evaluation of antishock MAST in post-traumatic hypotension, *J Trauma* 26: 779-786, 1986.

23. Mackenzie RC, Christensen BS, Lewis FR: The prehospital use of external counterpressure: does MAST make a difference? *J Trauma* 24: 882-888, 1984.

24. Gold CR: Prehospital advanced life support vs. "scoop and run" in trauma management, *Ann Emerg Med* 16: 797-801, 1987.

25. Mattox KL, Bickell WH, Pepe PE, et al.: Prospective MAST study in 911 patients, *J Trauma* 29: 1104-1112, 1989.

26. Cayten CG, Berendt BM, Byrne DW, et al.: A study of pneumatic antishock garments in severely hypotensive trauma patients, *J Trauma* 34: 728-735, 1993.

12

Trauma

Trauma is the leading cause of death for persons under the age of 45 and is the fourth leading cause of death overall in the United States.[1] Timely and skilled prehospital management of the trauma patient can greatly improve patient outcome. The first prehospital trauma course, BTLS, was introduced in 1982. BTLS, as well as other prehospital trauma courses, offers an organized and standardized approach to prehospital trauma care. It is essential that prehospital care providers recognize that trauma patients are not "treated" in the field. Definitive treatment occurs in the ED or operating room. Only a rapid, efficient primary survey and critical lifesaving interventions should be performed in the field. Time is a critical factor for the trauma patient. While ATLS teaches about the "golden hour" for trauma patients, prehospital educators should be speaking about the "golden 10 minutes."[2]

Prehospital trauma courses strongly support a "load and go" approach for the more critically injured patients (Box 12-1). The challenge to the prehospital care provider is to perform an efficient primary survey and identify the patient who requires critical intervention before or during transport. The prehospital treatment of the trauma patient must be tailored to the needs of a particular prehospital system. Critical factors in treatment decisions include the location of the trauma (distance from the trauma center) and the capabilities of the prehospital team. Most experts agree with the "load and go" philosophy when the trauma patient is within a 15-minute transport time to a trauma center. Each prehospital system must work with their particular strengths and weaknesses to achieve maximal efficiency while delivering optimal care.

Standing orders and protocols improve the prehospital care provider's ability to maximize efficiency and minimize field time. There is nothing more frustrating or time consuming for the field provider than trying to give a full report on a patient and waiting for orders while trying to comply with a "load and go" philosophy. Prehospital trauma courses define which penetrating and blunt trauma situations should be treated with a "load and go" protocol.

SUSAN M. DUNMIRE, MD, FACEP

Penetrating Trauma

The management of the trauma patient with a penetrating injury is fairly straightforward. These patients undergo a rapid primary survey by the EMT/paramedic followed by airway stabilization and spinal immobilization (if necessary). A "load and go" philosophy has proven beneficial in all patients with penetrating, chest, abdominal, and neck injuries.

Cervical spine immobilization is often forgotten during the prehospital treatment of the patient with penetrating trauma. Any patient who has received a direct force to the head or neck (e.g., gunshot wound to the head) or a fall should have spine immobilization before transport. In one retrospective study of patients with gunshot wounds to the head, 10% of those on whom x-rays were taken demonstrated cervical spine or spinal cord injury.[4]

Airway management in the patient with penetrating trauma may vary depending on the distance to the trauma center. If the patient is within a 15-minute transport time to the hospital and the EMTs/paramedics are able to maintain good oxygenation with a face mask or a bag-valve-mask and assisted ventilation, intubation may not be necessary on en-route. Intubation is indicated in a patient with an obstructed airway, acute respiratory distress, hypoventilation, or hypoxia that is uncorrected with oxygen. Intubation is not only time consuming, but it can frequently be difficult when there is blood in the airway or the patient is extremely combative. It is a much easier procedure in the controlled atmosphere of the ED to perform a rapid sequence induction and intubation of the patient. The ED has better lighting, more personnel, better suction equipment, and medications not available to the prehospital care provider that make intubation much easier. If there is difficulty in intubation in the ED, a surgeon or emergency medicine physician is present to obtain a surgical airway. If intubation is deemed necessary in the field, certain techniques can be very helpful. Orotracheal intubation is the preferred route in the trauma patient. Most trauma patients in whom the severity of injury warrants field intubation will be either minimally responsive or unresponsive and require no sedation. The major difficulty arises with airway secretions and bleeding. Visualizing the vocal cords is often impossible. A paramedic who is trained in digital intubation has an advantage in these situations. Digital intubation is often faster because no instruments are needed and with proper training and experience, can be a valuable airway skill.[5,6]

When possible, IV access should be established enroute to the hospital. Most experts agree that prolonging prehospital time to establish IV access in patients with penetrating trauma is unnecessary if the transport time is 15 minutes or less. If a patient is going to sustain an exsanguination arrest 10-15 minutes after injury, it is estimated that they have lost 2000-3000 cc of blood.[7] It is difficult to replace that volume during a short transport time, and the value of rapid crystalloid infusion to treat exsanguination is debatable. Recent studies suggest that vigorous volume resuscitation with crystalloid before surgical control of hemorrhage may be detrimental to the patient.[8-10] Several studies have demonstrated that aggressive crystalloid administration during massive uncontrolled hemorrhage may disrupt thrombus formation, increase blood loss by increasing blood pressure and diluting clotting factors, and ultimately decrease survival rates.[11,12] In one recent prospective randomized study of patients with penetrating trauma, there was a 70% survival rate in patients who did not receive crystalloid resuscitation before operative control of hemorrhage versus a 62% survival (p > 0.05) in patients who received fluid resuscitation immediately.[13] If the prehospital care provider has time during transport to the hospital, IV access can be attempted. In prehospital systems in which transport to the regional trauma center exceeds 15 minutes, IV access and crystalloid resuscitation may be of some benefit in the severely hypotensive patient who is at immediate risk of an exsanguination arrest. The goal of the prehospital care provider should not be to normalize blood pressure but to maintain tissue perfusion by carefully titrating crystalloid resuscitation to maintain a systolic blood pressure of 80-90 mmHg.

Blunt Trauma

The management of the blunt trauma patient often requires a more prolonged "scene time" than the patient with penetrating injuries. Not only is there frequently some extrication time but often a need for some definitive procedure(s) while preparing to transport. The importance of prehospital "scene" and transport times in blunt trauma is more controversial than with penetrating trauma. It is classically taught that the trauma patient should receive definitive therapy in a trauma center within the first or "golden hour". This implied that a rapid scene and transport time would improve the overall survival of the trauma patient. In a recent study of the Illinois Trauma Registry, no prehospital time of less then 90 minutes exerted a detrimental effect on patient survival.[14] In a retrospective study done in Portland, Oregon, unexpected death in trauma patients occurred more frequently in those with longer field times.[15] It is recommended that the prehospital care provider expedite transport of the trauma patient after the following crucial steps: a rapid primary survey followed by airway stabilization and spine immobilization.

Definitive airway management with orotracheal intubation, particularly in the patient with significant head trauma, is thought to improve the outcome of head trauma victims. It is recommended that an airway be established, if necessary, as rapidly as possible. In the blunt trauma situation, paramedics learn a variety of techniques and contortions while intubating patients who are entrapped. These patients are frequently combative enough to make intubation difficult but not alert enough to maintain their own airway. Sedation with opioids (fentanyl, morphine) and benzodiazepines is extremely controversial. All opioids will blunt a sympathetic response in a potentially hypovolemic trauma patient. Some prehospital systems have provided a "rapid sequence protocol" for intubation in the trauma patient. If a protocol is established, med-

ications to be considered would include fentanyl (Sublimaze™) for sedation and succinylcholine (Anectine™) for paralysis.

IV Line Placement and Fluid Resuscitation

The benefit of prehospital fluid resuscitation has been a hotbed of debate among trauma surgeons and emergency medicine physicians. The first question to be answered is whether rapid crystalloid fluid infusion is of benefit to the patient. The second question is whether the time for IV placement significantly prolongs the prehospital time. In a retrospective study from the San Diego Trauma Registry of 6855 patients, there was no influence on survival with the infusion of IV fluids during prehospital transport.[16] In a study of 176 trauma patients by Thal et al. in the Dallas system with an initial SBP < 80 in whom fluid resuscitation was begun in the prehospital arena, greater than 40% had a rise in SBP > 100 upon arrival to the hospital. In the patient group that did not respond to fluids, the mortality was 43%. In the patients with an arrival SBP > 100, the mortality was 6.1%.[4] As was discussed earlier, in the situation of massive uncontrolled hemorrhage, aggressive crystalloid resuscitation may be detrimental to the patient. The issue of to what degree to "fluid resuscitate" the blunt trauma patient is still being studied.

Many studies have quoted prehospital IV placement times in the range of 8-12 minutes.[17,18] Unfortunately, most of these studies are retrospective and the IV placement time has been equated with the total scene time. In a panel discussion by well-known trauma surgeons, Dr. Aprahamian states "the surgery community must get involved in medical control and paramedic training. Twelve minutes of an IV is a measure of incompetence."[4] This certainly exemplifies the dogmatic approach and misquoting of field statistics that has clouded the issue on the appropriate trauma patient care.

In a prospective study in Denver, a third person (nonparamedic) was assigned to determine time for IV access and total scene time. In trauma patients, 90% of IVs were successfully placed on the first attempt with an average time of placement of 2.2 minutes. Prehospital on-scene times for a trauma patient with an IV placed averaged 11 minutes.[19]

The value of IVs remains to be determined and is multifunctional. Little harm can be done to the patient if the IV is placed en-route to the hospital and fluids titrated to maintain tissue perfusion.

Pitfalls

A major pitfall in the prehospital evaluation is failure to recognize the severity of the trauma. Frequently, in the early stages of hemorrhagic shock, normal vital signs can be misleading. Major fractures (pelvis, femur) resulting in massive hemorrhage are often not evident to the prehospital care provider. The field provider must consider mechanism of injury, damage to the vehicle (if MVA), and death or major injury of any other individuals in the accident. It is extremely important not to minimize potential injuries.

Another pitfall occurs when the prehospital care provider gets "lost" in his or her stabilization and treatment of the trauma patient, thus wasting valuable time. As time has already been discussed earlier in this chapter, it will suffice to mention that training and retraining with an emphasis on the expeditious evacuation philosophy is extremely valuable in combating this pitfall.

Evaluation of the trauma patient under the influence of alcohol or drugs can be misleading to the prehospital care provider. These patients often do not localize pain appropriately and can appear deceivingly "normal". In addition, these patients add to an already difficult situation by frequently being combative and uncooperative with examination and procedures. It is helpful to educate the EMT/paramedic on how to deal with the combative trauma patient. A protocol should be developed for treating combative, disruptive trauma victims. Rapid tranquilization can be achieved with drugs, such as Haldol or Droperidol, that many EMS systems do not currently use.

Finally, a common pitfall for both prehospital and hospital personnel is the failure to recognize the trauma victim as a person. In hurrying to assess, stabilize, and transport the patient, there is often a failure to talk to the patient, reassure him or her, and explain what can be expected during the trauma resuscitation. Thus a frightening experience reaches terrorizing proportions. A few moments of reassurance and explanation go a long way toward making the trauma patient's experience tolerable.

Does the Patient Need a Trauma Center?

With the creation of regional trauma centers in the 1970s, it has become the role of the prehospital care provider to rapidly and accurately identify those patients whose severity of injury warrants the resources of a trauma center. Treatment of trauma patients in hospitals that are specifically equipped and staffed for the treatment of the trauma patient (trauma center) has been shown to reduce morbidity and mortality.[20,21] While an effective prehospital system delivers major trauma victims to a trauma center, it should also avoid overloading the trauma centers with minor injuries. The accurate triage of trauma victims is often challenging in that it must be done rapidly and is often based on information that may not be readily available at the scene. Many parts of the country are rural and do not offer alternatives to taking a patient to a trauma center. The decision is most difficult when the trauma center would require a much longer transport and longer field time. In these situations the decision must be made by discussion with the medical command physician.

Trauma Scoring

A variety of trauma scoring systems have been used in the prehospital setting. Although trauma scores are useful in predicting who will die, they do not identify possible survivors of major trauma and cannot be used alone to identify those patients who will benefit from care in a trauma center.[22]

Text continued on p. 169.

SAMPLE STANDING ORDERS / PROTOCOLS

Protocols and standing orders are crucial in the timely care of the trauma patient. During a "load and go" situation, the prehospital care provider cannot take time to contact the medical command facility and wait for orders. Standing orders for trauma patients should remain simple and straightforward, enabling the EMT/paramedic to minimize scene time. As stated previously, the EMT/paramedic has few responsibilities to the trauma patient before initiating transport. The standing orders/treatment protocols must provide for airway management, spine immobilization (may be optional in some penetrating trauma patients), and possibly establishment of IV access en-route to the hospital. Some examples of potential protocols are as follows:

S A M P L E   P R O T O C O L S
TRAUMA

GENERAL GUIDELINES FOR ALL TRAUMA PROTOCOLS:

1. MAXIMUM allowable time on-scene for all trauma protocols is 10 MINUTES. Scene times over 10 minutes MUST have documentation on trip sheet explaining circumstances (e.g., extrication or access problem).
2. Patients who meet regional trauma triage guidelines as listed below MUST be transported to the appropriate trauma center, considering patient preference, transport time, and specific specialty services.
3. TRAUMA CENTER NOTIFICATION—It is the responsibility of the field team to ensure trauma centers are given ample warning of the impending arrival of these patients. Trauma teams require some minutes to assemble, prepare equipment, ensure blood is immediately available, etc. Neglect of the important function of notification may jeopardize the patient's welfare and lead to major complications.

REGIONAL PREHOSPITAL TRAUMA TRIAGE GUIDELINES

Time and distance are extremely important variables to consider when triaging injured patients to local hospitals or trauma centers. Patients who meet the following guidelines and are within 15-minutes transport time to an accredited trauma center should be strongly considered for transport directly to that center. In the rural environment, an injured patient may be at a substantial distance from a trauma center. Such patients may be treated initially at the nearest JCAHO-approved (24-hour physician coverage) emergency facility.

PROTOCOL: MAJOR OR MULTI-SYSTEM TRAUMA

INDICATIONS

All patients who meet trauma triage guidelines.

EXCLUSION

Cardiac Arrest—use Traumatic Cardiac Arrest Protocol.

TIME

10-minute on-scene time maximum unless extrication or other extenuating circumstances.

PROTOCOL

1. Ensure SAFETY of personnel at scene.
2. PRIMARY TRAUMA SURVEY—Treat critical conditions:
   A. AIRWAY: ENSURE PATENCY—INTUBATE if obstructed or patient unable to protect. Maintain in-line stabilization of C-spine—use orotracheal, nasotracheal (only if no evidence of mid-facial or basilar skull fracture), digital (only if totally unresponsive), or lighted-stylet methods.
   B. BREATHING: OXYGEN face mask at 10-15 L. ASSIST VENTILATION and INTUBATE as appropriate.
   C. CIRCULATION: CONTROL *SEVERE* EXTERNAL BLEEDING with constant direct pressure. In case of life-threatening hemorrhage, tourniquet is appropriate only as a last resort.
3. IMMOBILIZE patient on long spine board with rigid cervical collar and head immobilizer.
   NOTE In cases of blunt trauma, place PASG on long spine board before patient and finish applying while en-route. The PASG should *not* be used in cases of penetrating chest trauma. Command physician discretion will determine use for penetrating trauma to the abdomen.
4. INITIATE RAPID TRANSPORT IF "LOAD and GO" SITUATION EXISTS:
   - Unrelieved airway obstruction
   - Major chest injury or respiratory distress
   - Shock
   - Decreased level of consciousness
   - Cardiac or respiratory arrest
5. SECONDARY SURVEY (Perform en-route if "load and go" situation present.)
6. IV 14 G or 16 G LR Maxidrip—two lines if possible.

(continued)

(continued)

A. Run wide open under pressure for 1 L if tachycardic or signs of poor perfusion, then reassess. Pressure infuse if patient is hypotensive.

B. If no signs of poor perfusion, no tachycardia, and no hypotension, give 250 cc bolus then run IV at KVO.

7. CONTACT MEDICAL COMMAND
   - Command MD will advise regarding—
     - Airway management
     - IVF administration
     - PASG inflation
     - Use of ANALGESIA when appropriate.
       (This will usually be nitrous oxide per investigational protocol)

8. RE-EVALUATE patient every 3-5 minutes en-route and update Command before arrival.

PROTOCOL: HEAD TRAUMA

NOTE

The goals of this protocol are—

1. To maintain the airway and circulatory status of the head-injured patient and protect the spine.
2. To record an initial neurological examination.
3. To institute measures that may reduce intracranial pressure.
4. To rapidly transport patients who may require neurosurgical intervention.

INDICATIONS

All patients with head injuries who—

1. Are unresponsive to verbal stimuli or exhibit major alteration in mental status.
2. Have a Glasgow coma score (GCS) of 13 or less or deteriorate more than 1 point on the GCS.
3. Exhibit unilateral or bilateral flexor response (decorticate posturing) or extensor response (decerebrate posturing) to pain.
4. Develop unequal pupils with a decreased level of consciousness.
5. Exhibit focal neurological deficits.

EXCLUSIONS

Systolic blood pressure less than 100 or other signs of poor perfusion or significant bleeding, of if any evidence of major non-CNS injury, use Protocol Major Trauma.

PROTOCOL

1. AIRWAY: Ensure airway patency and adequate ventilation. OXYGEN 15 L/min. Suction must be readily available. INTUBATE immediately if unable to maintain airway patency or adequate ventilation. (Use Endotracheal Intubation procedure protocol.) Give LIDOCAINE 1 mg/kg IV push 3 minutes before attempt whenever possible. Maintain in-line stabilization of cervical spine.
2. IMMOBILIZE C-spine with rigid collar, head immobilization device, and backboard.
3. BEGIN TRANSPORT to closest trauma center.
4. CONTACT COMMAND. Request EMS physician response if warranted.
5. IV LR Maxidrip KVO—unless patient develops hypotension or other sign of shock, then run IVF 500 cc and contact Command Physician. Check Chemstrip.
6. Document SERIAL VITAL SIGNS, GCS, and NEUROLOGICAL EXAMS. Monitor pulse oximetry and ECG.
7. If patient has signs of brain herniation (unresponsive or progressively decreasing level of consciousness with unilateral dilated, non-reactive pupil or asymmetric motor function), gently HYPERVENTILATE (about 16 ventilations/minute) with 100% oxygen. INTUBATE as soon as possible.

PROTOCOL: SPINAL CORD INJURY

NOTE

The goals of this protocol are—
1. Maintenance of ventilation and perfusion.
2. Prevention of further injury by proper handling.
3. Transport of the patient to a trauma center.

INDICATIONS

1. Neck pain or any loss of motor or sensory function after any trauma or injury.
2. Decreased level of consciousness with evidence of head injury or other trauma.
3. Mechanism suggestive of potential spine injury, such as—
   - MVA
   - Blunt facial trauma
   - GSW near midline
   - Fall

EXCLUSION

Patients who meet criteria for Protocol Major Trauma.

PROTOCOL

1. SUPPORT AND REASSURE PATIENT. Explain all procedures. Make no definitive comments regarding prognosis, extent of injury, etc. MANUALLY IMMOBILIZE C-spine until adequately secured.
2. AIRWAY—OXYGEN face mask at 10-15 L. ASSIST VENTILATION and INTUBATE as appropriate. Maintain strict in-line stabilization during procedure.
3. ASSESS PERFUSION:
   - ADEQUATE PERFUSION—IV large bore LR at slow-moderate rate.
   - POOR PERFUSION (altered mentation, cool extremities, hypotension), then immediately institute following measures:
     A. Apply and inflate PASG suit.
     B. Run LR wide open for 2 L; start second IV if possible. Monitor lung sounds and respiratory status.
     C. Rapidly but carefully IMMOBILIZE and EXPEDITE TRANSPORT to nearest trauma center.
4. EXTRICATE WITH CARE—IMMOBILIZE with rigid C-collar and head immobilization device on long spine board with PASG.
5. DOCUMENT carefully initial and subsequent neurological exam findings.
6. TRANSPORT gently to closest trauma center.
7. Contact medic command to notify trauma center and command physician. Possible further orders include—
   - Dopamine drip.
   - Additional IVF.
   - Small dose of epinephrine IV.

PROTOCOL: CHEST TRAUMA

PROTOCOL: FLAIL CHEST

INDICATIONS

Patients with blunt chest trauma who have—
1. Tachypnea, dyspnea, or respiratory distress, *and*
2. Paradoxical motion of a segment of their chest wall or other evidence of multiple rib fractures.

PROTOCOL

1. OXYGEN face mask at 15 L if airway patent and air exchange adequate. Otherwise INTUBATE with in-line

(continued)

(continued)

cervical stabilization.

2. MONITOR for TENSION PNEUMOTHORAX:
   - Decreasing blood pressure associated with worsening dyspnea, unilateral decreased breath sounds, and often increasing resistance to ventilation.

   If signs of tension pneumothorax present, perform NEEDLE DECOMPRESSION of chest (per procedure protocol).
3. PERFORM SPINAL IMMOBILIZATION AND EXPEDITE TRANSPORT to nearest trauma center.
4. STABILIZE the flail segment using pillow, folded sheet, towel and tape, or sandbags.
5. IV LR large-bore KVO; run wide open if hypotension or signs of shock.
6. Contact medical command.

PROTOCOL: SUCKING CHEST WOUND

INDICATIONS

Patient with any penetrating chest wound.

PROTOCOL

1. OXYGEN face mask at 10-15 L as needed to maintain pulse oximetry > 94%. ASSIST VENTILATION and INTUBATE as appropriate. In-line cervical stabilization if appropriate.
2. SEAL WOUND with occlusive dressing at end of exhalation. Leave one side of dressing untaped to function as a one-way pressure relief valve.
3. MONITOR FOR TENSION PNEUMOTHORAX: Decreasing blood pressure associated with worsening dyspnea, unilateral decreased breath sounds, increasing resistance to ventilation.
   A. If signs of tension pneumothorax develop, LIFT OCCLUSIVE DRESSING to allow air to escape.
   B. If this does not relieve the tension pneumothorax, perform NEEDLE DECOMPRESSION of chest (per procedure protocol).
4. PERFORM SPINAL IMMOBILIZATION IF INDICATED AND EXPEDITE TRANSPORT to nearest trauma center.
5. IV LR large bore KVO; run wide open if hypotensive or signs of shock.

PROTOCOL: TENSION PNEUMOTHORAX

INDICATIONS

Patients with signs of PNEUMOTHORAX associated with SHOCK or HYPOTENSION.

NOTE

Pneumothorax should be suspected in patients with chest trauma with dyspnea, tachypnea, or respiratory distress and any of these conditions:
1. Absent or diminished breath sounds on one side.
2. Tracheal deviation.
3. Subcutaneous emphysema, rib fracture, or chest wall deformity.
4. Worsening compliance while assisting ventilation.

PROTOCOL

1. OXYGEN face mask at 10-15 L as needed to maintain pulse oximetry > 94%. ASSIST VENTILATION and INTUBATE as appropriate.
2. Perform NEEDLE DECOMPRESSION of chest per procedural protocol.
3. Reassess ventilation. INTUBATE if inadequate airway or air exchange.
4. PERFORM SPINAL IMMOBILIZATION AND EXPEDITE TRANSPORT to trauma center.
5. CONTACT medical command.
6. IV LR large bore—run wide open if signs of inadequate perfusion; otherwise KVO.
7. Frequently reassess patient for recurrence of pneumothorax. Repeat needle decompression may be necessary.

PROTOCOL: EXTREMITY FRACTURE/DISLOCATION

INDICATIONS

Suspected fractures or dislocation in extremity.

EXCLUSIONS

1. Major trauma
2. Acute medical problem
3. Airway compromise or signs of shock

PROTOCOL

1. PERFORM PRIMARY AND SECONDARY SURVEY, including neurological and vascular exam of extremity distal to injury.
2. If patient stable, use NITROUS OXIDE (per Investigational Protocol) for ANALGESIA BEFORE SPLINTING or MANIPULATION of the injured area.
3. IV LR large bore KVO if femur fracture, multiple fractures, or if needed to administer analgesia.
4. SPLINTING: Attempt to splint in position found, particularly if the fracture is open and there is gross deformity. If grossly deformed limb cannot be splinted in place, apply traction until sufficient reduction to permit splinting.
   A. TRACTION splint for isolated femur fracture
   B. PASG (inflated) for pelvis or femur fracture
5. CHECK DISTAL CIRCULATION (color, temperature, capillary refill, and pulses) BEFORE AND AFTER SPLINTING.
6. Remove all rings and constricting clothing on the affected limb if possible.

7. ANALGESIA option:
   A. Morphine Sulfate 2-5 mg IV per dose, titrated to effect.
8. If vascular compromise exists distal to injury, command physician may instruct on application of traction and reduction (straightening) of injured limb to improve perfusion.

PROTOCOL: AMPUTATIONS

NOTE

This protocol addresses the problem of amputation of body parts and attempts to facilitate the preservation of tissue and the delivery of the patient to a trauma center with expertise in microsurgical techniques for replantation. Although great advances have been made in reconstructive techniques, field team members are reminded that only the surgical team is qualified to estimate the outcome of reconstruction. This often requires microscopic examination in the operating room. Therefore, EMS personnel must not make any comment to the patient concerning the possible outcome of the patient's injury.

INDICATION

Amputation or large avulsion of any body part.

EXCLUSIONS

Major trauma to other body systems—use other appropriate protocol and have other personnel retrieve amputated part.

PROTOCOL

1. OXYGEN 4 L NC or face mask at 10-15 L as needed to maintain pulse oximetry > 94%. ASSIST VENTILATION and INTUBATE as appropriate.
2. If patient stable, use NITROUS OXIDE (per Investigational Protocol) for ANALGESIA BEFORE SPLINTING or MANIPULATION of the injured area.
3. Control bleeding:
   A. Direct pressure and elevation.
   B. Proximal pressure point.

(continued)

(continued)

C. If profuse or if significant bleeding persists after 10 minutes of above measures, apply blood pressure cuff proximal to injury and inflate to 20 mmHg above systolic blood pressure.

4. PRESERVE ALL TISSUE, particularly amputated parts:
   A. Wrap part in sterile gauze slightly moistened with sterile saline solution and place in plastic bag.
   B. Place this bag in ice water (if available).
   C. Transport the part with the patient.
      DO *NOT*:
         Immerse parts directly in ice, saline, water, or preservative.
         Wash the part with antiseptic, e.g., Betadine, etc.
         Use dry ice for preservation.
         Place ice or cold packs directly against the part—immerse them in the water.

5. NOTIFY MEDIC COMMAND to alert receiving facility and contact command physician.
6. Monitor bleeding and vital signs en-route to the hospital.
7. Do not delay transport while searching for lost amputated part; have another crew or other responsible personnel do this.
8. IV LR Maxidrip KVO.

9. ANALGESIA option:
   A. Morphine Sulfate 2-5 mg IV per dose, titrated to effect.

PROTOCOL: EXTRICATION

INDICATIONS
All patients who are trapped, impaled, or who are at risk of the crush syndrome.

PROTOCOL
1. ENSURE safety of all personnel at scene.
2. OXYGEN face mask at 10-15 L as needed to maintain pulse oximetry > 94%. ASSIST VENTILATION and INTUBATE as appropriate.
3. SUPPORT cervical spine with rigid collar or manual stabilization if indicated (neck pain or tenderness or mechanism of injury).
4. PROTECT PATIENT from weather, rescue operations, and other hazards as possible.
5. Initiate IV LR large bore with regular drip tubing at moderate flow rate.
6. CONTACT MEDICAL COMMAND
   ■ Command MD will advise regarding—
   ■ Airway management
   ■ IVF administration
   ■ PASG inflation
   ■ Use of ANALGESIA when appropriate. (This will usually be Nitrous Oxide per Investigational Protocol)
   ■ SODIUM BICARBONATE for large crush injuries (before release)
7. If limb entrapped and crushed, place BP cuff (inflated to 20 mmHg above systolic pressure) proximal to injury before releasing.
8. During extrication, monitor vitals, level of consciousness, respiratory and cardiovascular status, and ECG as possible.
9. If cardiovascular collapse occurs following release of crushed area, give SODIUM BICARBONATE 100 mEq IV push.
10. Upon extrication, IMMOBILIZE on long spine board with rigid cervical collar and head immobilization device if any potential of spinal injury. Apply but do not inflate PASG.
11. Expedite transport to Trauma Center and provide update on patient status while en-route.

Text continued from p. 162.

Most prehospital systems base the trauma triage decision on a combination of an injury score with the mechanism of injury and the judgment of the EMT/paramedic.

The CRAMS (circulation, respiration, abdomen, motor, speech) scale is a popular prehospital trauma scoring system. It is easy to remember and can be applied rapidly. Most major systems that use the CRAMS score as part of the triage decision use a score of 8 or below to determine which patients should be transferred to a trauma center. Patients with a CRAMS score of 4 or below have been shown to have a higher survival rate when treated at a trauma center.

THE CRAMS SCORE

	Score
Circulation	
normal capillary refill and SBP > 100	2
delayed capillary refill or SBP 85-100	1
no capillary refill or SBP < 85	0
Respiration	
normal	2
abnormal (labored or shallow)	1
absent	0
Abdomen	
abdomen and thorax nontender	2
abdomen and thorax tender	1
abdomen rigid or flail chest	0
Motor	
normal	2
responds only to pain	1
no response (or decerebrate)	0
Speech	
normal	2
confused	1
no intelligible words	0

The Revised Trauma Score (RTS) by Champion is another prehospital scoring system for trauma.[23] It is based upon the GCS in combination with respiratory rate and systolic blood pressure. The revised trauma score provides more accurate scoring for patients with severe head trauma; however, it is more difficult than the CRAMS score for prehospital care providers to remember and calculate.

REVISED TRAUMA SCORE

GCS	SBP	RR	Value
13-15	>89	10-29	4
9-12	76-89	>29	3
6-8	50-75	6-9	2
4-5	1-49	1-5	1
3	0	0	0

Mechanism of injury is an important component of the triage decision on trauma patients and should be used in combination with the trauma score. Some of the more common mechanisms used as indicators for patients requiring a trauma center include[24]—

- Major damage to vehicle
- Falls > 15 feet
- Space intrusion
- Vehicle rollover
- Pedestrian struck
- Motorcycle with injury
- Extrication > 20 minutes
- Death of other passenger

A study by the San Diego Trauma Registry found increased sensitivity for predicting the injury severity score (ISS > 15) when one of the above mechanisms was combined with a CRAMS score <8.[25] The mechanism alone that was most sensitive in predicting severe injury was death of a passenger.

An underappreciated and underemphasized factor in trauma triage decision making is the judgment of both the prehospital care provider and the medical command physician. As the EMT/paramedic gains experience in the field, he or she learns to rely as much on judgment as on trauma scoring to aid in triage. Although judgment is useful in triaging a patient to a trauma center who otherwise would not have met criteria, the reverse is not true. Judgment should never override trauma scoring and mechanism in diverting a patient away from a trauma center.

Summary

Management of trauma in an efficient, well-organized fashion by prehospital care providers can have a major effect on patient morbidity and mortality. Only two factors have ever been shown to improve the trauma patient's survival rate: airway management and rapid transport to a trauma center. Above all else, it is the responsibility of the medical command physician to stress the importance of time and provide personnel with concise standing orders and protocols. Only then can we strive to reach the ultimate goal of the "golden 10 minutes" of prehospital care and optimize the trauma patient's chance of survival.

SAMPLE CASES

CASE #1

A 54-year-old male sustains a gunshot wound to the neck. Upon arrival of prehospital team (1 paramedic, 1 EMT), the patient is lying supine, unresponsive. A large wound is noted over the left lateral neck and a smaller wound in the right posterior neck. On primary survey, respirations are shallow but there are equal breath sounds bilaterally. A large amount of blood is exiting the wound on the left neck. Although the patient moans occasionally, there is no response to painful stimuli. A carotid pulse is present in the right neck. No brachial pulse is palpable. ETA to the hospital (driving time) = 5 minutes.

MANAGEMENT

Using standing orders, the patient is placed on a stretcher, supine and ventilation is assisted while in-line stabilization is applied to the neck. The primary survey is completed by one of the paramedics, and the EMT has realized that the patient's airway seems to be secured and intubation is attempted. It is realized that there is significant blood in the posterior pharynx. It is a relatively short distance to the trauma center and transport is done expeditiously while direct pressure is applied to the neck to minimize bleeding.

The patient is also placed in a slightly head-down position to prevent the possibility of an air embolus occurring from the large veins in the neck.

Scene time: 6 minutes
Transport time: 4 minutes

DISCUSSION

Overall, the treatment in this case was fairly good. Any patient who has sustained the force of a gunshot wound to the neck or face should have C-spine immobilization performed. In this case, it would have been easiest for the person at the head to apply in-line stabilization, since a collar would have prevented them from being able to apply direct pressure to the wound. An attempt at intubation is not unreasonable; however, with the transport time less than 5 minutes to the trauma center, it would have been most efficient to bag the patient until a controlled intubation could have been performed in the ED.

CASE #2

A 23-year-old female is the unrestrained driver in a single vehicle MVA. No other victims are present. The patient is entrapped on the driver's side. Her head is slumped back against the headrest and she is moaning. She does respond to questioning, but her answers are slurred. She spontaneously complains of her chest hurting. The rescue unit and 2 paramedics are at the scene. While the rescue team works on freeing her legs from under the dashboard, a paramedic opens the passenger door and slides across the seat to perform a primary survey. There is crepitance of the right chest wall with marked tenderness. The patient has decreased breath sounds on the right. The patient does respond spontaneously, but there is a strong odor of alcohol on her breath. There is a palpable brachial pulse, rate 140, blood pressure of 80 dilatation, and respiratory rate of 36.

MANAGEMENT

While extrication is in progress, the paramedic applies oxygen by face mask to the patient and initiates a 14 gauge IV with LR running wide open. Once extrication is completed, the patient is immobilized. At this time, her respiratory distress has worsened. The paramedic prepares to intubate. The patient is orotracheally intubated, and placement of the tube is confirmed. There are absent breath sounds on the right. The patient is loaded into the ambulance. Estimated transport time is 15 minutes. Repeat SBP in vehicle is 70/P. Report is given to the command physician. Understanding that the paramedics still have 15 minutes with the patient and the clinical picture is that of a tension pneumothorax, the command physician orders the paramedics to insert a 14 gauge IV catheter into the third intercostal space at the midclavicular line on the right. Although uncomfortable with this procedure, the medics proceed and the lung is decompressed with marked hemodynamic improvement. The remaining transport is without incident.

Scene time: 18 minutes
Transport time: 16 minutes

DISCUSSION

This blunt trauma case was managed appropriately by both the paramedics and the medical command physician. The primary survey was performed efficiently while the patient was still being extricated. The paramedics took advantage of the extrication time to initiate therapy with oxygen and IV fluids. Although the protocol calls for initiation of an IV en-route to the hospital, the paramedics were thoughtful enough to use time that would otherwise have been wasted to begin fluid resuscitation. A definitive airway was placed before initiating transport. En-route, they encountered a tension pneumothorax. Although needle decompression is not part of the standard protocol, with encouragement and directions from the command physician, they were able to successfully complete the procedure. This flexibility on the part of both the pre-hospital team and the command physician is important due to the variety of situations encountered. It is essential that the command physician remain calm and give simple, straightforward instructions.

References

1. Budnick LD, Chaiken BP: The probability of dying of injuries by the year 2000, *JAMA* 254:3350-3352, 1985.

2. Stewart RD: Prehospital care of trauma: The Golden Ten Minutes ... 55th Annual Meeting of The Royal College of Physicians and Surgeons of Canada.

3. Campbell JE: Critical trauma situations: Load and go. In Campbell JE, Alabama ACEP, editors: *Basic trauma life support for paramedics and advanced EMS providers,* ed 3, Englewood Cliffs, NJ, 1995, Brady.

4. Kennedy FR, Gonzalez P, Beitler A, et al.: Incidence of cervical spine injury in patients with gunshot wounds to the head, *South Med J* 87(6):621-623, 1994.

5. Stewart RD: Tactile orotracheal intubation, *Ann Emerg Med* 13(3):175-178, 1984.

6. Murray J, Thomas S, Weebel S: Digital endotracheal intubation for patients unsuitable for laryngoscopy in the EMS helicopter, *PDM* 10(Suppl):S70, 1995.

7. Border JR, Lewis FR, Aprahamian C, et al.: Panel: pre-hospital trauma care: stabilize or scoop and run, *Trauma* 23:708-711, 1983.

8. Goss E, Landau E, Assalia A, et al.: Is hypertonic saline resuscitation safe in uncontrolled hemorrhagic shock?, *J Trauma* 28:751-756, 1988.

9. Bickell WH, Bruttig SP, Millnamow GA, et al.: The detrimental effects of intravenous crystalloid after aortotomy in swine, *Surgery* 110:529-536, 1991.

10. Kowalenko T, Stern S, Dronen S, et al.: Improved outcome with hypotensive resuscitation of uncontrolled hemorrhagic shock in a swine model, *J Trauma* 33:349-353, 1992.

11. Stern SA, Dronen SC, Birrer P, et al.: Effect of blood pressure on hemorrhage volume and survival in a near-fatal hemorrhage model incorporating a vascular injury, *Ann Emerg Med* 22:155-163, 1993.

12. Gross D, Landau EH, Klin B, et al.: Quantitative measurement of bleeding following hypertonic saline therapy in "uncontrolled" hemorrhagic shock, *J Trauma* 29:79-83, 1989.

13. Bickell WH, Wall MJ, Pepe PE, et al.: Immediate versus delayed fluid resuscitation for hypotensive patients with penetrating torso injuries, *N Engl J Med* 331:1105-1109, 1994.

14. Petri RW, Dyer A, Lumpkin J: The effect of prehospital transport time on the mortality from traumatic injury, *Prehosp Disaster Med* 10(1):24-29, 1995.

15. Ferro S, Hedges JR, Simmons E, et al.: Does out-of-hospital EMS time effect trauma survival?, *Am J Emerg Med* 13:133-135, 1995.

16. Kaweski SM, Sise MJ, Virgilio RW: The effect of pre-hospital fluids in trauma patients, *Trauma* 30:1215-1219, 1990.

17. Gervin AS, Fischer RP: The importance of prompt transport in salvage of patients with penetrating heart wounds, *J Trauma* 22:443-448, 1982.

18. Smith JP, Bodai BI, Hill AS, et al.: Prehospital stabilization of critically injured patients: a failed concept, *J Trauma* 25:65-70, 1985.

19. Pons PT, Moore EE, Cusick JM, et al.: Prehospital venous access in an urban paramedic system: a prospective on-scene analysis, *J Trauma* 28:1460-1463, 1988.

20. Cales RH: Trauma mortality in Orange County: the effect of implementation of a regional trauma system, *Ann Emerg Med* 13:1-10, 1984.

21. West JG, Trunkey DD, Lim RC: Systems of trauma care: a study of two counties, *Arch Surg* 114:445-460, 1979.

22. Kilberg L, Clemmer TP, Claussen J: Effectiveness of implementing a trauma triage system on outcome: a prospective evaluation, *J Trauma* 10:1493, 1988.

23. Champion HR, Sacco WJ, Copes WS: A revision of the trauma score, *J Trauma* 29:623, 1989.

24. Alred L: Role of EMS helicopter. In Campbell JE, editor: *Basic trauma life support: advanced prehospital care,* Englewood Cliffs, N.J., 1988, Prentice Hall.

25. Baxt WG, Berry CC, Epperson MD, et al.: The failure of prehospital trauma prediction rules to classify trauma patients accurately, *Ann Emerg Med* 18(1):1-8, 1989.

13

Obstetrical and Gynecological Prehospital Emergencies

It is important for the medical command physician to have a well-established knowledge of obstetrics and gynecology to appropriately guide treatment and management of these patients in the field. Most prehospital obstetrical cases will be unremarkable with minimal interventions required, such as oxygen and an IV line. Some cases however, such as imminent delivery or severe vaginal bleeding, can be very challenging clinical encounters. For the prehospital care provider, prehospital deliveries are not uncommon and can have the potential for significant complication with associated morbidity and mortality.[1]

Training of most EMT-Ps is minimal for obstetrical emergencies, and their field experience is variable, especially for complicated cases. Taking care of an obstetrical or gynecological emergency can be stressful and demanding on the prehospital personnel. The amount of stress and anxiety that a situation produces will be dependent on the prehospital care provider's previous experiences, level of training, type of equipment carried, and medical command support. The tone of the prehospital care provider's voice over the radio can be the first indicator that a difficult situation is in progress. A knowledgeable medical command physician can alleviate some of the anxieties of the prehospital care provider, as well as provide needed medical guidance for these patients. Understanding these extreme situations can help to improve the patient's outcome and help prehospital personnel deal with the stressful and sometimes overwhelming situation.

Prehospital Evaluation

Important historical and physical information should be obtained by the prehospital care providers. If the patient is pregnant, information such as number of previous pregnancies and deliveries, due date, previous perinatal complications, membrane rupture, contraction onset, duration and interval, and vaginal bleeding should be sought. Physical findings, such as vital signs, fetal movement, and heart rate, should also be part of the

WILLIAM J. ANGELOS, MD, FACEP

TABLE 13-1 Differential Diagnosis of Vaginal Bleeding

Characteristic	Considerations
PREGNANT PATIENT	Ectopic pregnancy, threatened AB, placenta previa, abruptio placenta, bloody show
NONPREGNANT PATIENT	Ectopic pregnancy, dysfunctional uterine bleeding, degenerating fibroid, menses, trauma, cancer, hyperplasia

TABLE 13-2 Differential Diagnosis of Abdominal Pain

Characteristic	Considerations
OB/GYN RELATED	Ectopic pregnancy, PID, torsion of the ovary, degenerating fibroid, threatened AB, ruptured ovarian cyst, endometriosis
OB/GYN NON-RELATED	Gastroenteritis, appendicitis, cholecystitis, SBO, PUD, gastritis, diverticulitis, perforation, peritonitis

report that prehospital care providers obtain. If there is a history of precipitous delivery or the patient has the urge to push or is pushing, examination of the introitus should be performed. If there is a presenting part and the patient is pushing, delivery is imminent and the prehospital care provider should prepare to deliver the baby.

It is important for the prehospital care provider to recognize and treat problems that arise during pregnancy, labor, and delivery. Bleeding and abdominal pain are common complaints during pregnancy and can be from a variety of etiologies. Knowing what trimester the patient is in will help narrow the differential diagnosis (Table 13-1).[2] The medical command physician should aggressively treat bleeding in pregnancy (all trimesters) and consider the potential for hypovolemia.

Women of child-bearing age who present with abdominal pain can have a wide spectrum of etiologies (Table 13-2).[3] The physician who is giving medical command should develop a working diagnosis and supportive plan from the information that is supplied by the prehospital care provider. This plan should be explained to the field personnel caring for the patient, especially if subtle etiologies are being considered.

Pregnant Patient

Preeclamptic/Eclamptic Patient

The prehospital care provider has limited resources in the field to treat a preeclamptic or eclamptic patient. An IV line should be established, as well as oxygen by a non-rebreather mask. If the patient is seizing, 5-10 mg of diazepam should be ordered IV at a rate of 2 mg/min. If

there is no IV access, diazepam can be given rectally with a syringe and angiocath (5-10 mg). Newer formulations of diazepam can also be administered IM. If the medic unit carries magnesium, it should be given to all preeclamptic patients with a diastolic pressure of greater than 100 with symptoms (headache, visual complaints, RUQ pain) and all eclamptic patients (Box 13-1). Four grams of 10% magnesium sulfate in 250 cc of D5W IV can be given safely over 15 minutes.[4] Special attention should be made to maintaining an airway and for rapid transport to the hospital. If no IV access can be established, 5 grams of magnesium can be given IM.[5]

Pregnant Trauma Patient

The pregnant trauma patient should be treated with special consideration. BTLS should be carried out accordingly with high-flow oxygen, immobilization, and large bore IVs. The pregnant patient's physiology is different from that of a non-pregnant patient, and these differences should be known to the medical command physician. In the last trimester the blood volume has increased 50% above

BOX 13-1 Signs and Symptoms of Preeclampsia

- Systolic blood pressure greater than 160
- Diastolic blood pressure greater than 110
- Increasing pedal edema
- Headache
- Epigastric/RUQ abdominal pain

baseline, the heart and respiratory rate have also increased by 10% to 15%, blood pressure is lower, and cardiac output is increased (Box 13-2).[6] Because of the increase in blood volume, signs of shock may occur later than normal or be absent with considerable amount of blood loss.[7,8] Gastric motility is also decreased, which increases the risk of vomiting and aspiration.

All pregnant trauma patients in the second and third trimester should be transported in the left lateral decubitus position. This can be accomplished after the patient is immobilized on a long spine board by lifting the right side of the board approximately 15 degrees with blankets or sand bags. This position allows for the uterus to be moved off the inferior vena cava and facilitates blood return to the heart to maintain uterine flow.[8,9] If at all possible, fetal heart tones should be assessed by the medics without delaying transport. Usually the heart tones can be heard with a stethoscope after 20 weeks of gestation. Variation of normal fetal heart tones (normal = 120-160) may be the first sign that maternal circulation is compromised, as well as indicate fetal hypoxia. If vaginal bleeding is present, the possibility for uterine rupture or placental separation is likely.[7,9] In this situation the prehospital care provider should not perform a digital vaginal exam because of the potential to aggravate the condition.

Use of PASG has a limited role in the trauma pregnant patient. If there are signs or symptoms of hypovolemia, the PASG can be inflated on the legs only but are of unkown value in this situation. PASG can also be used to splint lower extremity fractures as needed.[7,9]

Arrested Pregnant Patient

Resuscitation methods for the arrested pregnant patient are different for the nonpregnant patient. The prehospital care provider should "load and go" with interventions and resuscitation measures en-route. The success of emergent cesarean section in the ED correlates directly with the length of time the patient has been in arrest. Communication with the obstetrician and a neonatal resuscitation team should be made regarding the possibility of a C-section. If available, subspecialty team members should be prepared to meet the patient in the ED. Being prepared and ready in the ED will give the neonate every possible chance of survival. There are reported cases of good neurological outcome of the neonate if the C-section is done promptly within the first 15 minutes of the arrest.[10-12]

Imminent Delivery

All women who are in active labor should have oxygen by face mask applied and a large bore IV line of a crystalloid solution established, which usually can be done en-route to the hospital. Every effort should be made to ensure delivery in the hospital. When the prehospital care provider calls for command, it is important for the physician to get the appropriate information, as well as remind the field team to expedite transport if possible. Understandably, not all patients will be amenable to being moved to the back of the ambulance as the delivery is advancing; however, it should be explained to the patient that if there is a problem with the delivery, help is only a drive away. Only truly imminent deliveries justify prehospital deliveries. All too often the prehospital care provider will state that they have an imminent delivery and call back to command 45 minutes later when the infant is born! Paramedics should not wait around for delivery but should be reminded what constitutes a true imminent delivery (Box 13-3). The practice of waiting for the "delivery" should be discouraged.

If a delivery is about to take place, it is important for the prehospital care providers to be prepared emotionally and technically. Most experienced paramedics will have been involved in some aspect of a delivery in the past. Although they may have previous knowledge and expe-

---

BOX 13-2 Physiological Changes in Pregnancy

- Blood volume increased greater than 50% of baseline
- Heart rate increased 10% to 15%
- Respirations increased 10% to 15%
- Cardiac output increased
- Blood pressure lower or normal

BOX 13-3 Signs and Symptoms of Imminent Delivery

- Presenting part is visible at the introitus
- Patient has urge to push
- Increasing bloody show
- Bulging perineum

rience, a delivery can be challenging, and the physician giving medical command must help alleviate anxiety, as well as give technically accurate information. An area should be designated for resuscitation of the neonate, and appropriate airway equipment should be ready.

The delivery in most cases will progress with little intervention. Once the head is delivered, the nares and mouth should be suctioned out with a bulb syringe unless there is meconium. The umbilical cord should be double clamped and divided after the remaining body is delivered. The baby should be immediately dried and evaluated.

Prolapse of the Umbilical Cord

There are several potential complications associated with vaginal deliveries. One such complication is the prolapse of the umbilical cord.

If the prehospital care provider reports the umbilical cord is prolapsed while the patient is in labor, the provider should be instructed not to push the cord back into the vagina. The prehospital care provider should wrap the cord in sterile gauze, which should be moistened with sterile saline or water. It is recommended to keep the presenting part off the pelvic brim.[13] You can instruct the prehospital care provider to insert two fingers of a sterile gloved hand into the vagina and lift the presenting part off the bony pelvis. The patient should be placed in a knee-chest position to allow gravity to help take pressure off the cord. This will improve umbilical blood flow and reduce the chance of hypoxia to the neonate. This maneuver should be done while in transit to the hospital and by no means should it delay transportation. It is important to remind the prehospital crew to stabilize the patient on the stretcher when in the knee-chest position. If the delivery is imminent, then the prehospital care providers should proceed as discussed earlier.

Nuchal Cord

Another complication of vaginal deliveries is a nuchal cord. If there is an umbilical cord wrapped around the fetus' neck, the prehospital care provider should be instructed to attempt to gently lift the cord over the head. If the cord is tight and cannot be lifted over the neonate's head, the prehospital care provider should suction out the oral pharynx and nares before double clamping and cutting the cord. By doing this maneuver, the airway is cleared and allows the neonate to breathe on its own.

Meconium

If thick meconium is present, the prehospital care provider should be instructed to suction out the hypopharynx with a bulb syringe. The prehospital care provider should be told not to stimulate the neonate so that respirations are not initiated. Once the delivery is complete the prehospital care provider should intubate the neonate and suction through the endotracheal tube as it is being withdrawn from the airway. This procedure should be continued until the majority of the meconium has cleared or the newborn becomes bradycardic (<80 bpm). The provider should not bag the neonate or stimulate it until the meconium is cleared. In some cases the provider will be in a situation where meconium is not totally clear and the neonate has become bradycardic. In this case the prehospital care provider will need to ventilate and oxygenate the infant. Endotracheal intubation is not required if watery or thin meconium is present. The provider's skill and the equipment available will determine how much airway control will be achieved. The medical command physician should know in advance what the prehospital system is capable of and make medically sound decisions based on this information.

Breech

The problem that arises with a breech presentation is that the presenting part does not adequately dilate the cervix, making spontaneous delivery difficult. Morbidity and mortality is significantly higher even if delivery occurs in the labor and delivery room of a hospital.[14] It is almost impossible to give proper instructions over the radio for a breech delivery. The best approach is to have the paramedics support the presenting part, letting the delivery occur spontaneously. When the head presents, the paramedics can place two fingers forming a V into the vagina to allow the neonate to breathe. Simultaneously, the paramedics should move the patient into the back of the ambulance for expeditious transport. Oxygen should be administrated to the mother, and an IV line should be established en-route to the hospital. They should not push the presenting part back into the vagina but allow the delivery to proceed spontaneously.

Shoulder Dystocia

In most deliveries the shoulders will be delivered easily. If the shoulders by chance become impeded, the prehospital care providers can apply mild suprapubic pressure (not fundal pressure). This maneuver alone will occasionally relieve the dystocia. If suprapubic pressure by itself does not work, you can instruct the prehospital care provider to rotate the shoulders while suprapubic pressure is being applied. This can be accomplished by having the provider apply two fingers on the front part of the top shoulder (anterior) and rotate the neonate toward the back into an oblique position.[15,16] The success of freeing of the shoulders will depend primarily on the experience of the prehospital care provider and the ability of the physician to provide precise instruction.

If at all possible, have the prehospital care provider get the patient into the ambulance early before delivery problems arise. This will allow him or her to drive for help and experience.

Post Delivery

Care of the Neonate

Once the umbilical cord is divided, the neonate should be placed in a supine, head-down position with the head turned to the side. Normally, the newborn begins to breathe and cry almost immediately after birth. If respirations do not occur or are infrequent, suction of the mouth and pharynx should be performed. Also, stimulating the feet or back may initiate breathing. The neonate should be dried and kept warm. If the neonate is stable, the infant can be held close to the mother's chest to decrease heat loss.

A helpful method in evaluating the newborn's condition is using the 1- and 5-minute Apgar scores (Table 13-3). Scores between 4 and 6 at 1 minute may indicate a mildly- to moderately-depressed infant; whereas scores below 3 represent a severely depressed infant.[17] If warming and stimulating the neonate do not initiate the infant's respirations, the prehospital care provider will need to resuscitate the infant. First, the prehospital care provider should place the infant on oxygen and assess the patient's color and respiratory status. If respiratory status does not pick up, it may be necessary to start bag-valve-mask ventilation of the neonate until spontaneous respirations occur. If a bradycardia exists despite adequate ventilation, chest compression should be initiated. Chest compressions can be performed by having the provider place both thumbs on the lower third of the sternum with fingers wrapped around the torso in support of the back.[18] The thumbs should be positioned side by side on the sternum just below the line of the two nipples. The sternum is compressed, ½ to ¾ of an inch downward and at a rate of approximately 120 times per minute. If the neonate's respiratory and heart rates and color do not improve with chest compression, the neonate will need to be intubated. If this does not correct the situation, medications may be warranted. Epinephrine is indicated if spontaneous heart rate is less than 80 beats per minute despite adequate ventilation with 100% O_2 and chest compressions. The dose is 0.01 to 0.03 mg/kg of 1/10,000 solution. This can be given down the endotracheal tube.

TABLE 13-3 Apgar Chart

Sign	0	1	2	Score 1 minute	Score 5 minutes
Appearance (skin color)	Blue, pale	Body pink, extremities blue	Completely pink		
Pulse rate (heart rate)	Absent	Below 100	Above 100		
Grimace (irritability)	No response	Grimaces	Cries		
Activity (muscle tone)	Limp	Some flexion of extremities	Active motion		
Respiratory (effort)	Absent	Slow and irregular	Strong cry		
			TOTAL SCORE =		

IV access is difficult in the prehospital setting on a neonate, and time should not be delayed trying to establish IV access. An alternative would be to establish an IO line if drugs and fluid are needed to resuscitate. The prehospital care provider should be reminded that if he or she is having difficulties with the infant or mother, get the patient into the vehicle and transport to the closest appropriate facility.

Postpartum Hemorrhage

Blood loss greater than 500 cc after the third stage of labor is considered abnormal. Even after delivery, bleeding can occur anywhere along the reproductive tract. Bleeding at the placenta is usually controlled by uterine contractions. Usually, early postpartum bleeding is either from uterine atony or lacerations to the genital tract (Box 13-4).[19] If bleeding is significant, the providers should establish a line of crystalloid and give a large bolus of fluid with reassessments of the patient's vitals.

A quick abdominal exam should be performed to evaluate the uterus. If the uterus is soft and boggy, this suggests uterine atony. If the uterus is firm and contracted, the source of bleeding is most likely a laceration of the genital tract. Unfortunately, these findings are often difficult to discern in the field. Prehospital treatment is mainly IV crystalloids and oxygen. The prehospital care provider should expedite transportation of the patient to the hospital.

Delivery of the Placenta

In most cases, the placenta will deliver spontaneously. The prehospital care provider should not wait around for delivery of the placenta but transport the mother and neonate to the hospital. Physical signs that the placenta is about to be delivered are that the uterus becomes globular in shape, the umbilical cord lengthens, and there may be a gush of blood just before to the delivery. If the placenta is delivered before arrival at the hospital, the placenta should be saved for pathological evaluation.

Vaginal Bleeding

The Pregnant Patient

As mentioned earlier, all pregnant patients should be placed on high-flow oxygen and have an IV line of a crystalloid solution. The amount of bleeding and the change in vital signs will determine how much fluid you will need to give. If the vital signs are stable (appropriate for pregnancy) and minimal blood loss has occurred, a 300-400 cc bolus should be ordered. If there are unstable vitals, moderate-to-severe bleeding, or even subjective complaints (i.e., lightheaded, dizzy), a larger bolus, preferably using a pressure bag, should be given until the vital signs are corrected or symptoms improved. Instruct the prehospital care provider to recheck vitals after the fluid bolus and report the results. It is important to err on the side of too much volume than not enough in these patients. Supportive care is the major prehospital concern, and transport to an appropriate hospital should be expedited for the unstable patient.

Abdominal Pain With Vaginal Bleeding

All patients of child-bearing years with abdominal pain and vaginal bleeding should be treated as possible ectopic pregnancies until proven otherwise.[20-22] The prehospital care provider should be instructed to establish two large bore IV lines with LR or NS and to administer oxygen by mask. A modest bolus of 500 cc during transport is good prehospital care as long as there is no underlying cardiac or renal disease, and it should be ordered even if vitals are within normal limits. Evidence of bradycardia on physical exam may be a sign of intraperitoneal blood and would warrant more aggressive fluid resuscitation. If there are signs of hypovolemia, the PASG suit would be another alternative to increase blood pressure and possibly reduce the amount of intraperitoneal bleeding.

Vaginal Bleeding Without Pain

The lack of abdominal pain with vaginal bleeding does not mean that the patient has no urgent condition. Vaginal bleeding alone can be lifethreatening, and this should be explained to the paramedics. All patients should be

---

BOX 13-4   Differential Diagnosis

Early Postpartum Hemorrhage
- Uterine atony
- Laceration of the genital tract
- Retained placenta
- Uterine rupture
- Uterine inversion

placed on oxygen and an IV line established with a crystalloid solution. A fluid bolus of 500 cc should be given en-route depending on the estimated blood loss and the vital signs. Remember that for every 1 cc of blood loss, 3 cc of crystalloid is needed to replace intravascular volume. Obviously if vitals are unstable or there are symptoms of hypovolemia, a larger fluid bolus should be given.

Pitfalls

1. Allowing prehospital deliveries to take place when an imminent delivery is not present is a common pitfall. It is important to ask specific questions to the prehospital care providers to determine if the delivery is truly imminent. If the patient is pushing and there is a presenting part that can be seen at the introitus, then it is justified to proceed with the delivery in the field. Even if this scenario were present, it is recommended to at least have the patient in the back of the ambulance. If there is a problem with the delivery, the prehospital care provider can drive to the hospital expeditiously.

2. If a delivery is to take place out of hospital, not having the prehospital care provider equipped for airway management or resuscitation could be problematic. The airway kit should be open with the appropriate blades and endotracheal tubes. Also remind them to have the suction readied. A card with neonatal doses of medications should be with the paramedics and physician. If there is a need for an airway and resuscitation, everything should be immediately available.

3. Failure to consider ectopic pregnancy in women of child-bearing years with abdominal pain with or without vaginal bleeding can be a serious oversight. All women of child-bearing years with abdominal pain should have oxygen and an IV line established. Not all ectopic pregnancies will initially have vaginal bleeding. Also the blood pressure and pulse can be normal initially and signs of shock delayed. Giving a modest fluid bolus to a young healthy woman will not be harmful.

4. Failure to transport a pregnant third trimester trauma patient in the left lateral decubitus position. There will be a time when a prehospital care provider consults you panicked with a trauma patient who is pregnant and has a blood pressure of 70/40. Granted there is always the potential for hypovolemia, but the simple maneuver discussed here may be all that is needed.

5. The medical command physician inappropriately triaging the patient is another potential pitfall. If a situation occurs where your facility is not capable of handling the patient and there is a facility that can (without significant transport delay), the patient should be diverted. It is extremely important that communicate immediately with the receiving facility.

6. Failure to communicate early with the obstetrician or the neonatal personnel can also be problematic. In certain situations, (i.e., abnormal presentation) it is important that the obstetrician, as well as the neonatologist, be contacted immediately so that they are ready and hopefully waiting for the patient when the ambulance arrives. Time should not be wasted by waiting for the patient to arrive first. It is better to overestimate the situation than to underestimate and waste valuable minutes.

Summary

Most prehospital management of obstetrical and gynecological problems in the field will be uneventful but have potential for complications. It should be made routine that oxygen be administered and an IV line established on all women of child-bearing age who have symptoms of gynecological or obstetrical origin. All effort should be made to have in-hospital deliveries. In some instances, it will be unavoidable to have a prehospital delivery. The EMS command physician can reduce the prehospital complication with good judgment and direction. Also the EMS command physician can be involved with continuing education for the prehospital care provider with reviewing obstetrical and gynecological emergencies, as well as neonatal resuscitation with both formal and informal lectures.

S A M P L E   C A S E S

CASE # 1

A 23-year-old female GIPO who is 38 weeks pregnant with no prenatal complications and noticed contractions 3 hours ago that are now 3 minutes apart. The prehospital care provider states that there is no presenting part and the membranes haven't ruptured.

Command physician responds: Establish an IV line of LR at KVO en-route, administer high-flow oxygen by mask, and expedite transport.

DISCUSSION:

This case is an example of uncomplicated, early labor. The patient is a primigravida with only contractions and no sign of impending delivery. The paramedics should expedite transport and can perform their interventions on the way to the hospital.

CASE # 2

27-year-old female G5P4 who is 39 weeks pregnant and has a history of precipitous deliveries and now has the urge to push. The infant's head can be seen at the introitus. The membranes ruptured 30 minutes ago with the onset of contractions.

Command physician responds: Instruct the prehospital care provider to set up for an imminent delivery. High-flow oxygen by mask should be administered and, if possible, an IV of crystalloid solution. Also the prehospital care provider should be instructed to have an area set up for neonate resuscitation. After delivery, the cord should be double clamped and cut, and the neonate should be wrapped in a blanket and given to the mother. If the infant is stable, the mother should be instructed to hold it close to her chest to diminish heat loss. The prehospital care providers should expedite transport after delivery. The placenta can be delivered en-route or at the hospital.

DISCUSSION:

It is obvious that the delivery is going to occur within minutes. It cannot be stressed enough that the prehospital care providers should be prepared for this event. If possible, have the paramedics get the patient into the back of the ambulance so that if any problems arise, they can easily begin transport to the hospital.

CASE # 3

25-year-old female GOPO who developed abdominal pain and slight vaginal bleeding. This pain and bleeding

is not typical for her menses and her last period was 7 weeks ago. All vital signs are stable.

Command physician responds: Establish a large bore IV line of crystalloid and run in 500 cc en-route. Also administer oxygen by mask and reconsult if there is a change in vitals or new symptoms.

DISCUSSION:

All women of child-bearing years with abdominal pain with or without vaginal bleeding should be considered to have an ectopic pregnancy. Remember that most ectopic pregnancies present with normal blood pressure and heart rate. Don't be fooled! Have your prehospital care providers start a large bore IV and give a modest bolus of fluid. If the vital signs are unstable, the PASG suit would be appropriate.

CASE #4

35-year-old female restrained driver who is 35 weeks pregnant and is complaining of lower extremity pain and neck pain after hitting a telephone pole. Vitals—BP 70/P HR 100 RR 24.

Command physician responds: Immobilize the patient with a cervical collar and long spine board, establish 2 large bore IVs of crystalloid, high-flow oxygen by mask and expedite transport. Instruct the prehospital care provider to place the patient in the left lateral decubitus position while transporting and to reassess the vitals. Also a bolus of fluid would be appropriate and the amount would depend on whether the BP corrected with moving the patient in the left lateral decubitus position.

DISCUSSION:

All pregnant trauma patients in the second and third trimester should be transported in the left lateral decubitus position. Also the pregnant patient's physiology is different, which can confuse the picture. Remember that blood volume and blood cells are increased and signs of shock may appear late.

CASE #5

23-year-old female GIPO who is 36 weeks pregnant notices that her legs are more swollen over the past few days and complains of a headache. The BP is 160/100 HR-100 RR-24 and has no previous history of hypertension.

Command physician responds: place the patient on high-flow oxygen by face mask and establish an IV of crystalloid. Caution should be made not to load the patient with fluids. Explain to the prehospital care provider that this is a serious condition and transport should be done expeditiously with seizure precautions.

DISCUSSION:

It is difficult to make the diagnosis of preeclampsia in the field. There are no medications that most prehospital care providers carry that are approved for lowering the BP in a pregnant patient. If the diastolic blood pressure is above 100 and the patient has no prior history of hypertension, the prehospital care provider can give magnesium if their unit carries it and the transport time is long (> 30 mins). For the most part, the prehospital care is rapid transport with interventions en-route.

CASE #6

27-year-old female G1P0 whom the prehospital care provider found seizing at home. The seizures have been going on for 15 minutes. The blood pressure is 220/110.

Command physician responds: The prehospital care provider should be instructed to maintain an airway and to administer high-flow oxygen by mask. An IV line should be rapidly started, and 5 mg of Valium should be given through the IV line over 2½ minutes. If the seizures do not stop after 2 minutes, another 5 mg should be given. Special attention should be made for maintenance of the airway, as well as rapid transport to the hospital.

DISCUSSION:

Lifesaving interventions for the mother and fetus are to control the seizure and reduce the blood pressure. Valium and magnesium are temporizing measures. The patient needs to be transported to the hospital as rapidly as possible. The definitive treatment for eclampsia is delivery of the baby. Communication should be made early with the obstetrician and neonatal team while the patient is being transported.

REFERENCES

1. Verdile VP, Tutsock G, Paris PM, et al.: Out of hospital deliveries, a five-year experience, *Prehosp Disaster Med* 10:10-13, 1995.

2. Green-Thompson RW: Antepartum hemorrhage, *Clin Obstet Gynecol* 9(3):479-515, 1982.

3. Staniland JR, Ditchburn J, DeDombal FT: Clinical presentation of acute abdomen: study of 600 patients, *Br J Med* 3:393-398, 1972.

4. Pritchard JA: Management of preeclampsia and eclampsia, *Kidney Int* 18:259-266, 1980.

5. Sibai BM, Graham JM, McCubbin JH: A comparison of intravenous and intramuscular magnesium sulfate regimens in preeclampsia, *Am J Obstet Gynecol* 150:728, 1984.

6. Cruikshank DP: Anatomic and physiologic alterations of pregnancy that modify the response to trauma. In Buchsbaum HJ, (editor): *Trauma in pregnancy,* Philadelphia, 1979, WB Saunders.

7. Pearlman MD, Tintinalli JE: Evaluation and treatment of the gravida and fetus following trauma during pregnancy, *Obstet Gynecol Clin North Am* 18:371, 1991.

8. Lavery JP, Staten-McCormick M: Management of moderate to severe trauma in pregnancy, *Obstet Gynecol Clin North Am* 22:69, 1995.

9. Neufield JD, Moore EE, Marx JA, et al.: Trauma in pregnancy, *Emerg Med Clin North Am* 5:623, 1987.

10. Weber CE: Postmortem cesarean section: review of the literature and case reports, *Am J Obstet Gynecol* 110:158, 1971.

11. Katz VL, Dotters DJ, Droegemueller W: Perimortem cesarean delivery, *Obstet Gynecol* 68:571, 1986.

12. Lopez-Zeno JA, Carlo WA, O'Grady JP, et al.: Infant survival following delayed postmortem cesarean delivery, *Obstet Gynecol* 76:991, 1990.

13. Barnett WM: Umbilical cord prolapse: a true obstetrical emergency, *J Emerg Med* 7(2):149-152, 1989.

14. DeGrespigny LJC, Pepperell RJ: Perinatal mortality and morbidity in breech presentation, *Obstet Gynecol* 53:141, 1979.

15. Resnik R: Management of shoulder girdle dystocia, *Clin Obstet Gynecol* 23:559-564, 1980.

16. Woods CE: A principle of physics as applicable to shoulder delivery, *Am J Obstet Gynecol* 45:796, 1943.

17. Drage JS, Berendes H: Apgar scores and outcome of the newborn, *Pediatr Clin North Am* 13:635-642, 1966.

18. Todres ID, Rogers MC: Methods of external cardiac massage in the newborn infant, *J Pediatr* 86:781-782, 1975.

19. Watson P: Postpartum hemorrhage and shock, *Clin Obstet Gynecol* 23:985-1001, 1980.

20. Jones EE: Ectopic pregnancy: common and some uncommon misdiagnoses, *Obstet Gynecol Clin North Am* 15:55, 1991.

21. Abbott JT, Emmans L, Lowenstein SR: Ectopic pregnancy: ten common pitfalls in diagnosis, *Am J Emerg Med* 8:515, 1990.

22. Gonzales FA, Waxman M: Ectopic pregnancy: a prospective study on differential diagnosis, *Diag Gynecol Obstet* 3:101-109, 1981.

SUGGESTED READINGS

Carson BS, Losey RW, et al.: Combined obstetric and pediatric approach to prevent meconium aspiration syndrome, *Am J Obstet Gynecol,* 126:712-715, 1976.

Farnell RG: *OB/GYN emergencies: the first 60 minutes,* Rockville, MD, 1986, Aspen Publications.

Higgins SD: Emergency delivery: prehospital care, emergency department delivery, perimortem salvage, *Emerg Med Clin North Am* 5(3):540, 1987.

Taber B: *Manual of gynecological and obstetric emergency,* Philadelphia, 1984, WB Saunders.

SAMPLE PROTOCOLS
OBSTETRICAL EMERGENCIES

DEFINITIONS

Crowning: Bulging of fetal head through perineum such that the cervix is stretched around the entire circumference of the fetal head. This should be evaluated *during a contraction.*

Eclampsia: Preeclampsia associated with generalized seizure(s); seizure may be preceded by hyperreflexia or visual changes.

First trimester: First 3 months of pregnancy.

Hypertension of pregnancy: Blood pressure ≥ 140/90 in pregnant woman not previously hypertensive; usually occurs in third trimester of first pregnancy and may progress to preeclampsia or eclampsia.

Labor: Regular, rhythmic cramping pains in back and abdomen due to uterine contractions that occur at least every 5 minutes and last at least 30 seconds. The three stages of labor are—
1. Cervical dilation.
2. Delivery of fetus.
3. Delivery of placenta.

Malpresentation: When presenting part (i.e., first part of fetus to deliver out the birth canal) is not the head.

Meconium: Fetal feces present in amniotic fluid; if aspirated by fetus can cause airway obstruction or severe pulmonary complications.

Placenta previa: Part or all of placenta lies over cervical opening of uterus; this may lead to catastrophic hemorrhage (without pain) when labor begins or if disrupted by manual examination.

Placental abruption (abruptio placentae): Premature separation of placenta from uterine wall, usually in late third trimester or early labor; very painful; bleeding may be contained inside uterus; may lead to catastrophic hemorrhage.

Preeclampsia: Condition of unknown etiology that generally occurs in third trimester of first pregnancy, involving new onset of hypertension (>140/90) during pregnancy associated with protein loss in urine and edema of hands and face. May lead to renal, liver, and CNS dysfunction.

Rupture of membranes: Painless breakage of amniotic sac before birth leading to small, uncontrollable gush of fluid from vagina. Also called "bloody show" or "water broke".

Third trimester: Last 3 months of pregnancy.

PROTOCOL: LABOR PAINS

NOTES:
1. The important differential in these patients are—
   ▪ If first trimester, threatened abortion vs. ectopic pregnancy.
   ▪ If third trimester, imminent vs. delayed delivery and preterm vs. full term.
   ▪ Complications—prolapsed cord, malpresentation, meconium aspiration, excess hemorrhage.
2. Thus, the following must be determined quickly in all patients:
   A. Number of previous pregnancies.

B. Gestational age.

C. Complications of this pregnancy.

D. Presence of vaginal bleeding and nature of pain.

E. Frequency, duration, and time of onset of contractions.

F. Whether rupture of membranes (water broke) occurred. If so, determine color of fluid—thick, dark green indicates meconium.

3. Predicting the time of delivery is virtually impossible. Because of this, the potential necessity for surgical intervention for complications of pregnancy and delivery, and the need for patient privacy, the patient should be transferred to the ambulance as quickly as feasible.

PROTOCOL: FULL-TERM—IMMINENT DELIVERY

INDICATIONS

Presence of *all* following conditions:

1. Gestation of 36 or more weeks.

2. Contractions consistently less than 3 minutes apart (measure interval between *start* of contractions) and last at least 1 minute.

3. Either crowning is present or mother feels strong urge to push (feels like she will have a bowel movement).

EXCLUSIONS

1. Prolapsed cord—see Protocol 602-A.

2. Malpresentation—see Protocol 602-B.

PROTOCOL

1. Place mother supine, OXYGEN by nasal cannula and, if time and personnel allow, initiate IV LR KVO. If mother's "coach" or significant other present, position him or her at mother's head.

2. Remove pants and undergarments, place pillow under mother's buttocks, or position buttocks near edge of bed to allow room for delivery.

3. Explain delivery process to mother and ensure her of your competence and readiness.

4. Visually EXAMINE PERINEUM for crowning, prolapsed cord, malpresentation, bleeding (crowning can only be determined during contraction).

5. Coach mother to bear down during contraction.
Use one hand, covered with clean towel, to apply gentle upward pressure on posterior perineum/anus of mother. Place other hand over vagina to exert gentle downward pressure on head to avoid explosive delivery.

6. After head delivers, it will spontaneously turn to one side. During this phase, USE BULB SYRINGE TO SUCTION *MOUTH FIRST* THEN *NARES,* and wipe face with towel.

   * Purpose is to clear airway before first breath. Do mouth first since doing nares stimulates respiration.

   * Do *not* suction *nares* if meconium present. This is so trachea can be suctioned before first breath—see Protocol 602-C—Meconium Aspiration.

7. Use index finger to CHECK FOR NUCHAL CORD (umbilical cord encircles neck). If present, gently unwrap it before fetus delivers further. If cannot unwrap, clamp and cut cord at this time.

8. Assist delivery of anterior shoulder by gentle downward traction on head, then posterior shoulder by elevating the head.

9. Carefully maintain hold on infant as delivery is completed. Hold infant slightly below mother's vagina for about 20 seconds to allow full infusion of blood from placenta, then clamp and cut cord.

   *Do not raise infant above level of placenta until cord clamped.
PROCEDURE FOR CUTTING CORD:
Place one clamp about 8 inches from newborn and second clamp about 2-3 inches further away from newborn. Use sterile scissors or scalpel to cut cord between clamps. Inspect ends of cord for bleeding, and apply additional clamps if needed.

(continued)

(continued)

10. CARE OF NEWBORN:
    A. Ensure adequate respiratory effort—STIMULATE by rubbing back or tickling feet if necessary. Administer blow-by OXYGEN. If central cyanosis or poor respiration persists, SUCTION airway and assist ventilation. First few ventilations may require relatively high pressure. INTUBATE if unable to adequately ventilate.
    B. Gently wipe entire body DRY and WRAP in warm blankets.
    C. Position on side, head slightly down to allow drainage of secretions; allow mother to hold if possible.
    D. Assess APGAR (1 and 5 minutes, if possible) and pulse oximetry.

Apgar Chart

Sign	0	1	2	Score 1 minute	Score 5 minutes
Appearance (skin color)	Blue, pale	Body pink, extremities blue	Completely pink		
Pulse rate (heart rate)	Absent	Below 100	Above 100		
Grimace (irritability)	No response	Grimaces	Cries		
Activity (muscle tone)	Limp	Some flexion of extremities	Active motion		
Respiratory (effort)	Absent	Slow and irregular	Strong cry		
			TOTAL SCORE =		

11. POST-DELIVERY CARE OF MOTHER:
    A. Observe for massive hemorrhage. Monitor vital signs. IV LR regular drip 250 cc bolus then slow drip. If signs of hypovolemia, give IVF wide open and contact command physician.
    B. Observe for delivery of placenta—usually 5-10 minutes after delivery of fetus but may be 20-30 minutes.
       *Do not delay transport while waiting for placenta to deliver.
    C. Signs of placental separation are a spontaneous lengthening of cord and small gush of blood. At this time, *gentle* traction can be applied to umbilical cord as placenta delivers. Place placenta in plastic bag and give to hospital personnel.
       DO NOT PULL ON CORD.
12. Contact command physician as early as possible; request response of EMS physician if needed.
13. Transport to appropriate facility.

PROTOCOL: FULL-TERM—NON IMMINENT DELIVERY

INDICATIONS
1. Gestation of more than 36 weeks.
2. Contractions *more* than 3 minutes apart.
3. *Absence* of crowning or strong urge to push.

EXCLUSIONS
1. Prolapsed cord—see Protocol 602-A.
2. Vaginal hemorrhage—see Protocol 602-B.

PROTOCOL

1. Obtain baseline OBSTETRICAL HISTORY as described in introduction to Protocol 601.
   If patient feels abnormal sensation or foreign body in perineal area, contractions occur more frequently than every 3 minutes, or vaginal bleeding or ruptures of membranes occurs, then with precautions to protect patient privacy, *VISUALLY* EXAMINE PERINEUM for prolapsed cord, crowning, malpresentation, hemorrhage (crowning can only be determined during contraction).
2. TRANSPORT in position of comfort. If patient prefers to lie down or if evidence of supine hypotensive syndrome, place in left lateral recumbent position or elevate right side.
3. En-route, apply OXYGEN and initiate IV LR regular drip KVO.
4. Contact command physician.

PROTOCOL: PRETERM LABOR

INDICATIONS

1. Gestation less than 36 weeks.
2. Sustained contractions (at least every 5 minutes).

EXCLUSIONS

1. Prolapsed cord—see Protocol 602-A.
2. Vaginal hemorrhage—see Protocol 603-B.

PROTOCOL

1. Obtain baseline OBSTETRICAL HISTORY as described in Introduction to Protocol 601. *VISUALLY* EXAMINE PERINEUM for prolapsed cord, crowning, malpresentation, hemorrhage.
2. If more than 20 weeks gestation, place in left lateral recumbent position.
3. Initiate IV LR regular drip KVO and administer OXYGEN.
4. Contact command physician and TRANSPORT to appropriate facility.
5. If delivery occurs, provide neonatal care per Protocol 601-A, step #10.
   A. Protect against hypothermia, respiratory depression, and hypoglycemia.
   B. Viability is considered 500 gm—if status in doubt, initiate resuscitation.

6. Possible orders (designed to inhibit labor):
   A. IVF bolus (1-2 L).
   B. Morphine sulfate 3-5 mg IVP.
   C. Albuterol 2.5-5.0 mg aerosol.
   D. Magnesium sulfate 4 gm in D_5W 250 cc IV over 20 minutes.

PROTOCOL: COMPLICATIONS OF DELIVERY

PROTOCOL: PROLAPSED UMBILICAL CORD

NOTE

When umbilical cord precedes fetus through birth canal, it is likely to be compressed between fetal head and maternal pelvis, leading to severe fetal ischemia.

INDICATIONS

Any pregnant patient with protrusion of any part of umbilical cord through cervix.

PROTOCOL

1. Place mother in TRENDELENBURG OR KNEE-CHEST POSITION. Apply high-flow OXYGEN.
2. Insert two fingers of gloved hand into vagina, and lift fetal head off cord; head may be pushed *gently* back up into birth canal slightly.

(continued)

(continued)

Ensure effectiveness of maneuver by palpating pulse in cord.

NOTE: Pulse in cord represents *fetal* heart rate. Rate *less than 120* indicates fetal distress.

Do not remove hand until transfer of care to hospital personnel.

3. IMMEDIATE, RAPID TRANSPORT TO APPROPRIATE FACILITY.
4. En-route:
   A. Contact command physician and consider rendezvous with EMS physician if long transport.
   B. Cover exposed cord with saline-moistened dressings.
   C. Initiate IV LR regular drip KVO.

PROTOCOL: MALPRESENTATION (BREECH OR LIMB PRESENTATION)

INDICATION

1. Patient in labor with visible malpresentation.
2. Patient in labor with malpresentation suspected through prenatal care.

PROTOCOL

1. Obtain OBSTETRICAL history per Protocol 601.
2. *If delivery is not in progress,* TRANSPORT RAPIDLY TO APPROPRIATE FACILITY in Trendelenburg position with elevation of the right side.
3. *If delivery has begun or is imminent,* position patient as for normal delivery (Protocol 601-A):
   Contact command physician and request EMS physician response.
   A. *BREECH (buttocks or lower extremities first):*
      - Support buttocks/legs as delivered. Be patient—do not pull.
      - Once body is delivered, apply gentle upward traction to body to assist delivery of head.
      - If head does not deliver in 5 minutes, place two fingers of gloved hand between neonate's face and birth canal to allow air entry for neonate to breathe.
        If this occurs, transport rapidly to high-risk neonatal facility.
        Maintain "airway" en-route and provide supplemental oxygen (place end of O_2 tubing in vagina between fingers).
   B. *FACE/BROW/SHOULDER/ARM PRESENTATION:*
      - Face first *may* proceed as normal delivery.
        Any other presentation (and face first if delivery does not progress as usual) requires RAPID TRANSPORT TO HIGH-RISK OBSTETRICAL FACILITY.

PROTOCOL: MECONIUM ASPIRATION

INDICATIONS

Meconium in amniotic fluid before delivery of fetus; this appears as dark green, thick material in amniotic fluid or on infant upon delivery.

PROTOCOL

1. Upon noting presence of meconium, contact Command and request EMS physician response.
2. Upon delivery of head, SUCTION MOUTH *but not nares* with bulb syringe. Avoid stimulating neonate to breathe.
3. Upon completion of delivery, INTUBATE (tube size = 3.5, blade size = 1) and SUCTION through endotracheal tube BEFORE VENTILATION.
4. Carefully check for proper tube placement and VENTILATE neonate. First few breaths may require higher than expected pressure.
5. Carefully SUCTION nares and oropharynx.
6. Assess APGAR (see Chart in Protocol 601-A) and pulse oximetry.
7. TRANSPORT to appropriate facility.

PROTOCOL: MASSIVE VAGINAL HEMORRHAGE

INDICATIONS
Persistent active large volume vaginal bleeding after or during delivery.

NOTE
This is usually due to uterine atony, uterine rupture, birth canal trauma, or retained products of contraception.

PROTOCOL
1. Place in Trendelenburg position.
2. High-flow OXYGEN and IV LR regular drip large bore—begin 500 cc bolus wide open.
3. Gently MASSAGE UTERUS (one hand above fundus near umbilicus, other hand below fundus above pubic symphysis).
4. Assist with delivery of placenta per Protocol 601-A.
   Be sure to collect all tissues delivered for inspection at receiving facility.
5. RAPID TRANSPORT to appropriate facility.
6. If patient develops clinical signs of hypovolemic shock, continue IVF wide open. Start second IV if possible.
7. Contact command physician as early as possible.

PROTOCOL: COMPLICATIONS OF PREGNANCY

PROTOCOL: HYPERTENSIVE EMERGENCIES: PREECLAMPSIA AND ECLAMPSIA

INDICATIONS
Patients in third trimester of pregnancy who were normotensive before pregnancy and now have BP >140/90; this may be associated with edema of hands and face. This usually occurs during patient's first pregnancy.

NOTE
Definitive treatment is delivery of fetus. Thus, rapid transport indicated.

PROTOCOL
1. Take OBSTETRICAL HISTORY per Protocol 601 and inquire whether patient has been diagnosed with hypertension of pregnancy or preeclampsia. Perform neurological exam (hyperreflexia and visual changes indicate imminent seizure).
2. Place patient in comfortable position—elevate right side if supine.
   Administer OXYGEN and initiate IV saline lock. Check glucose level by Chemstrip.
3. If patient has generalized (grand mal) seizure:
   A. Ensure adequate ventilation and oxygenation. Protect airway.
   B. Administer MAGNESIUM SULFATE 1 g/min IV push until seizure stops. Dilute each gram in 10 cc IVF. Maximum dose is 4 gm.
4. Initiate transport and contact command physician.
   Monitor vitals, airway and neurological status en-route.

5. Possible additional orders include—
   A. For uncontrolled seizure:
      - Valium 5 mg IV slow push (may be repeated as needed).
      - Additional magnesium sulfate.
      - Intubation.
   B. For BP >160/110 (not seizing):
      - Magnesium sulfate 4 gm in D_5W 250 cc IV over 10-20 minutes.
      - NTG 0.4 mg sublingual or spray.

(continued)

(continued)

PROTOCOL: BLEEDING/ABDOMINAL PAIN DURING PREGNANCY:

INDICATION

Patient in any stage of pregnancy who has vaginal bleeding *or* steady (nonlabor) abdominal pain.
First trimester: Ectopic pregnancy, miscarriage.
Third trimester: Placenta previa, placental abruption.

NOTE

Bleeding or abdominal pain during any stage of pregnancy may involve life-threatening hemorrhage. Etiology depends on the stage of pregnancy:

PROTOCOL

1. Take OBSTETRICAL HISTORY per Protocol 601.
2. Place supine (right side elevated if >20 weeks gestation).
   VISUALLY EXAMINE PERINEUM for prolapsed cord, crowning, malpresentation. If bleeding present, assess rate and nature (venous vs. arterial) of active bleeding and presence of any tissues.
3. Administer OXYGEN and IV LR regular drip KVO.
4. *If signs of shock present,* initiate RAPID TRANSPORT to nearest appropriate facility. Start IVs en-route and run IVF WIDE OPEN.
5. Contact Command Physician.
   Start second IV en-route if possible.
   Monitor patient and vitals closely for signs of shock.

14

Pediatric Emergencies

Although pediatric calls account for only 10% of ambulance runs[1], they provoke a disproportionate degree of concern and anxiety for prehospital care providers and, in turn, the medical command physician. Approximately one half of pediatric ambulance runs are for trauma: motor vehicle accidents and other injuries, with the other half for medical complaints: seizures, respiratory illnesses, fever, ingestions, altered mental status, and arrests.[1-3] There is also a bimodal age distribution of the calls: 0-3 years and 13-18 years.[1] The majority of calls for children under 3 years are medical, whereas the majority of adolescent calls are trauma.[1,3]

Prehospital care providers are often uncomfortable with pediatric patients due to limited training, experience, variation in drug doses based on weight (Table 14-1), and, sometimes, inappropriate equipment. Empathy in treating ill and injured children also plays a large role. Therefore their anxiety is often expressed during radio communications, making it difficult to obtain a clear picture of the severity of the patient's condition. A medical command physician can provide guidance, improve patient outcome, and ultimately alleviate some of these anxieties.

As a medical command physician, one should also recognize that there is an underuse of medical direction for prehospital pediatric calls. Some of the reasons include lower acuity level of many younger patients, inability to recognize severity of illness, and lack of specialized call-in requirements for children.[4] A knowledgeable medical command physician should realize the problematic areas in prehospital care provider training that leads to these problems. National curricula have focused on specific illnesses (e.g., dehydration, meningitis) rather than assessment-based protocols (e.g., recognition of shock).[5] Decisions about whether rapid transport ("load and go") versus field treatment and intervention ("stay and play"), as well as triage decisions, are in a constant state of flux.[5] As the medical command physician, one should know the particular EMS system's patient illness/injury algorithms and triage rules so that cases are managed properly and consistently.[5]

Rather than concentrate on algorithms and protocols, this chapter will highlight some important issues regarding pediatric patients including patient assessment, recognition of respiratory distress, prevention of respiratory arrest, recognition and treatment of shock, trauma and trauma triage, and seizures.[6]

SUSAN M. FUCHS, MD, FAAP

Table 14-1 Emergency Medications

Medication	Dose	Maximum Single Dose	Route/ Comment
Activated charcoal	< 1 Year 1-2 gm/kg > 1 Year 25-50 gm	n/a	PO, NG tube
Adenosine	0.1 mg/kg if not effective, 0.2 mg/kg	12 mg	IV, IO rapidly
Albuterol™	unit dose vial (2.5 mg)	n/a	aerosol inhalation
Alupent™	unit dose vial (15 mg) or 0.3 cc in 2.0 cc NS	n/a	aerosol inhalation
Atropine	0.02 mg/kg	0.5 mg 0.1 mg minimum	IV, ET, IO
Benadryl™	1 mg/kg	50 mg	IV, IO, IM
Bretylium	5 mg/kg if not effective, 10 mg/kg		IV, IO
Calcium chloride (10%)	20 mg/kg	500 mg	IV, IO slowly
Dextrose (25%) Newborn (10%)	2-4 ml/kg 1-2 ml/kg		IV, IO IV, IO
Epinephrine 1:10,000 (0.1 mg/ml) 1:1000 (1 mg/ml)	IV/IO 0.01 mg/kg (1:10,000) *2nd dose 0.1 mg/kg (1:1000) ET 0.1 mg/kg (1:1000) 2nd dose 0.1 mg/kg (1:1000) SQ 0.01 mg/kg (1:1000)	0.5 mg 0.35 mg	IV, IO ET SQ
Lasix	1 mg/kg	40 mg	IV, IO
Lidocaine (1%)	1 mg/kg	100 mg	IV, IO, ET
Naloxone	0.1 mg/kg	n/a	IV, IO, ET
Sodium bicarbonate (8.4%) Newborn (4.2%)	1 mEq/kg 2 mEq/kg	n/a n/a	IV, IO IV, IO slowly
Syrup of ipecac	30 ml	n/a	PO
Valium™	IV/IO 0.1-0.3 mg/kg PR 0.5 mg/kg initial 0.25 mg/kg subsequent	10 mg 10 mg	IV, IO slowly rectal

*For cardiac arrest.

Patient Assessment

This is one area where children are truly different. An accurate assessment of a pediatric patient is the key to proper field evaluation and treatment and, in turn, appropriate on-line medical control. Initially, important (verbal) information can be obtained from the parent, child, or guardian while assessing the child's general appearance. This information is best obtained at a distance from a young child, preferably while in the parent's arms, due to stranger anxiety. A child who is smiling and playing with toys is probably not in need of aggressive ALS interventions, whereas a lethargic infant with a weak cry who doesn't react to your presence may need treatment at the scene as well as rapid transport.[7] The next steps in patient assessment are the ABCs:

A-Airway: Assessment of the patient's airway should answer the following questions: Is it patent? Is the child maintaining his or her own airway, or is assistance needed in the form of airway positioning-jaw thrust, chin-lift, oral airway, nasal airway, bag-valve-mask, or endotracheal tube?

B-Breathing: This involves obtaining a respiratory rate. The rate varies with age (it decreases with increasing age) and can be very difficult to determine in a crying child. A child in respiratory distress will usually breathe fast, but as they tire, the respiratory rate will decrease, which is an ominous sign. Note the effort the child needs to breathe, as well as the child's position. Are there nasal flaring or retractions (e.g., subcostal, intercostal, supraclavicular, suprasternal)? Is the child more comfortable sitting upright than supine? What is the child's color? Always remember that a child can be hypoxic without being cyanotic.

When one listens to the chest, are there any adventitious sounds—grunting, stridor, wheezing, rales, rhonchi, or no sounds (no air movement)?

C-Circulation: The heart rate and strength of peripheral pulses (radial) can be accomplished at the same time. Heart rate varies with age (it decreases as children get older) and can also increase with fever and anxiety. A heart rate below the normal range is worrisome and can imply impending arrest. If peripheral (radial or brachial) pulses are weak, central pulses (femoral or carotid) should be checked as a means of assessing circulation. Capillary refill, which should be less than 2 seconds in a healthy child, can be assessed with the evaluation of the temperature and color of the extremity. Cold, blue, pale, or mottled extremities indicate poor circulation and shock (note: hypothermia can also cause this). Although obtaining a blood pressure is part of the vital signs, in children it is often inaccurate because of a wrong size cuff or an uncooperative child. A normal blood pressure in the face of some of the above abnormalities should not make a prehospital care provider comfortable. In fact, hypotension in a child is a late finding of shock.

Pediatric advanced life support (PALS) includes assessment of level of consciousness (mental status) in circulatory assessment. The key is a quick assessment that is done initially as general appearance—this is a recheck. It is not necessary to memorize a pediatric (or adult) Glasgow Coma Scale, since a rapid assessment can include alert and playful, crying but consolable, crying and unconsolable even by parents, responsive to painful stimuli, alternating level of consciousness.[8]

Based on the above assessment, it should be possible for prehospital care providers to relay some useful information to the medical command physician. From this it may be possible to group the child into one of several assessment-based categories that can guide appropriate field therapy and transport guidelines.

A few points to remember regarding prehospital treatment:

1. BLS is all that is required for the majority of prehospital pediatric care. In fact, one study demonstrated that 75% of pediatric calls required evaluation and BLS care only.[1]
2. There should be frequent updates of prehospital pediatric protocols based on recent advances in pediatric emergency care.[9]
3. Often the best field ALS treatment decision is no treatment at all. When patient assessment is confusing, rapid transport with BLS interventions to a facility that can manage the patient may be the best idea.[9]

Pitfalls

1. Vital signs must be interpreted carefully in the field. Although there is great emphasis on vital signs, they can vary widely, so an overall patient assessment (respiratory effort, breath sounds, pulse quality, skin color and temperature, level of consciousness) is more sensitive and useful. If vital signs are available, they should be compared with age-related norms (Table 14-2).[9]

2. The treatment should be no worse than the disease, and field ALS treatment should avoid causing unnecessary distress or patient anxiety.[9] (While all children in respiratory distress or shock require oxygen, an IV is not required in most patients with respiratory complaints).

Recognition of Respiratory Distress: Prevention of Respiratory Arrest

In the majority of infants and children, the cause of cardiopulmonary arrest is usually respiratory in origin. Therefore, if one can learn to recognize a child in respiratory distress, the respiratory, and then cardiac, arrest can be prevented. Recognition that a child is in respiratory distress is more important than making a specific diagnosis. While there are many respiratory diseases unique to chil-

Table 14-2 Vital Signs

Age	Weight (kg)	Respiration Min–Max	Heart Rate Min–Max	Systolic Blood Pressure Min–Max	Distance (cm) Mid-Trachea to Teeth	Endotracheal Tube (Uncuffed)	Laryngoscope Blade	Suction Cath.
Premie	1-2	30-60	90-190	50-70	8	2.5-3.0	0 straight	5-6 F
Newborn	3-5	30-60	90-190	50-70	10	3.5	1 straight	6 F
6 MO	7	24-40	85-180	65-106	12	4.0	1 straight	8 F
1 YR	10	20-40	80-150	72-110	12	4.5	2 straight	8 F
3 YR	15	20-30	80-140	78-114	15	5.0	2 straight	8 F
6 YR	20	18-25	70-120	80-116	16	5.5	3 straight	10 F
8 YR	25	18-25	70-110	84-122	18	6.0 (cuffed)	3 straight/curved	10 F
12 YR	40	14-20	60-110	94-136	20	7.0 (cuffed)	3 straight/curved	12 F
15 YR	50	12-20	55-100	100-142	21	7.0 (cuffed)	3 straight/curved	12 F
18 YR	65	12-18	50-90	104-148	22	7.0-8.0 (cuffed)	3 straight/curved	12 F

dren, the underlying approach is the same: maintenance of the airway with oxygenation and ventilation.

If a child is not breathing, simple BLS procedures should be performed following current AHA guidelines for pediatrics.

1. Determine responsiveness.

2. Position child ("sniffing position").

3. Open airway (chin lift, jaw thrust).

4. Give 2 breaths.

5. If there is no chest movement, reposition the airway.

6. Give 2 breaths.

7. If there is no chest rise and fall, suspect foreign body obstruction.

8. Give 5 back blows then 5 chest thrusts in infants <1 year or 5 Heimlich maneuvers (abdominal thrusts) in children ≥1 year.

9. Remove the foreign body if visualized.

10. Open the airway and resume rescue breathing.[10]

Evaluation of the respiratory rate and effort are the first keys to determining respiratory distress. Tachypnea is often an early sign of respiratory distress. However, the normal respiratory rate varies with age, and it can also increase due to fever or fear.[8] Therefore assessment of res-

piratory mechanics and effort is also important. (It should be stressed that as much of the evaluation of the infant and young child in respiratory distress should be performed while the patient is in the parent's/guardian's arms when possible.) A child with nasal flaring or retractions (intercostal, subcostal, supraclavicular) is in distress, as is an infant (or any child) with grunting respirations. Auscultation of the chest may reveal wheezing, rales, rhonchi, or prolonged expirations (lower airway disease). The presence of stridor is a clue to upper airway problems. High-flow oxygen should be provided to all children in respiratory distress, in a manner that does not agitate the child. Even if these children are not cyanotic, they all require supplemental high-flow oxygen (simple face mask at 12-15 L/min). If the child is cyanotic, oxygen with assisted ventilation may be required. A pulse oximeter (if available), is useful to determine if the child is receiving adequate oxygen en-route. If low (saturation <94%), this should prompt an increase in oxygen flow or an alternate delivery method, such as a non-rebreather mask. Frequent reassessment is required en-route, with decisions for additional therapy based on prehospital care provider reports (e.g., bronchodilator therapy for wheezing).

Another important factor to assess is mental status, since a child who is becoming tired due to increased effort of breathing or hypoxia will not be able to breathe as fast or as hard as needed, so a decreasing respiratory rate is an ominous sign. On the other hand, an anxious child (due to fear or hypercapnia) may resist therapy and become more distressed. As many interventions as possible should be non-anxiety producing and may be accomplished easily with the parent's assistance. This includes the administration of oxygen by "blow-by"—holding the face mask 1-2 inches in front of the child's face, but slightly above the nose and mouth. Another option is placing the oxygen tubing through the bottom of a paper or plastic (not styrofoam) cup and holding it in a similar location. If aerosol nebulization set-ups are available, 3 cc of saline can be placed in the nebulizer (instead of medication) and administered by the parent.

The key is not to worry if the child has asthma, bronchiolitis, croup, or epiglottitis but to ensure an open airway and provide supplemental oxygen.

Pitfalls

1. Oxygen should be given to any child with tachypnea, retractions, or grunting respirations. Do not wait for cyanosis!

2. Do not force a child to lie supine if he or she prefers to sit upright. Infants and children in respiratory distress will often assume a position of comfort to help them maintain their own airway.

3. Do not focus your decisions on a specific diagnosis (e.g., croup vs epiglottitis or asthma vs bronchiolitis), since the basic prehospital management is no different.

4. IV access is not required in most cases of respiratory distress and may actually lead to worsening distress secondary to agitation and crying.

Recognition and Treatment of Shock

What is "shock"? In simple medical terminology it means failure to perfuse vital organs.[8] How is this assessed in children in the field? Many prehospital care providers equate shock with hypotension or low blood pressure. While this may be useful for adults, it provides many problems when caring for a child. What is a normal blood pressure for a child? It would be hard to argue with a systolic pressure below 70 mmHg in anyone, but the normal systolic blood pressure of a 2 year old can be 90 mmHg, which is low for most adults. The next problem is obtaining an accurate blood pressure in a child. This requires the proper-sized cuff, a cooperative child, a quiet environment,

and knowledge of the various age-based norms. Obviously, there are easier and more accurate methods to assess a child's circulatory status available to prehospital care providers.

Heart rate is a key parameter initially and on reevaluation. A child who is in shock has an elevated heart rate long before his or her blood pressure begins to drop. Therefore tachycardia mandates further investigation for some of the underlying causes, such as fever, anxiety, hypovolemia, or hypoxia.[8] It should also be remembered that heart rate, like respiratory rate and blood pressure, varies with age, so knowledge of the norms is needed to determine if tachycardia is present in the first place (Table 14-2). Clinical assessment of stroke volume is easily performed by assessing pulse quality (strength) and comparing peripheral and central pulses. The presence of a strong radial pulse means that a child probably is not in shock. On the other hand, a weak, thready radial pulse should mandate a comparison with a brachial or carotid pulse. A discrepancy can be due to peripheral vasoconstriction, as in hypothermia, but it can also be a sign of diminished stroke volume.[8] Since decreased skin perfusion is another early sign of shock, another reliable sign is the assessment of peripheral circulation. This can be done in several ways: by determining capillary refill, skin color, and skin temperature. Delayed capillary refill (> 2 seconds) and mottled skin (uneven or marbled appearance) indicate low cardiac output and shock (in the absence of hypothermia). The presence of cool extremities and pallor would also support the above findings.[11]

Inasmuch as shock affects all vital organs, the effects on the brain are demonstrated by a change in the level of consciousness. While this may be subtle, it is often useful in children. A child over 2 months old should be able to recognize and respond to his or her parents' faces. Therefore failure to recognize one's parents may be an early sign of brain ischemia.[8] A decreasing level of consciousness from awake, to responsive to voice (sleepy), responsive to pain, and finally unresponsive is an ominous sign. Other parameters to assess should include muscle tone and pupillary responses. While blood pressure is often difficult to obtain, if one is obtained, it can be used as a baseline and taken again when the providers reassess the child, since it may identify trends along with the other parameters listed.

While identification of shock is the primary goal, it is often beneficial to determine the cause of shock, since it may modify some of the prehospital treatment. Pediatric shock tends to result from hypovolemia due to fluid or blood loss. This commonly occurs in gastroenteritis/dehydration and trauma respectively. Another form of shock is distributive, caused by a maldistribution of blood such as would occur in septic or anaphylactic shock. The least common form of shock in children is the most common in adults—cardiogenic shock. Just as in adults, this can result from an arrhythmia, CHF, or congenital heart disease (both known and unknown).[11] However, after a cardiopulmonary arrest in a child, the heart often acts as if it were in cardiogenic shock.

The goal of therapy in shock is the restoration of adequate blood volume. This can be done in the field by IV or IO administration of 20 cc/kg of a crystalloid such as RL or NS as fast as possible (<20 minutes). After this is done, patient reassessment should be performed, focusing on the parameters mentioned above. This fluid bolus should be repeated if there is not an adequate response, such as decreased heart rate or improved capillary refill. After the next bolus and patient reassessment, further management should be based upon the child's status, etiology of shock (if known or suspected), and transport time. One additional therapy that should be given to all children in shock is high-flow oxygen.

Obviously, the major difficulty in these situations may be the ability of the prehospital care provider to establish intravascular access. It is very difficult and time consuming to establish IV access in ill young children.[12] In some situations, rather than waste precious moments of transport time, it may be useful to "load and go" and search for access en-route. Another method is to limit the number of attempts (3) or time allowed for IV access (90 seconds) before IO placement is attempted in the appropriate patient less than 6 years old.[13]

Although PASG may be of benefit in some cases, in children, only the legs should be inflated.

As medical command physician, the decisions regarding initial (and subsequent) interventions and treatment should be based upon the reports received from the field, provider skills and training, accepted protocols for the region, and repeated patient assessment once therapy is initiated.

Pitfalls

1. The assessment of shock in a child is not based solely upon blood pressure, since hypotension is a late finding. If the report you receive reveals an ill or injured child with tachycardia and a normal blood pressure, the child may still be in shock.

2. While IV access and fluids are the first-line treatment for children in shock, if transport time is short, scene time should not be delayed to obtain IV access. The prehospital care providers should "load and go" and attempt IV or IO access en-route. On the other hand, if transport time is long, IV access (or IO access) should be attempted before transport, so therapy can be given en-route.

3. Basic treatment is no different from that for adults and involves the administration of crystalloids at 20 cc/kg as fast as possible. If rapid fluid infusions are needed, do not assume that a wide open rate will do the job. Infuse the fluid under pressure (pressure bag, squeezing, or 60 cc syringe).

4. Do not be afraid to give an infant or child too much fluid, since very few conditions will put them into pulmonary edema. What fluid they do not need will be excreted in the urine.

5. If a PASG is used, inflate the legs only, not the abdominal compartment.

Trauma and Trauma Triage

Some of the differences between pediatric and adult trauma have to do with the mechanism of injury. Most pediatric trauma is blunt injury, (e.g., motor vehicle accident) rather than penetrating. Head trauma is more common in pediatric patients, with over 60% of children with major trauma having a significant head injury.[14] In addition, children often have occult injuries, especially involving the liver and spleen. The basic approach and treatment of a pediatric trauma patient varies little from that of an adult. The keys remain: airway control with cervical spine stabilization, breathing, circulation, disability, and exposure (full head-to-toe examination).

The initial approach to a pediatric trauma patient is the same as that of an adult: airway with cervical spine stabilization, breathing, circulation, disability, and exposure. All trauma patients should receive supplemental high flow oxygen and immobilization. If an appropriate sized cervical collar is not available, use towels and tape, NOT sandbags or IV fluid bags. The most important factor is to ensure that the airway is open and the child is breathing.

Suctioning the airway and positioning (jaw thrust) may accomplish this task. Supplemental oxygen (high flow) is best given by a pediatric face mask, but since this is often difficult, blow-by oxygen may be sufficient. If bag-valve-mask ventilation is required, be sure to watch for the rise and fall of the chest, in addition to improvement in the patient's color. Circulatory assessment should include heart rate, capillary refill, peripheral pulse strength, skin color and temperature of extremities, and level of consciousness. IV fluids should be administered to any victim of multiple trauma with hypotension and any child with poor circulation (as assessed previously). The decision whether to start an IV at the scene should be based upon patient condition and the anticipated transport time. The sooner IV access can be obtained, the sooner 20 cc/kg of crystalloid (LR or .9 NS) can be infused. It can be very difficult to start an IV in a child, so if valuable time is being wasted at the scene, it is often beneficial to transport and attempt IV access while en-route. Once the initial fluid bolus has been administered, the child should be reassessed and an additional bolus (20 cc/kg) given as warranted. While concerns have been raised in adult patients that aggressive fluid resuscitation for uncontrolled bleeding will result in normalization of the blood pressure and increased bleeding, due to different mechanisms and types of injury, this does not hold true for children.

The use of a PASG remains controversial, however, it can be used in a child to immobilize extremity and pelvic fractures by inflating the legs only, NOT the abdominal compartment. Disability assessment should include level of consciousness and a check of the pupils. Exposure refers to a complete rapid secondary survey. It should be stressed that if a life-threatening injury is found during the initial assessment, the injury should be evaluated and treatment begun and then "load and go". If no such injury is found and time permits (scene times on trauma patients should be less than 10 minutes), the child can be fully examined (this can also be done en-route). Take care to keep the child warm during this time, since the large body surface area allows him or her to become hypothermic easily, which can complicate resuscitation.

When a prehospital care provider calls for medical command regarding a pediatric trauma patient, besides the above information, a trauma score is helpful so that medical command can direct the patient to the appropriate facility, such as a pediatric trauma center. An ideal trauma score should be reliable, reproducible, simple, and able to predict patient outcome. It should be able to categorize patients so that severe injuries are not missed and the score obtained by one observer is the same as another observer using the same information.[15] This information can then be used by prehospital care providers to communicate to command physicians the severity of injury, which should then indicate to which hospital a patient should be transported (based on previously existing trauma triage criteria).

Several adult scores exist (trauma score, revised trauma score, injury severity score, CRAMS score), but it was difficult to apply these scores to pediatric patients. The Pediatric Trauma Score (PTS) was developed to overcome this problem, since this score combines anatomical variables and physiological variables.[15] The components include size, airway, systolic blood pressure, CNS (level of consciousness), skeletal injury, and cutaneous injury. Each is scored from -1 to $+2$, with a range of scores from -6 to $+12$ (Table 14-3).[15] Research has demonstrated that a PTS of 8 or below will identify those patients in whom mortality is likely to occur (inverse relationship between decreasing PTS and increasing mortality).[15] From this information, prehospital decisions about pediatric trauma patient transport can be made for the region and reinforced by the medical command physician.

Pitfalls

1. Since the majority of childhood trauma is blunt injury, there may be multisystem injury, as well as occult abdominal injury. Infants and children can have serious internal injuries without evidence of external trauma.

2. If the appropriate size cervical collar/immobilization equipment is not available, towels and tape can be used to secure the head; do not use IV bags or sandbags. A car seat, if intact, can be used to immobilize an infant or child. A cervical collar should still be applied, and towels can be used a padding along the head. Tape should then be used across the forehead to secure the infant.

3. If there is evidence of severe head injury (unequal pupils, seizures, unresponsive patient), assist ventilation with bag-valve-mask and 100% oxygen and hyperventilate (normal rate +25%) (see Table 14-2).

4. Children can easily become hypothermic if left exposed. After a full evaluation, the child should be covered and the transporting vehicle warmed to avoid hypothermia.

Table 14-3 Pediatric Trauma Score

Component	+2	+1	−1
Size	> 20 kg	10-20 kg	< 10 kg
Airway	Normal	Maintainable	Unmaintainable
CNS	Awake	Obtunded	Comatose
Systolic BP	> 90 mmHg	50-90 mmHg	< 50 mmHg
Open Wounds	None	Minor	Major or penetrating
Skeletal	None	Closed fracture	Open/multiple fractures
			Total

If proper sized BP cuff is not available, BP can be assessed by assigning—
+2 pulse palpable at radial or brachial artery
+1 pulse palpable at groin
−1 no pulse palpable.

5. IV access and the administration of crystalloids (20 cc/kg) should be done quickly and should not prolong scene time.

Seizures

Due to the high incidence of febrile seizures in children under 7 years old (1 in 20), it is not surprising that seizures account for many prehospital transports.[16,17] Prehospital care providers are often anxious about the call for several reasons: Will the child still be seizing when they arrive? What ALS interventions will be needed? As the prehospital command physician, you will need to be concerned about the cause of the seizure, as well as field treatment. However, it is important to realize that prehospital care providers should not have to diagnose the cause of the seizure, so appropriate therapy and transport should not be delayed.

Although there are many causes of seizures, the basic prehospital management remains the same: assessment of airway, breathing, and circulation. If a child is still seizing, the first priorities are ensuring a patent airway and breathing, and BLS procedures such as chin-lift, jaw thrust may be required. Suction should be available, and the crew should be ready to assist ventilations with a bag-valve-mask if the respiratory rate is slow or absent or the child is cyanotic, even just around the lips. All patients should also have supplemental oxygen administered during a seizure. The decision to use anticonvulsants should be based upon several factors: the length of the seizure, patient history (e.g., known seizure disorder), patient

medications, possible etiology (e.g., low blood sugar), transport time, and ability and comfort level of the providers to provide adequate or additional airway support (intubation if needed). A fingerstick glucose level (Dextrostix, Chemstrip) should be performed before initiating anticonvulsants. The providers should reassess the patient frequently en-route, even if the seizure stops. They should also be made aware that the seizure may recur en-route.

If upon the providers' arrival the child has stopped seizing, more time can be spent obtaining information from the parents or caretakers after the child has been assessed and found to be in stable condition. Because of the possibility of a fall during or after the seizure, this should be determined quickly so that appropriate immobilization can be performed if necessary. Information regarding the presence of fever before the seizure, recent illness, type of movements (jerking, rigid, flaccid), extremities involved (legs or arms, both sides or one side), eye movements (staring, rolling back), loss of continence (urine or stool), underlying medical problems, medications, allergies, and family history of seizures will provide help in establishing the etiology once the child is seen and evaluated at the hospital.[18] During transport it will be necessary to perform repeated evaluations of the child with regard to airway and breathing, reporting any changes to you en-route.

If the seizure is prolonged (>15 minutes) or persistent, the use of an anticonvulsant is warranted. Diazepam (Valium) can be administered by several routes: IV or IO 0.1-0.3 mg/kg IV slowly (no greater than 1 mg/min) with maximum single dose of 10 mg; this can be repeated up to three times with doses spaced 10 minutes apart. Rectal administration, 0.5 mg/kg for the first dose, 0.25 mg/kg for any subsequent dose, can be done by attaching a syringe (of the IV formulation of the drug) to a 16 or 18 g plastic IV catheter (needle removed) or a 10 Fr suction catheter and advancing it 4-6 cm into the rectum. This should be flushed with air (keep the catheter in place and fill the syringe with air) or 5 cc of saline. Since the major side effect of diazepam is respiratory depression, it is mandatory to have airway equipment (bag-valve-mask ventilation) ready before its administration and to reassess the patient frequently after its use.

Pitfalls

1. During a seizure, control of the airway with proper head position, suctioning, oxygen, and assessment or assistance of breathing are more important than stopping the seizure.

2. After a seizure, if a child is postictal, airway positioning and oxygen remain a priority.

3. Not all seizures require anticonvulsant therapy. If a decision is made to use anticonvulsants (especially benzodiazepines such as diazepam), as medical command physician, you should make sure the crew is aware of the side effect of respiratory depression and

has the necessary equipment and training to manage the patient should this occur.

4. Transport of a child after a seizure is mandatory, since the etiology cannot be determined from the field.

Summary

While pediatric calls account for only a small percentage of runs, they cause an inordinate amount of anxiety. Some of the factors, such as training, appropriate equipment, and prehospital protocols[19] can be addressed beforehand; other aspects cannot. Your level of comfort giving command on pediatric calls can be discerned by the prehospital care providers as well.

Patient assessment skills are the cornerstone of therapy, since treatment and triage decisions should be based on this information. At a minimum, all ill or injured infants and children should be transported on oxygen, but further decisions regarding IV access or medications should be based upon the age of the child, transport time, and the information you are given by the prehospital care providers. Frequent reassessment should be performed en-route, and in many cases, a child will have "turned around" by the time he or she arrives at the ED due to the providers' and your prehospital care and expertise.

SAMPLE CASES

CASE #1

A 9-month-old male has had a cold for 3 days. The prehospital care providers report that he is breathing at 60 times a minute, pulse is 160, and he feels a bit warm. They are unable to get an accurate pressure, since the cuff is too big.

The command physician should ask a few more questions: Is the child grunting or wheezing? Are there retractions? What is the child's level of consciousness? As long as the child's level of consciousness is adequate (awake, even if irritable), high-flow oxygen should be provided. This can be done by blow-by or mask, if tolerated by the infant. On the other hand, if the child is very sleepy, difficult to arouse, or the respiratory rate begins to decrease (inappropriately), the providers may have to provide assisted ventilation en-route, using a bag-valve-mask device.

DISCUSSION:

This infant is in respiratory distress, the cause is not important at this point. Providing high-flow oxygen is the key. An IV is not necessary and may agitate the infant, causing increased respiratory distress.

CASE #2

A 6-year-old has had vomiting and diarrhea for 2 days.

Her pulse is 130, respiratory rate 24, blood pressure 110/70 mmHg. She is sleepy but easily arousable, her radial pulse is strong.

Command physician: Depending upon the transport time, all that may be needed is expeditious transport. On the other hand, if transport time is long (>20 minutes), if the providers can establish an IV route, they can start a crystalloid fluid bolus (20 cc/kg) of RL or NS. If possible, a fingerstick glucose test should be performed and a level <60 should be treated. (For children <6 years, 25% dextrose is recommended: 0.5-1 gm/kg of glucose is equivalent to 2-4 cc/kg of D25. If only D50 is available, mix D50 1:1 with sterile water). In any case, repeated assessment of the patient en-route is required, and if the heart rate increases or blood pressure drops, rapid fluid replacement is required.

DISCUSSION:

This child is not in shock but is dehydrated (note the elevated heart rate). An IV is not needed and may waste time if transport time is short. For prolonged transport time, an IV would be beneficial but should not delay scene time, and an IO is inappropriate due to the child's age and level of consciousness.

CASE #3

A 14-year-old was riding his bike when he was struck by a car traveling about 35 mph. He was thrown across the road, and witnesses say he lost consciousness for 1 minute. He is now able to say his name but is confused. He has a deformity of this right thigh and right forearm. He has abrasions to his abdomen and a large laceration of his scalp. His pulse is 140, respiratory rate is 20, blood pressure is 100/60. He is currently immobilized on a backboard with head restraints, and a cervical collar has been applied. The scalp laceration stopped bleeding with direct pressure and is covered with a dressing. The right forearm is immobilized, and there is a strong radial pulse, but the pulse at the right ankle is weak and the foot is cool. (The left pulse is strong.) The providers are asking if they can apply and inflate the PASG.

Command physician: Splinting the leg as it currently lies in PASG will not correct the circulation problem in the leg or for the youth in general. Slight manipulation and straightening of the thigh and rechecking the pulses (if improved) may allow application and inflation of the affected PASG leg. The providers should be told that inflation of the other leg may be beneficial, but they should pay careful attention to the child's respiratory and neurological status while this is done. This child definitely needs a rapid infusion of IV fluids, as well as high-flow oxygen since he is in shock. Rapid transport to an appropriate trauma facility should not be delayed. The crew should be instructed to keep you posted of any changes in the patient's condition while en-route.

DISCUSSION:

This child has multisystem injuries: head, abdomen (possibly liver or spleen), and extremity trauma.

His pulse is elevated and his blood pressure low, which indicate shock (most likely hypovolemic) due to blood loss. The scalp laceration alone is not causing this; he could lose a large amount of blood into his thigh, but another hidden area is a liver or spleen injury. Keys points are immobilization with cervical spine stabilization and assessment of the child's airway and breathing: both of which are OK. Circulatory status of his leg is questionable without some manipulation (traction would be another option). Assessment of disability (level of consciousness) reveals that he is awake but confused, so it is not normal. IV fluids, oxygen, and rapid transport with repeated assessments should be stressed. Based upon this youth's injury and PTS (+1), transport should be to a pediatric trauma facility if available and if it will not unduly increase transport time.

CASE #4

A 3-year-old has had a seizure, which lasted 5 minutes. She has never done this before and was well earlier today. Now she is sleepy but arousable and recognizes mom. She feels very warm, her heart rate is 120, respiratory rate 22 and unlabored, and blood pressure is 96/60.

Command physician: As long as she did not fall and strike her head or neck, the child can be transported without immobilization. No specific therapy is required, such as an IV, but oxygen and suction equipment should be readily available in case the child has another seizure en-route.

DISCUSSION:

This child is probably postictal, which can explain her sleepiness. Although this was probably a febrile seizure, that diagnosis cannot be made in the field. A thorough examination by a physician is required to make this diagnosis and exclude other causes.

References

1. Tsai A, Kallsen G: Epidemiology of pediatric prehospital care, *Ann Emerg Med* 16:284-292, 1987.

2. Meador SA: Age-related utilization of advanced life support services, *Prehosp Disaster Med* 6(1):9-14, 1991.

3. Kallsen GW: Epidemiology of pediatric prehospital emergencies. In Dieckmann RA, editor: *Pediatric emergency care systems: planning and management,* Baltimore, 1992, Williams & Wilkins, pp. 153-158.

4. Dieckmann RA: Medical direction. In: Dieckmann RA, editor: *Pediatric emergency care systems: planning and management,* Baltimore, 1992, Williams & Wilkins, pp. 139-152.

5. Luten RC, Stenklyft, PH: Early recognition of illness. In Dieckmann RA, editor: *Pediatric emergency care systems: planning and management,* Baltimore, 1992, Williams & Wilkins, pp. 101-108.

6. Fuchs S, Paris PM: EMS physicians. In Dieckmann RA, editor: *Pediatric emergency care systems: planning and management,* Baltimore, 1992, Williams & Wilkins, pp. 405-412.

7. Simon JE, Goldberg AT: *Prehospital pediatric life support,* St Louis, 1989, Mosby, pp. 1-13.

8. Chameides L, Hazinski MF: Recognition of respiratory failure and shock: anticipating cardiopulmonary arrest. In *Textbook of pediatric advanced life support,* Dallas, 1994, American Heart Association, pp. 2-1 — 2-10.

9. Hoffman SH, Dieckmann RA: Prehospital illness treatment. In Dieckmann RA, editor: *Pediatric emergency care systems: planning and management,* Baltimore, 1992, Williams & Wilkins, pp. 178-202.

10. Emergency Cardiac Care Committee and Subcommittees, American Heart Association: Guidelines for cardiopulmonary resuscitation and emergency care, V: pediatric basic life support, *JAMA* 268:2251-2261, 1992.

11. Simon JE, Goldberg AT: *Prehospital pediatric life support,* St Louis, 1989, Mosby, pp. 34-41.

12. Rossetti VA, Thompson BM, Aprahamian C, et al.: Difficulty and delay in intravascular access in pediatric arrests, *Ann Emerg Med* 13:406, 1984.

13. Chameides L, Hazinski MF: Vascular access. In *Textbook of pediatric advanced life support,* Dallas, 1994, American Heart Association, pp. 5-1 — 5-17.

14. Simon JE, Goldberg AT: *Prehospital pediatric life support,* St Louis, 1989, Mosby, pp. 70-81.

15. Tepas JJ: Prehospital trauma scoring and triage, In Dieckmann RA, editor: *Pediatric emergency care systems: planning and management.* Baltimore, 1992, Williams & Wilkins, pp. 169-177.

16. Nelson K, Ellenberg J: Prognosis in children with febrile seizures, *Pediatrics* 61:720-727, 1978.

17. Nelson K, Ellenberg J: Antecedents of seizure disorders of early childhood, *AJDC* 140:1053-1061, 1986.

18. Fuchs S: Managing seizures in children, *Emergency* :47-52, 1990.

19. Luten R, Foltin GL, editors: *Pediatric resources for prehospital care,* Arlington, VA, 1993, National Center for Education in Maternal and Child Health.

15

Poisoning and Drug Overdose

In 1993, the American Association of Poison Control Centers (AAPCC) reported over 1.8 million poisonings in the United States.[1] Of these, over 1.5 million calls were directed to the poison control center (PCC) from the prehospital setting and 626 fatalities were reported. Interventions in the prehospital setting by physicians, paramedics, and other prehospital care providers may have a significant impact on the outcome of these patients. Although field interventions are extremely important, prolonged scene times may be detrimental, especially in critically ill patients.

Poisonings are classified as accidental or intentional. Accidental exposures may include pediatric ingestions, misuse of medications, and occupational and environmental exposures. Intentional exposures most commonly involve suicidal attempts by adolescent or adult patients. Two thirds of exposures are in patients less than 12 years old. Pediatric exposures most commonly involve accidental ingestion of medications, household cleaning products, and plants. Toddlers can also become intoxicated by eating or sucking on transdermal formulations such as Catapres® (Clonidine). Exposures in children frequently occur in the summer and during the holidays when children are home from school. Intentional overdoses in adolescents and adults generally involve multiple medications, such as benzodiazepines, barbiturates, cyclic antidepressants, and acetaminophen. In some situations, poisonings occur without the victim's knowledge or recognition. Application of topical medications, such as lindane and diphenhydramine, may lead to severe systemic toxicity. Exposure to carbon monoxide from automobiles, space heaters, and malfunctioning furnaces may lead to serious sequelae, including death. Cyanide and carbon monoxide are potential toxins in victims of fire. Inhalation of methylene chloride, frequently used as floor stripper, causes carbon monoxide poisoning, including headache, nausea, and changes in level of consciousness.

General Approach

Prehospital care providers and command physicians have several responsibilities in the management of poisoning. First, the potential for poisoning must be recognized. An

SANDRA M. SCHNEIDER, MD   DANIEL J. COBAUGH, PHARM D

assessment of the physical environment in which a comatose patient is found may lead the prehospital care provider to suspect that a drug overdose has occurred. In other environments, prehospital care providers need to be cognizant of the potential for toxicity. Second, the prehospital care provider needs to provide initial treatment in the management of the poisoned patient. This may include, but is not limited to, administration of syrup of ipecac to induce emesis, administration of naloxone to reverse the effects of opioids, or dermal decontamination of the hazardous materials exposure. Prehospital care providers must also be prepared to manage the life-threatening sequelae of poisonings, such as respiratory hypotension or depression or dysrhythmia. It is impossible for any physician to have a working knowledge of all environmental and pharmacological toxins. A PCC can assist in identification of substances, assessment of potential toxicity, and treatment guidelines for the toxic manifestations. They also monitor the incidence of exposures/poisonings, providing important epidemiological information, and should be informed of all patients.

Diagnosis

The diagnosis of most patients with overdoses or poisonings may be obvious. Patients are sometimes found with suicide notes, empty medication containers, or in suspicious circumstances that allow prehospital care providers to conclude that an overdose or poisoning has occurred. It is important for prehospital care providers to

determine if such evidence exists. Often the patient may have attempted to dispose of medication containers immediately after the ingestion, or family members may try to disguise an overdose scenario. Once an overdose or poisoning is suspected, the degree of toxicity should be established rapidly. The toxicity can be estimated from the patient's symptoms and physical condition, as well as the toxins involved, the amount (or concentration), the time since exposure, and in some cases the length of exposure. Sustained release formulations, commonly used for calcium channel blockers and theophylline medications, may cause delayed onset of symptoms for 4-16 hours after ingestion. Patients may then deteriorate rapidly. Acetaminophen, mushroom poisoning, carbon tetrachloride, or chloroform toxicity may take days to become apparent. In some patients, there is suspicion of an overdose, but the substance involved is unknown. In others, symptoms do not correlate with the medication identified. Patients with immediate outward symptoms probably have a significant overdose, but it may not have reached full effect. If the patient is having symptoms that do not go along with the toxins identified, believe the symptoms. Some patients take a polypharmacy overdose; different pills get mixed in different bottles. Tables 15-1 and 15-2 describe several toxidromes helpful in identifying toxicity in these cases.

At times an overdose or poisoning may be totally unsuspected, particularly in the trauma patient. In a recent study, nearly 50% of fatal motor vehicle accidents

Table 15-1   Toxidromes

Syndrome	Symptoms	Agents

Cholinergic
    Muscarinic
    Nicotinic
	"Sludge" — Salivation lacrimation, urination, defecation (diarrhea), GI pain, emesis Tachycardia, hypotension, hypertension	Organophosphates, carbamates, some wild mushrooms, carbachol Tobacco, insecticides

Anticholinergic	Dry mucous membranes, dilated pupils, tachycardia, delirium, coma	Cyclic antidepressants, diphenhydramine, antihistamines, some plants (Jimson weed)
Sympathomimetic	Seizures, tachycardia, hypertension	Cocaine, theophylline, caffeine, phenylpropanolamine (diet pills)
*Opioid	Coma, respiratory suppression, pinpoint pupils	Heroin, morphine, fentanyl, diphenoxylate, propoxyphene, dextromethorphan
Late hepatotoxicity	Mild initial symptoms, late onset jaundice, hepatic coma	Acetaminophen, some wild mushrooms, carbon tetrachloride, chloroform

This term is used for all natural, semi-synthetic, and synthetic drugs that work at opiate receptors.

involved alcohol or drugs.[2] Trauma patients with unexplained hypotension, respiratory depression, seizures, or agitation should be investigated for a possible overdose. A widened QRS, bradycardia, hypotension, and severe

Table 15-2 Common Toxins and Symptoms

Clinical Effect	Agent Involved	Clinical Effect	Agent Involved
Hypotension	Clonidine Beta blockers Calcium channel blockers Barbiturates Opioids Cyclic antidepressants Iron Cyanide Organophosphates Phenothiazines MAOIs	**Pupillary Changes**	
		Dilation	Amphetamines Caffeine Cocaine LSD MAOIs Nicotine PCP
		Constricted	Barbiturates Clonidine Benzodiazepines Opioids Phenothiazines Organophosphates
Hypertension	Amphetamines Cocaine Ephedrine/Pseudoephedrine LSD MAOIs Phencyclidine	**Cardiac Changes**	
Decreased LOC	Barbiturates Benzodiazepines Alcohol Cyclic antidepressants Clonidine Opioids Lithium Carbon monoxide Cyanide Calcium channel blockers Beta blockers	Bradycardia/Block	Barbiturates Carbamazepine Phenytoin Organophosphates Phencyclidine Beta blockers Calcium channel blockers Digitalis Cyclic antidepressants
		Sinus Tachycardia/SVT	Amphetamines Cocaine Decongestants Antihistamines Antipsychotics Antidepressants Caffeine Theophylline
Agitation	Amphetamines Antihistamines Anticholinergics Caffeine Cocaine LSD PCP Theophylline Cyclic antidepressants	Ventricular Tachycardia	Amphetamines Caffeine Digitalis glycosides Phenothiazines Tricyclic antidepressants
Seizures	Amphetamines Cocaine Decongestants LSD Cyclic antidepressants Camphor Organophosphates Isoniazid	QRS and QT Prolongation	Beta blockers Quinidine Procainamide Tricyclic antidepressants Lithium Phenothiazines

agitation, unexplained by the patient's trauma, should lead to treatment of possible toxicity (such as cyclic antidepressant toxicity). A decreased level of consciousness in adolescent and adult patients is often assumed to be drug induced. In the absence of other physical evidence of overdose, other causes should be considered: hypoglycemia, infectious causes such as meningitis, and cerebral vascular accidents. A useful mnemonic when considering the differential diagnosis of decreased level of consciousness is **AEIOU TIPPS**.

A- **A**irway - hypoxia and postanoxic encephalopathy
E- **E**ndocrine and metabolic
I- **I**nsulin - hypoglycemia
O- **O**verdose, opioids
U- **U**remia and Hepatic encephalopathy
T- **T**rauma, Tumor
I- **I**nfection - meningitis, encephalitis, brain abscess
P- **P**rimary Neurological - seizures, tumors, strokes
P- **P**sychological
S- **S**hock

Treatment

The standard care for an overdose patient includes stabilizing the patient, limiting absorption, increasing elimination, and providing specific antidotes. Early attempts at gastric decontamination are helpful in decreasing systemic toxin absorption. Some decontamination measures can be instituted in the prehospital setting, such as emesis (with syrup of ipecac) or administration of activated charcoal, dermal decontamination (washing), and ocular irrigation. Activated charcoal may be given to limit absorption of retained drugs. Aggressive gastric decontamination is not indicated in asymptomatic patients with known nontoxic ingestions.

The alkaloids in syrup of ipecac, emetine, and cephaeline induce emesis through local irritation of gastric mucosa along with stimulation of the chemoreceptor trigger-zone in the brain. Use 15 ml ipecac for children less than 1 year old and 30 ml for any patient older than 1 year, followed by 180-240 ml of fluid. Emesis is expected within 30 minutes of administration.[3] If emesis does not occur within 30 minutes, more fluid is encouraged and the dose of ipecac repeated. Ipecac is contraindicated in patients who have a decreased level of consciousness, who

have ingested agents that may cause a rapid decrease in level of consciousness, such as the cyclic antidepressants, have ingested hydrocarbons, or who have ingested caustic substances. As a rule, induction of emesis with syrup of ipecac is contraindicated in adult overdose patients due to the potential for inaccurate histories. Syrup of ipecac is often suggested for home use by PCCs for pediatric poisonings.

Boxes 15-1 and 15-2 list some common field contraindications and adverse effects of ipecac. Adverse effects after acute administration of ipecac are limited but may include protracted vomiting, diarrhea, drowsiness, and, rarely, Mallory-Weiss syndrome. The cardiac and neurological toxicities associated with ipecac are due to accumulation of these alkaloids after long-term misuse.[4]

Activated charcoal, as a gastric decontaminant, is probably underused in the prehospital management of toxic ingestions. Charcoal adsorbs nearly all commonly ingested substances. Substances such as lithium, iron, and the toxic alcohols including ethanol, isopropanol,

Box 15-1	**Agents Where Emesis is Contraindicated in the Field**

- Cyclic antidepressants
- Calcium channel blockers
- Beta blockers
- Theophylline
- Strychnine
- Camphor
- Isoniazid
- Sedative hypnotics including benzodiazepines barbituates all sleeping medications
- Ammonia
- Batteries, battery acid
- Corrosives—including drain openers, automatic dishwashing detergent, oven cleaners
- Hydrocarbons— especially mineral seal oil (furniture polish), gasoline, kerosene

Box 15-2	**Adverse Effects Associated with Syrup of Ipecac**

Adverse Effect	Classification
Protracted vomiting	Acute
Diarrhea	Acute
Drowsiness	Acute
Mallory-Weiss syndrome	Acute
Neuropathics	Chronic
Cardiomyopathies	Chronic

methanol, and ethylene glycol are not adsorbed by charcoal. In some cases, even injected drugs that undergo enterohepatic circulation can be adsorbed by oral activated charcoal. An initial dose of activated charcoal is 1 gm/kg in pediatric patients and 50-100 gm in adolescents and adults. Premixed aqueous suspensions of activated charcoal are easiest to use in the prehospital setting. Combination products of charcoal and sorbitol should be avoided in the field setting due to the risk of over-medication with sorbitol in pediatric patients, and its use should be withheld until arrival in the ED. Adverse effects associated with charcoal are limited but may include vomiting, aspiration pneumonia, and decreases in gastrointestinal motility. Administration of activated charcoal is contraindicated in patients with altered levels of consciousness who do not have protected airways, in the absence of bowel sounds, and following a caustic ingestion, since it may interfere with later endoscopic visualization of burns.

When faced with a topical agent, such as organophosphate pesticides and hydrofluoric acid, dermal decontamination is indicated. The prehospital care provider should first protect himself or herself with gloves, gown, and protective face mask, when indicated, to prevent self-intoxication. Contaminated clothing should be removed and all exposed skin irrigated with copious amounts of water for at least 15 minutes. If solid or powdered toxins are present on the patient's skin, these should be removed before irrigation, since dilution with water may hasten absorption and potential for toxicity. The drainage water should be handled as contaminated waste. If ocular exposure occurs, the affected eye(s) should be irrigated with a gentle stream of lukewarm water for at least 15 minutes.

There are few specific pharmacological antidotes or antagonists that may decrease the potential for or reverse the effects of certain toxins. Naloxone has withstood the test of time as an opioid antagonist. Nalmefene has a longer duration of action but may have a slower onset. Flumazenil, the benzodiazepine antagonist, may have some role, although very limited in the field. Oxygen, which we identify as a very necessary component of supportive care, may also quickly reverse the effects of toxins such as carbon monoxide and carbon tetrachloride.

Age Considerations

Toddlers generally take small amounts of medications (with the possible exception of iron-containing vitamins). Histories are often more accurate after pediatric ingestions. Parents or grandparents are, at times, unable to give

appropriate histories due to hysteria, or in some cases very young mothers may be unable to communicate a history of the ingestion. Adolescents and young adults commonly have suicidal gestures (or attempts) or experiment with mind-altering drugs. Teenagers often ingest over-the-counter medications, such as acetaminophen and iron, that may not manifest severe toxicity for 48-72 hours. Experimentation with some mind-altering agents may result in immediate severe, life-threatening sequelae. An example of this would be the teenager who inhales solvents that cause cardiac catecholamine sensitization. This can result in immediate onset of cardiac arrest. Often friends of the victim will try to conceal the fact that abuse preceded the event. The prehospital care provider is then faced with ruling out all causes of sudden cardiac arrest in an adolescent patient. Older adults or elderly patients may have toxicity from a therapeutic misadventure (i.e., taking too many drugs, double-dosing through the day) or a change in their physiological status (e.g., hepatic failure, renal failure, dehydration) that allows toxicity to build. Changes in neurological function secondary to toxicity in older adults may be missed and attributed to worsening dementia, etc. They also take overdoses in suicide attempts. Often they are reluctant to discuss their intoxication.

Children are at risk for developing seizures after ingestion of over-the-counter cold preparations that contain antihistamines such as diphenhydramine. Without an adequate history, the toxic etiology of this new onset of seizure activity may be missed. Toddlers tend to take medications that do not cause CNS depression. Adults tend to take medications that cause seizures and CNS toxicity. Although these are *gross* generalizations, they have been used to support the notion that pediatric patients can safely be given syrup of ipecac in the field, while adult patients should usually undergo alternate means of gastric decontamination. Pediatric patients exposed to even small doses of calcium channel blockers, diphenoxylate, or clonidine may have a *precipitous* decline in CNS function and hemodynamic function. Withhold syrup of ipecac in these situations. In general, syrup of ipecac has little usefulness in the teenager or adult in the prehospital setting.

Even in pediatric patients, there is a certain degree of risk associated with administration of ipecac. If the history was not accurate, that is, if different medications were ingested or larger amounts were ingested, the patient could experience a decrease in level of consciousness after ipecac administration.

Cardiac Arrest

Cardiac arrest is an ominous event in the overdose patient. However, some patients have been resuscitated despite very prolonged CPR.[5] Unlike patients with coronary artery disease, overdose patients generally have normal coronary arteries, normal myocardial function, and normal pulmonary function before their ingestion. In many of these patients, normal function can be restored if the patient survives the toxicity and arrest. Therefore prolonged resuscitation may be indicated, particularly in young overdose patients. Cardiopulmonary bypass (CPB) has been successfully used in a small number of arrested overdose patients[5-7], particularly patients who have taken lethal amounts of calcium channel or beta blocker medications. Patients with serious calcium channel blocker, or beta blocker overdoses and overdose patients in cardiac arrest should be taken to institutions with emergency CPB capabilities, where available.

Specific Common Toxins

Box 15-3 lists the most common poisonings reported by the National Database of the AAPCC.[1] Note that most of these are benign substances involving accidental exposures in small children. Box 15-4 lists the most common substances used in fatal poisonings.[1] The figures used are for incidents reported and are not accurate for drugs of abuse, such as cocaine and opiates.

To get a better idea of the relative risk associated with substances, a ratio of fatalities to exposures can be calculated. Table 15-3 lists fatality ratios for common

Box 15-3 Most Common Poisonings as Reported by AAPCC

Household Products
Household cleaners
Cosmetics
Plants
Pesticides
Hydrocarbons

Pharmaceuticals
Acetaminophen (including combination preparations)
Alcohols
Benzodiazepines
Antihistamines
Cyclic antidepressants

Box 15-4 Most Common Agents Taken in Fatal Poisonings as Reported by AAPCC*

- Cyclic antidepressants
- Ethanol
- Acetaminophen
- Aspirin
- Aminophylline/Theophylline
- Calcium antagonists
- Cocaine
- Carbon monoxide

*As reported to the AAPCC National Data Collection System.

Table 15-3 Agents Most Likely to Cause Fatalities if Exposure Occurs

Agent	% Cases Fatal*
Strychnine	15.4
Cyanide	3.2
Paraquat	2.3
Morphine	1.6
Arsenic	1.3
Glutethimide	1.3
Methanol	1.0
Calcium antagonists	0.8
Cardiac glycosides	0.8
Chloral hydrate	0.6

*As reported to the AAPCC National Data Collection (street drugs eliminated).

poisonings. Again, the values calculated for opioids and cocaine are not accurate but reflect reported exposures.

Cyclic Antidepressants

Cyclic antidepressant drugs, such as amitriptyline and imipramine, are a common cause of death after intentional drug overdose. Patients often become combative and delirious and experience a rapid decrease in level of consciousness. Other anticholinergic effects include sinus tachycardia and decrease in gastrointestinal motility. The tricyclic antidepressants have quinidine-like cardiac membrane stabilizing effects, which are due to a blockade of sodium channels. This often manifests as a conduction disturbance and sudden life-threatening ventricular arrhythmias. Hypotension is secondary to norepinephrine depletion and alpha-1 adrenergic blockade. Seizure activity occurs due to excessive release of catecholamines from nerve terminal sites. Due to a rapid decrease in level of consciousness, ipecac administration is contraindicated. Activated charcoal may be administered to an awake patient in the prehospital setting. Since changes in level of consciousness may occur rapidly, protection of the patient's airway should be of primary concern to the prehospital care provider. Seizure activity should be managed with traditional agents such as diazepam and phenytoin. Ventricular dysrhythmias should be managed with lidocaine and phenytoin. Procainamide should be avoided, since its pharmacological mechanism is similar to the cardiotoxic mechanisms of the cyclics. Bretylium may cause hypotension in a manner similar to the cyclics. Hypotension is often resistant to fluids and dopamine and may require norepinephrine.

Sodium bicarbonate has been effective in controlling the cardiovascular toxicities of the cyclic antidepressants.[8] It is theorized that alkalosis causes an increase in protein binding of the antidepressants and decreases the amount of free drug available for toxic effects. The sodium loading that occurs with sodium bicarbonate administration may reverse the effect of the antidepressants on rapid sodium channels. Alkalization is appropriate in patients with evidence of significant toxicity, such as QRS widening > 0. 10 msec or dysrhythmias. In the field, begin alkalization by administration of a 1 mEq/kg bolus of sodium bicarbonate. This bolus dose may be repeated in 10 minutes. Arterial blood gas levels are monitored after arrival in the ED to maintain a pH of 7.5-7.55. Inability to monitor arterial blood gas levels in the field limits the prehospital care provider's ability to aggressively treat with sodium bicarbonate.

Calcium Channel Blocking Agents

Over the past several years, prescribing of calcium channel blockers, such as diltiazem, nifedipine, and verapamil has increased dramatically. Along with the increase in the use of these agents, there has been a dramatic increase in the number of accidental and intentional ingestions involving them. These agents may cause profound life-threatening hypotension, bradycardia, and asystole. Calcium channel blockers interfere with conduction through sinuatrial and atrioventricular nodes, resulting in bradyarrhythmias, conduction disturbances, and a decrease in cardiac output.

Even small quantities (1-2 pills) may cause death in a pediatric patient. Asymptomatic patients who claim to have ingested these agents should be treated seriously.

These drugs are commonly prescribed in sustained release preparations, which will have *delayed onset* (several hours) of symptoms, such as an extremely precipitous decrease in blood pressure to severe hypotension.

Syrup of ipecac should be *avoided* due to the potential for rapid decrease in level of consciousness. Activated charcoal is effective and can be used as long as the patient is conscious. Symptomatic bradycardia may be treated with atropine and isoproterenol and when necessary a transcutaneous pacemaker. Calcium chloride is a potential antidote for calcium channel blocker toxicity. One gram of calcium chloride (the preferred calcium salt) should be administered as a 10% solution. Doses should be repeated 2-3 times until symptoms subside. Very large doses may be necessary (> 10 amps).[9] Glucagon (1-10 mg) IV has also been beneficial in some patients.[10] If further research confirms anecdotal reports, this drug should be added to prehospital protocols.

Sedative-Hypnotics

The sedative-hypnotics include several classifications of drugs — benzodiazepines, barbiturates, and several older agents such as chloral hydrate. Ingestion of a benzodiazepine alone will usually result in mild symptomatology. When these agents are ingested along with other CNS depressants, such as ethanol or barbiturates, profound CNS depression and respiratory depression may occur. The prehospital presentation most commonly involves drowsiness, lethargy, and ataxia. Coma that does not respond to painful stimuli, or that involves hyporeflexia or hemodynamic instability suggests the involvement of other CNS depressants. Ipecac is best avoided. Activated charcoal is effective in adsorbing the benzodiazepines in the gastrointestinal tract.

Flumazenil is a specific benzodiazepine antagonist that competes with benzodiazepines at the benzodiazepine receptor site. Administration of flumazenil may result in reversal of the toxic effects of the benzodiazepine, but seizures may occur if the patient has long-term benzodiazepine abuse (withdrawal) or co-ingested a seizure-provoking drug, such as theophylline, isoniazid, or a cyclic antidepressant (lowers the seizure threshold). Flumazenil dose for overdose is a maximum of 0. 5 mg IV q 1 minute up to 5 mg.[11]

Opioids

Prehospital exposure to opioids can occur in a variety of situations, such as abuse of heroin and fentanyl derivatives or opioids used for pain control. Agents such as diphenoxylate, clonidine, and dextromethorphan may have opioid-like effects. Physicians and prehospital care providers may not consider opioid toxicity in a patient taking over-the-counter cough preparations. In meperidine overdose, pupils may be dilated rather than constricted. Anticholinergic effects will predominate in diphenoxylate ingestions.

Treatment of exposure to these substances includes supportive care, consideration of gastric decontamination, and the use of specific opioid antagonists. Administration of naloxone will result in rapid reversal of opiate/opioid toxicity, often precipitating opioid withdrawal. Usual initial adult dose of naloxone is 2 mg, although massive doses (10-20 mg) have been required to manage exposure to the fentanyl derivatives, diphenoxylate, and clonidine. Repeat doses of naloxone may be necessary to manage recurrence of toxic effects due to the short half-life of naloxone. Patients who respond to naloxone should be encouraged to come to the hospital for an observation period. Nalmaphene, also an opioid antagonist, has a half-life longer than that of naloxone and therefore may not require repeat administration in the management of uncomplicated patients.

Cocaine

The recreational use and abuse of cocaine continues to become more common in the United States. Typical effects observed in cocaine toxicity are the result of the sympathetic storm from cocaine's potentiation of the neurotransmitters, epinephrine, and norepinephrine. In the early stimulation phase, neurological effects observed include hyperexcitability, euphoria, muscle twitching, irritability, headache, and hallucinations. Cardiovascular effects include bradycardia, tachycardia, chest pain, and hypertension. Seizure activity may advance to status epilepticus. Agitation and seizures in the cocaine-toxic patient can be treated with benzodiazepines, such as lorazepam or diazepam.

Since cocaine is most often abused by inhalation and IV injection, gastric decontamination is often not necessary. The exception to this is the case of the individual who is a body-packer or body-stuffer. The body-packer ingests bags of cocaine (containing huge amounts of drugs) as a means of transporting the drugs. These bags are usually of high quality and difficult to break. The body-stuffer is a person who swallows bags of cocaine to rid himself/herself of evidence. These bags or balloons are often thin, prone to breakage, and may contain enough

cocaine to cause serious toxicity. Activated charcoal should be administered in the field, if possible, to either a body-packer or a body-stuffer. In the case of bag breakage, the charcoal will absorb cocaine in the gastrointestinal track.[12] Administration of activated charcoal can be followed later by irrigation and cleansing of the gastrointestinal tract to eliminate the bags of cocaine. The patient should be monitored since ventricular dysrhythmias are common.

Foreign Body Ingestion

Foreign body ingestion is common, particularly in small children. The child is usually seen playing with a coin, only later to have the coin disappear. Because they are frequently asymptomatic, there is an inclination to leave children at home and allow nature to take its course ("this too shall pass"). However, esophageal erosion can occur, particularly with button batteries. Therefore, all children, even though asymptomatic, should be brought to the hospital for x-ray localization. Once the foreign body is in the stomach, it will generally pass into the feces without further difficulties.

Hazardous Materials

Hazardous materials are a potential threat, not only to workers, but to prehospital care providers and the population at large. Large communities can afford to have specialized Hazmat teams, but smaller communities rely on their EMS services. Some basic principles for handling hazardous materials are discussed in this section; however, it is not meant to be a thorough description.

A hazardous material incident is any situation that may cause harmful contamination to the environment (air, water, or soil) or to personnel. In many cases the substance involved is unknown. Extreme caution should be used when approaching a scene. Realize that contamination flows downstream and by air currents. Areas where the chances of contamination are high are considered "hot." Hot zones should be entered only by a limited number of personnel equipped with protective gear. A secondary area around the hot zone, a "contamination reduction zone" should be established for basic decontamination. Basic decontamination facilities need not be fancy—a water supply, a kiddie inflatable pool (to collect run off), and plastic bags to double-bag exposed clothing and jewelry are often all that is necessary. Treatment should take place beyond the contamination reduction zone unless a critical condition exists.

Identification of toxic substance may be aided by labels, placards, and shipping papers. The U. S. Department of Transportation uses a 4 digit identification code.[13] A similar code by the National Fire Protection Association is described in Table 15-4.[14] A patient decontaminated at the scene may still have the potential to contaminate an ambulance or ED. Vomit, urine, etc. may add to the contamination risk. Additional decontamination outside the ED is appropriate. The prehospital care providers should have protective gear, and the ambulance itself may require decontamination.

Prehospital Triage Criteria

There is a growing trend to develop specialized centers for handling Hazmat victims and victims of poisoning and overdose. Adequate treatment and decontamination facilities are essential, as well as immediate access to antidotes and laboratory support. Guidelines for facilities wishing to become regional toxicology treatment centers have been established[15] and endorsed by several organizations,

Table 15-4   National Fire Protection Association Classification of Hazardous Materials

Blue = Health Hazard
4 - Short exposure can be critical.
3 - Short exposure can be serious — temporary or residual impairment.
2 - Prolonged exposure can be serious — temporary or residual impairment.
1 - Minor injury.
0 - No injury.

Red = Combustible
4 - Vaporizes in atmosphere conditions — burns easily.
3 - Can be ignited at high temperatures.
2 - Can be ignited at normal temperatures.
1 - Must preheat before ignited.
0 - Will not burn.

Yellow = Explosive Hazard
4 - Readily detonates.
3 - Requires strong initiating source to explode or will explode with water.
2 - Violent chemical reaction, but no explosion. May form explosive with water.
1 - Becomes unstable at high temperature.
0 - Stable.

including the American Academy of Clinical Toxicology. Few facilities specializing in the care of poisoning victims currently exist, but as these facilities become more common, appropriate triage in the field will become necessary. Unstable patients (hemodynamically unstable, respiratory distress) may be more appropriately handled in a regional center, should one be close. In addition, patients who ingest unusual materials, victims of major industrial exposures, and patients ingesting drugs with high lethal potential (like those listed in Table 15-2) may be triaged to centers with special abilities when and where these exist. Local capabilities will determine local triage criteria.

Pitfalls

One of the primary pitfalls in prehospital management of overdose patients is the inability to obtain an accurate history of the exposure. Patients who are truly suicidal are notoriously unreliable historians. In addition, the medications or drug of abuse cannot be identified or the time of the ingestion cannot be estimated. Also, in situations where multiple medications are involved, it is difficult to determine which medication(s) was taken in a quantity significant enough to contribute to toxicity.

In many circumstances, the prehospital care provider may be at risk for physical harm due to the combative or violent behaviors exhibited by overdose patients. One example of this would be the patient who becomes violent after exposure to cocaine or LSD. Two paramedics may not be capable of restraining this patient long enough to sedate before transport. Another example would be the patient who has experienced a decrease in level of consciousness and respiratory depression secondary to an opioid exposure. If naloxone is administered in doses capable of completely reversing the effects of the opioids, the patient may become violent upon arousal or experience opioid withdrawal.

Another pitfall that should be considered is a situation in which toxicity is masked or forgotten due to the presence of trauma. Examples include the burn trauma patient who may have been exposed to both carbon monoxide and cyanide in a fire. These life-threatening toxicities may be overlooked when providing initial stabilization and burn care. Often in cases of blunt and penetrating trauma, toxins such as ethanol, opioids, and cocaine may cause confusing symptoms (unexplained tachycardia or coma) and complicate care.

A growing number of adults mix several medications in their suicide attempt, often as many as 3-4 different medications plus alcohol. The paramedics gather huge bags of medications and recite long lists of potential toxins. Medic command physicians spend precious minutes researching all potential toxicities. Some simple rules may apply. If it is several hours since ingestion and you have not heard about calcium channel blocker, beta blocker, tricyclic antidepressants, theophylline, or a sustained release medication, then the patient can usually be treated according to presenting symptoms. If it has been less than 1 hour since ingestion, the patient should be treated with an IV and airway/hemodynamic monitoring, regardless of the suspected ingestant. Drug-drug interactions and significance of the ingestion can await discovery in the ED.

Refusals

There is considerable liability in not transporting potentially suicidal patients. Patients may take an overdose as a gesture, or they may have had earlier suicidal ideation, which they and the family now deny. On occasion, not only does the patient display dysfunctional behavior, but also the patient's family and friends can be more dysfunctional than the patient. Patients who cry "wolf" should be believed and brought to a facility for toxicologic analysis and medical observation. Such patients may need psychiatric referral. No potentially suicidal overdose patient should be able to refuse transport to the hospital. When appropriate, an involuntary commitment should be obtained through normal procedures.

SUMMARY

The overdose or poisoned patient can provide many challenges to the prehospital care provider and command physician. Sometimes the exposure is obvious, however, often the offending substance is unknown, occult, or masked by other trauma or exposures. Once an exposure has occurred, the role of the prehospital care provider and command physician is to establish the potential for toxicity. The toxicity can be estimated from the patient's symptoms, the toxins involved, and facts surrounding the exposure. The command physician must keep in mind that some patients may deteriorate rapidly (i.e., tricyclic overdoses, calcium channel blocker overdoses), while others may have delayed onset of symptoms (i.e., acetaminophen, mushroom poisoning).

The treatment of the overdose patient must include the evaluation and initial treatment by the prehospital care provider. This treatment must include ensuring the ABCs, as well as limiting toxin absorption, increasing elimination, and providing specific antidotes. The command physician must keep in mind several pitfalls associated with the care of the overdose patient, including the inability to obtain an accurate history, the potential masking of overdose symptoms due to the presence of trauma, or polydrug overdose. In addition, the prehospital care providers are at risk when treating the overdose patient due to violent patients or exposure to hazardous materials. The command physician must also remember that there is considerable liability in not transporting potentially suicidal overdose patients and in specific circumstances, prehospital care providers should be requested to transport patients against their will.

Since it is impossible for any command physician to have a working knowledge of all potential toxins, their local PCC can be a valuable resource for toxin identification, assessment of potential toxicity, and treatment guidelines.

SAMPLE CASES

CASE #1

Prehospital care providers state that they are on the scene with a 27-year-old female who recently ingested "a bottle of pills" in a suicide attempt. They note that the patient has a history of depression and was recently discharged from a psychiatric facility. The patient is now restless and slightly confused. She complains of a dry mouth and blurred vision. Vital signs include a BP of 96/60, a pulse of 140, and respirations of 18. Her pupils are dilated, lungs are clear, and her skin is warm and dry. She has no evidence of trauma or needle marks. The prehospital care providers are unable to find a pill bottle. The prehospital care providers have placed the patient on oxygen via face mask, have initiated an IV line of NS, and have placed the patient on a cardiac monitor. The monitor reveals a sinus tachycardia with a QRS width of 0.18.

What orders would you provide?
DISCUSSION:

Although the identity of the drug ingested is not known, the patient has a toxidrome consistent with that of a tricyclic antidepressant including the anticholinergic symptoms of dilated pupils, blurred vision, dry mouth, and tachycardia. The widened QRS and hypotension suggest that this is a serious and potentially life-threatening overdose. The prehospital care providers have initiated their care by addressing the ABCs (airway, breathing, and circulation). They should watch closely for a precipitous change in the patient's level of consciousness, seizures, arrhythmias, or hypotension. At this point, a fluid challenge of 300-500 cc of NS would be appropriate in light of the patient's hypotension. In addition, sodium bicarbonate should be administered in a loading dose of 1 mEq/kg. This may be repeated in 10 minutes. If the patient fails to respond to initial fluid challenge and sodium bicarbonate, additional fluid challenge should be administered. However, since the hypotension may be resistant to fluids, pressors may be required. Rapid transport to an appropriate facility should be accomplished, while police and other public safety officials search the patient's home for pill bottles and other evidence of drug ingestion.

CASE #2

Prehospital care providers are called to the home of 75-year-old female who has apparently ingested multiple digoxin tablets in a suicide attempt. The patient was distraught over the recent death of her husband and

decided to "end it all" by taking these pills. The prehospital care providers had found an empty digoxin bottle, which was filled yesterday for 100 tablets. The prehospital care providers note that the patient is awake and alert without significant complaints. Her medications include digoxin, furosemide, and potassium. She has no known drug allergies, and her past medical history is remarkable for heart disease and CHF. Currently her vital signs are BP 110/70, pulse of 58 and irregular, with respirations of 16. She is awake and alert with normal mentation. Her lung exam reveals scattered rales, and her heart rate is irregular. She has no peripheral edema or JVD. The prehospital care providers have placed the patient on oxygen and have initiated an IV line of NS at KVO. The monitor reveals a sinus bradycardia (rate of 58) with occasional PVCs, 1-2 per minute.

What additional orders would you provide?
DISCUSSION:

The patient has taken a massive digitalis overdose, and prehospital care providers should be aware of the potential toxicity including severe ventricular dysrhythmias, aggressive bradydysrhythmias, heart block, and cardiac arrest. If available, prehospital care providers should place pads for an external pacemaker, keeping it ready to be used if necessary. Prehospital care providers should also be prepared to administer antiarrhythmics should the ventricular ectopy worsen. Since Digibind® (digoxin immune Fab) may be used to reverse the effects of the addition of the massive overdose, the prehospital care providers should initiate rapid transport to an appropriate facility. This facility should be notified ahead of time by the command physician that the prehospital care providers are en-route with a patient suffering from a potentially massive digoxin overdose and that Digibind® should be immediately available.

CASE #3

The prehospital care providers are called to the home of a 3-year-old child who has ingested an unknown quantity of extra-strength acetaminophen tablets. The mother states that the bottle was inadvertently left within the child's reach and the child ingested multiple tablets. The ingestion occurred approximately 15 minutes ago. The child has no significant past medical history and is on no meds and has no drug allergies.

Prehospital care providers find the child awake and playful with age-appropriate vital signs.

(continued)

(continued)

What orders should be given to the prehospital care providers?
DISCUSSION:

In this situation, ipecac would be appropriate and the prehospital care providers should be instructed to administer 30 ml of ipecac followed by 180-240 ml of fluid. The prehospital care providers should expect emesis within 30 minutes of administration. If emesis does not occur within 30 minutes, more fluid should be encouraged and the dose of ipecac repeated.

CASE #4

A 35-year-old male has reportedly ingested a large quantity of alcohol along with multiple benzodiazepines and opioid pain relievers. He apparently was distraught over the recent break-up of his marriage. He is awake but drowsy. At this time, he agrees to paramedic evaluation but refuses transport.

How should the prehospital care providers proceed?
DISCUSSION:

If the patient allows, the paramedic should initiate an IV and place the patient on oxygen and cardiac monitor. If available, the patient's blood glucose level should be estimated via dextrose stick. If the patient's level of consciousness decreases, naloxone should be administered starting at a dose of 2 mg up to 10-20 mg .as required.

The prehospital care providers should also quickly initiate the appropriate legal proceedings for transporting the patient against his will. Although the exact procedure may vary by jurisdiction, often this includes a telephone call to the local mental health bureau and assistance from the police. This patient should not be allowed to refuse transport and must be transported to the hospital. If the patient's level of consciousness decreases, he should be treated and transported immediately without his verbal consent.

References

1. Litovitz TL, Holm KC, Clancy C, et al.: 1992 annual report of the American Association of Poison Control Centers toxic exposures surveillance system, *Am J Emerg Med* 11:494-555, 1993.

2. Lowenfels A, Miller T: Alcohol and trauma, *Ann Emerg Med* 13:1056-1060, 1984.

3. Bond GR, Requa RK, Krenzelok EP, et al.: Influence of time until emeisis on the efficacy of decontamination using acetaminophen as a marker in a pediatric population, *Ann Emerg Med* 22:1403-1407, 1993.

4. Wrenn K, Rodewald L, Dokstade L: Potential misuse of Ipecac, *Ann Emerg Med* 22:1408-1412, 1993.

5. Hendren WG, Schiever RS, Garrettson LK: Extracorporeal bypass for the treatment of verapamil poisoning, *Ann Emerg Med* 18:984-987, 1989.

6. McVey FK, Corke CF: Extracorporeal circulation in the management of massive propranolol overdose, *Anaesthesia* 46:744-746, 1991.

7. Larkin GL, Graeber GM, Hollingsed MJ: Experimental amitriptyline poisoning: treatment of severe cardiovascular toxicity with cardiopulmonary bypass, *Ann Emerg Med* 22:480-486, 1994.

8. Hoffman JR, Votey SR, Bayer M, et al.: Effect of hypertonic sodium bicarbonate in the treatment of moderate to severe cyclic antidepressant overdose, *Am J Emerg Med* 11:336-341, 1993.

9. Hattori VT, Mandel WJ, Peter T: Calcium for myocardial depression from verapamil, *N Engl J Med* 306:238, 1982.

10. Zaritsky AL, Horowitz M, Chernow B: Glucagon antagonism of calcium channel blocker induced myocardial dysfunction, *Crit Care Med* 16:246-251, 1988.

11. Spivey WH, Roberts JR, Derlet RW: A clintrial of escalating doses of flumazenil for reversing suspected benzodiazepine overdose in the emergency department, *Ann Emerg Med* 22:1813-1821, 1993.

12. Tomaszewski C, McKinney P, Phillips S, et al.: Prevention of toxicity from oral cocaine by activated charcoal in mice, *Ann Emerg Med* 22:1804-1806, 1993.

13. Research and Special Programs Administration: *Hazardous materials: emergency response guide book.* DOTP5800.2, U. S. Government Printing Office, 1984.

14. Fire protection guide to hazardous materials, ed 9, 1986, National Fire Protection Association.

15. Facility assessment guidelines for regional poison treatment centers, *Vet Hum Toxicol* 33:384-397, 1991.

16

Behavioral Emergencies

A behavioral emergency can be defined as an acute change in conduct that results in an intolerable behavior for the patient, family, or society.[1] These changes range from the inability to cope with a stressful situation to the agitated and violent patients that present a danger to themselves and others.

From a literature review, it is evident that very little has been written about behavioral emergencies in prehospital care. The "standard care" is mostly extrapolated from the experience in EDs and psychiatric wards. In general, prehospital care providers receive little training regarding these conditions during their initial or continuing education.[2,3] All these factors add up to make the encounter with the emotionally disturbed patient very difficult.

Facing a patient with a behavioral emergency is always a stressful situation. Even in the ED setting, these patients are difficult to evaluate. They are time consuming and often require special attention. For an EMS crew responding to the scene, the situation can be even more complicated. The patient can be non-cooperative, and frequently there are no reliable sources for history. Family members, if available, might be uninformed about the patient's medical or psychiatric history. The emotionally disturbed patient therefore requires a different approach than the routine patient.

The "standard" approach EMS personnel use may be inadequate for the assessment of these patients. They may feel uncertain and insecure on how to proceed given their training and limited treatment options.[4] They will contact direct medical control for help, but it can be even more difficult for the on-line physician to obtain a good assessment of the case. Under these circumstances, it is very easy to make serious mistakes with terrible repercussions for the patient and the system. It is very important for the medical director to ensure that the prehospital care providers and the physicians to which direct medical control is delegated have the appropriate training in how to deal with these patients before they face them in the field. General guidelines should be provided by the system, although each situation should be evaluated individually.

Another important aspect in the care for these patients is to remember that they have a health problem, as does every other patient encountered by EMS. Unfortunately,

HECTOR M. ALONSO-SERRA, M.D.

patients with behavioral changes can be mislabeled by the prehospital care providers as "uncooperative patients", which may result in a lack of compassion. We need to keep in mind that their behavior is a manifestation of their disease. Compassionate care, understanding, and patience are essential if we want to make a difference in these patients' outcome.

The main objective for this chapter is to provide an overview on how to assess and treat the patient with a behavioral emergency in the prehospital setting. Some of the information discussed will not be given as a medical command order but is provided in an effort to help the command physician understand what is occurring at the other side of the radio. We will discuss and define the most common behavioral emergencies. Special attention is given to suicidal and violent patients, since they represent true emergencies and are usually one of the most challenging and demanding patients encountered in the prehospital domain. Specific risk factors are enumerated, which should help to predict the potentially violent or suicidal patient in the early phases of the evaluation. Also, pharmacological alternatives for rapid tranquilization of the agitated and violent patient are discussed.

Common Psychiatric Conditions in EMS

EDs and EMS systems are common points of entry for the psychiatric patient to the health-care system.[1] Emergency physicians acting as medical control should be familiar with the psychiatric terminology and be aware of common presentations, complications, and management. Although detailed descriptions of psychiatric disorders are beyond the scope of this chapter, the following are simple definitions of some of the most common conditions faced in the daily practice of EMS.

Anxiety Disorders

Anxiety is defined as the unpleasant emotional state consisting of psycho-physiological responses to anticipation of unreal or imagined danger, ostensibly resulting from unrecognized intrapsychic conflict. Physiological concomitants include increased heart rate, altered respiration rate, sweating, trembling, weakness, and fatigue; psychological concomitants include feelings of impending danger, powerlessness, apprehension, and tension.[5]

Some level of anxiety is a normal and necessary reaction to stressful situations. Patients with anxiety disorders show a disproportionate response that may preclude them from normal interaction with family, friends, or society. When these symptoms are directed to or produced by a specific object, activity, or situation, and as a consequence the patient consciously avoids the stimulus, it is then referred to as phobia. The phobic patient can usually recognize the problem but is unable to control the symptoms. A panic attack is an acute, extreme level of anxiety with disorganization of personality and function.[5] Attacks can last from a few minutes to hours and occur in patients with and without chronic anxiety.

Depression

Depression is defined as a mental state of depressed mood characterized by feelings of sadness, despair, and discouragement. It ranges from the normal feeling of "the blues" through dysthymia to major depression. There are often feelings of low self-esteem, guilt, and self-reproach, withdrawal from interpersonal contact, and somatic symptoms such as eating and sleep disturbances.[5]

Schizophrenia

Schizophrenia can be defined as a group of disorders comprising most major psychotic disorders and characterized by disturbances in form and content of thought (loosening of associations, delusions, and hallucinations), mood (blunted, flattened, or inappropriate affect), sense of self and relationship to the external world (loss of ego boundaries, dereistic thinking, and autistic withdrawal), and behavior (bizarre, apparently purposeless and stereotyped activity or inactivity).[5] The manifestation of symptoms varies from patient to patient. Even the same patient will show different levels of symptomatology during his or her lifetime.

Bipolar Disorder

A mood disorder characterized by the occurrence of one or more manic episodes; in almost all cases, one or more major depressive episodes will eventually occur. The manic phase is characterized by expansiveness, elation, agitation, hyperexcitability, hyperactivity, and increased speed of thought and speech.[5]

Initial Assessment and Intervention

When responding to a scene, EMS personnel rarely know the diagnosis for that patient. With the confusion commonly present when facing a disturbed patient, an accurate psychiatric diagnosis in the field is not only almost impossible but irrelevant. Protocols should describe how to assess and treat clinical symptoms and not a specific diagnosis.

The first step when facing a disturbed patient is to evaluate the scene. "Is the scene safe?" If not, EMS personnel should wait for the arrival of law enforcement authorities before any further intervention. This is particularly important when dealing with the violent patient. If the scene is safe, then prehospital care providers should carefully approach the patient and try to perform a quick medical assessment. They should evaluate if the behavioral changes are due to an organic etiology or if the patient is under imminent danger secondary to a medical emergency. It is extremely important to emphasize that there are multiple medical conditions that can present with behavioral changes (Box 16-1). Presentation may vary from lethargy and confusion to agitation and violence. Classic examples are the confused patient with acute hypoglycemia, the agitated patient with hypoxia, and the lethargic patient with shock. The initial evaluation must include history (medical and psychiatric) and physical exam, including measurement of blood sugar level and pulse oximetry. Mental changes of acute onset without previous history of psychiatric disorder are highly suggestive of an organic etiology. EMS personnel should ask specifically for prescribed medications or suspected drug abuse. Physical exam should pay special attention to neurological findings. If during the evaluation vital signs are abnormal, consider the patient to be medically unstable and his or her mental changes secondary to organic problems until proven otherwise. Promptly instruct the personnel in the field to execute appropriate interventions for the correction of abnormal vital signs. Delayed stabilization or even nontransport of patients with organic problems can be a dangerous mistake when dealing with a mentally disturbed patient.

Occasionally, the patient may not cooperate with initial assessment and stabilization. In these situations, EMS personnel should try to gain the patient's confidence by providing reassurance, explaining who they are, and describing every step before they do it. If the patient is still not cooperative, the presence of a physician (medical control) in the field is a figure of authority that could be of great help to have the patient cooperate. Unfortunately, this is typically not possible. One alternative is for the medical control physician to talk to the patient over the phone

Box 16-1 Organic Disorders with Behavioral Manifestations[7-9]

NEUROLOGICAL
CNS infections (meningitis, encephalitis, brain abscess)
Head trauma
Hypertensive encephalopathy
Stroke
Mass lesion
Seizure disorder
Dementia

DRUG INTOXICATION/POISONING
Alcohol
Amphetamines
Anticholinergic syndromes
Cocaine
LSD
Marijuana
Phencyclidine (PCP)

WITHDRAWAL SYNDROMES
Alcohol
Barbiturates
Opiates

METABOLIC
Hypoxia
Hypoglycemia
Renal failure (acidosis/electrolytes disbalance)
Hepatic failure

ENDOCRINOLOGIC
Hypothyroidism/hyperthyroidism
Addison's disease
Cushing's disease

or to try to reach the patient's primary care physician. If, in spite of every effort by EMS personnel, the patient does not cooperate with the initial assessment, physical or chemical restraints should be considered. No patient with behavioral changes should be left behind by EMS without an adequate assessment.

If the assessment is that the patient is medically stable, the next step is to decide whether his or her mental status represents a danger for himself or herself or others. Every case needs to be evaluated on an individual basis. Not every patient with abnormal behavior needs to be transported against his or her will. If the patient is refusing transport, he or she has to meet ALL of the following criteria for his or her request to be honored: 1) organic etiology has been ruled out by appropriate medical evaluation, 2) no evidence of suicidal or aggressive behavior, 3) known history of psychiatric disorders with similar behavior in the past, and 4) appropriate social or family support.

It is the responsibility of the on-line physician to ensure that a complete evaluation is done before EMS personnel leave the scene. Most adult patients who present to the ED with acute psychiatric symptoms have an organic etiology.[6] Evaluation and "medical clearance" in the field can be even more difficult than at the ED.

Suicidal and violent patients are the major behavioral emergencies for which the medical control physician and personnel in the field have to be ready to cope. Give special attention to the presence of risk factors for suicide or the development of violent behavior (discussed in the next two sections). If the patient shows potential for suicide or aggressiveness, EMS personnel should not leave him or her alone or without supervision under any circumstances. Carry out and document every possible effort to accomplish transport. Cooperation from the family, friends, co-workers, private physician, and law enforcement authorities, if available, can be of great value. Protocols with detailed descriptions of the role for interagency cooperation are very helpful in these situations.

The Suicidal Patient

Always take very seriously any patient who is making a suicide threat in the field. Suicidal statements indicate the presence of a crisis the individual feels he or she is unable to handle. Intervention by the EMS system and appropriate authorities may be the last opportunity to provide help to the patient. These patients should be treated with the same urgency as a patient in shock.

After arriving on the scene, EMS personnel should perform a complete assessment of the situation. They must explore the surroundings for weapons or potential weapons. If guns or knives are present, the EMS crew should stay back for their own safety and wait for trained personnel (usually police) to remove the weapon as soon as possible. If the patient voluntarily surrenders the weapon, he or she should be asked to drop it to the floor. Immediately remove any objects that the patient could use to inflict physical damage to himself or herself or others. If the patient locked himself or herself inside a room, prehospital care providers should be instructed to stand by the side of the door, never directly in front of it. Attempts to initiate communication with the patient should be

made as soon as possible. If he or she is conscious and willing to negotiate try to "talk him or her out." It is better to talk through closed doors than to try to break in, since this may produce further agitation and confusion from the patient. Direct communication with the on-line physician or the patient's family physician may have some impact for the patient who is asking for help. During the negotiations, you can also use friends or family members that the patient trusts and respects. If the patient identifies any individual present at the scene as being part of the crisis, that individual should be removed from the scene. Encourage the patient to discuss the situation and what is exacerbating this crisis. Most patients are relieved to discuss their thoughts.[10] Emphasize with the EMS crew to show sympathy and concern and do nothing that could frighten or agitate him or her. They don't have to agree or disagree with the patient, just listen to what he or she has to say. Avoid comments such as: "Don't do that!" or "You know it is not true!" The patient may consider these comments as a challenge or as members of the rescue team being judgmental and not supportive. If the patient perceives a negative attitude from the rescue team, it will worsen the patient's already low self-esteem. Provide reassurance that the crisis can be solved and that authorities are there only to help in any possible way. Do not make promises that you or the prehospital care providers cannot keep because the patient will likely become more suspicious.

Once the patient starts to cooperate and agrees with transport, everything that will be done should be explained to him or her. If possible, the patient should be fastened to the stretcher and never allowed to sit next to the exit door in the ambulance. Explain these are security measures for his or her own safety. The person who established the best rapport with the patient should ride along with him or her to the hospital. Members of the rescue team should then sit next to the exit. Do not allow patients to ride in the front seat, and again, never next to the door.

If all reasonable efforts by the rescue team fail to persuade the patient to cooperate, the issue of whether to commit the patient to an involuntary transport must be decided. This is a decision in which direct medical control must be involved. There are several factors that correlate with a higher risk for committing suicide. These are listed in Table 16-1. If the assessment is that the patient is in immediate danger for suicide, proceed with the transport and do not leave him or her alone under any circumstances. Laws pertaining to involuntary transport and admissions vary from state to state. Physicians involved in direct medical control need to be familiar with the specifics of these statutes in the local area. When in doubt, it is better to err on the side of involuntary transport and have the patient evaluated at an ED or psychiatric institution. If once the decision for involuntary transport has been made the patient becomes agitated or violent, consider physical or chemical restraints following the guidelines described in the violent patient section.

Table 16-1 Factors Associated with a Higher Risk for Suicide

Factors	High Risk
Suicide intentions	■ Affirmation of suicide intention ■ Detailed and violent plan with poor probability for rescue and accessible resources (e.g., gun) ■ History of previous attempts
Psychiatric diagnosis	■ Schizophrenia ■ Bipolar disorder ■ Major depression ■ Acute psychosis
Medical problems	■ Diagnosis of terminal diseases (e.g., cancer, AIDS) ■ Diagnosis of chronic illness (e.g., diabetes)
Drug abuse	■ Alcohol, cocaine, other illicit drugs
Social history	■ Marital status—widowed or divorced ■ Recent significant loss—death of a loved one ■ Unemployment ■ No family support
Family history	■ Suicide ■ Psychiatric disorders
Sex	■ Women—attempt suicide more often ■ Men—successful attempts more often
Age	■ Over 45 years old

The Violent Patient

Violence is like a spreading cancer reaching every aspect of today's society. As a result, the number of violence-related calls in the prehospital setting is increasing. Prehospital care providers deal with violence from different angles. They see victims of violent events (e.g., stab and gunshot wounds, domestic violence, rapes), but they are also confronting violent patients. Paramedics are generally very well-trained in how to deal with the wounded patient, but unfortunately they have significantly less training in the management of the aggressive patient.[2,3,11] These patients must be addressed with extreme caution, since minor pitfalls may lead to major tragedies. As always, when arriving on scene before any intervention, they should assess if the scene is safe. The first priority should always be to ensure their safety. They cannot assist the patient if they become victims themselves. If there are weapons in the surroundings, the EMS crew should wait for proper authorities to clear the scene before they proceed.

It is important that paramedics receive training not only on how to interact with the violent patient, but they should also be able to evaluate the potentially violent patient as well, before violence erupts.[12] When facing the patient, prehospital care providers should perform a quick assessment of his or her physical and emotional status. We already discussed Box 16-1, which lists organic conditions that could manifest as behavioral emergencies. It is very important to keep them in mind when building the differential diagnosis. Always give priority to vital sign stabilization. Once organic etiologies have been ruled out, there is valuable information that the EMS personnel can collect on scene that will help to assess the potential danger for violence. Ask them to observe and describe the patient's attitude. Patients who are talking in a loud voice, moving around constantly, gesticulating with arms, or showing closed fists should be considered potential aggressors.[3,11,13] Investigate if the patient has previous history of aggressive behavior. This is the single most important risk factor to predict the possibility of aggressiveness, especially if the previous history was against law enforcement officers or figures of authority.[14] Also, investigate for a history of psychiatric disorders. Psychosis, paranoia, manic-depressive disorder, and antisocial personality have been identified as diagnoses with a higher incidence of violent behavior.[14] The presence of drug paraphernalia or any indication of alcohol or illicit drug abuse are significant risk factors as well. Intoxicated patients have poor control of their emotions and become violent more easily.

After this quick evaluation the EMS crew should have a better understanding of the patient's condition. Even if the evaluation indicates low risk for aggressiveness, prehospital care providers should always be alert and ready to react. If the patient is considered to be at high risk for violence, the following measures should be taken immediately:[1,8]

- Never leave the patient alone. Keep a safe distance and have a member of the rescue team standing by the exit at all times. Never allow the patient to block the escape route!
- Any object at the scene that could be used by the patient as a weapon has to be removed.
- Nominate one individual to be the "negotiator". If the patient is medically stable, be prepared to spend a long time talking to him or her. If the negotiator seems to be losing patience, someone else should let him or her know and assume the role. It is better to spend the extra minute for a peaceful solution than to rush to a physical confrontation.
- When facing a violent individual, avoid prolonged eye contact since it may be considered as a challenge.
- Try to identify the reasons for this crisis and let the patient ventilate his or her thinking. Be supportive and never argumentative.
- A "show of force" with several members of the team backing the negotiator to let the patient know that he or she is outnumbered is usually enough to calm him or her down.

It is always possible that in spite of all reasonable preventive measures by the rescue team, the patient will become violent or will refuse transport even if it is medically or psychiatrically indicated. At this point, physical or chemical restraints may be necessary. In general, the on-line physician must be involved and decide if the patient should be transported against his or her will. This is a medical decision with heavy legal implications. This kind of decision should not be on the hands of the paramedics. The legal justification for this procedure is based in the professional judgment of the physician in charge that the patient is mentally incompetent.[15] You have to be involved, and you have to be familiar with the statutes in your area. Generally, the medicolegal risk of let-

ting a patient go who is at risk of harming others or himself or herself is much higher than the risk involved in the involuntary transport.

Physical Restraint

The major indication for restraining a patient is when he or she is considered incompetent to make decisions by himself or herself and his or her behavior precludes a good evaluation. It is important to document how the patient represents a threat to himself or herself or others. Before proceeding with physical restraints, the rescue team should identify a team leader. The leader should be the same person who has been the negotiator up to this point. Give the patient a last opportunity to cooperate and explain to him or her that otherwise he or she will be restrained for his or her own safety and to help him or her maintain self-control. The team has to be well-organized, and each member should have specific responsibilities. The ideal number of persons in the team is five, one for each extremity and one for the head and neck. The following is commonly recommended procedure for physical restraint:[1,16]

- The leader should continue to communicate with the patient.
- Two persons should approach the patient from behind, while two more approach from the front. This will make it difficult for the patient to concentrate and attack from one flank.
- If the patient attacks to one side, the persons left behind him should grasp both arms by the elbows simultaneously. The patient should be forced to the floor, face down, by locating the legs in front of his or hers and pushing forward.
- At this point the other two members of the team will hold the patient's legs by the knees while the leader restrains the head to prevent injury and precludes the patient from biting and spitting.
- Restrain the patient facedown to the stretcher using the four-point restraint technique. Leather restraints are recommended, but straps, towels, and other similar materials can be used to improvise if necessary.
- Restrain one hand over the patient's head and the other by the patient's side. This will decrease the amount of force in one direction that he or she can use.

- Once restrained, keep talking to the patient to try to calm him or her down. Do not leave him or her alone, and monitor neurovascular status distal to the restraints in all extremities closely. Search his or her clothes for any other potentially dangerous object (e.g., sharp objects, matches). If possible, this should be done in the presence of law enforcement authority.
- Do not negotiate the restraints with the patient during transport. Do not remove the restraints until arrival at the receiving facility.
- Once at the receiving facility, make sure they have all the necessary equipment and backup personnel before taking the restraints off.

Ideally, law enforcement officers should be involved in the procedure and stay during transport. They have better training and much more experience with these kinds of situations. EMS and law enforcement personnel should work together, but prehospital care providers should not allow police officers to influence the evaluation and treatment of the patient.[3] It is desirable to have frequent training sessions to practice these techniques. That would help to improve communication and cooperation between the agencies in the real situation.

Chemical Restraint

Sometimes physical restraint is not enough. Although they may be able to restrain the patient, it is impossible to perform a good evaluation if the patient is still agitated. The care the patient needs is obstructed by his or her behavior. It is now recognized that the use of chemical restraint is more effective and humane than physical restraint. Rapid tranquilization is the technique of giving a psychotropic drug to control behavioral disturbances.[17] The combination of physical and chemical restraints is the best approach to control the patient and proceed with the evaluation and transport. The medical control physician has to be directly involved in the decision making process. The use of drugs is indicated only when the clinical impression of the physician is that the patient is not competent to decide for himself or herself and his or her behavior represents an immediate danger for himself or herself and others or hinders a safe transport. The goal is to control agitation and psychotic symptoms. When considering medications for agitated patients in the

prehospital environment, certain characteristics are of vital importance:

- The medication should be available for IM administration. Frequently, in the field the patient will not have an IV line and will not cooperate to establish one.
- It should have a rapid onset of action, since we are waiting for the patient to calm down to accomplish transport.
- It should have a minimal effect on CNS depression and a short half-life so that a complete evaluation can be performed at the receiving facility.
- As with any other medication, we want it to have the lowest possible incidence of side effects.

Rapid tranquilization is a fairly common technique used in EDs and psychiatric wards. EMS personnel are extrapolating from the EDs experience and are using the same technique. The availability for appropriate medications can be limited by the state or regional list of approved drugs for EMS personnel to administer.[16] Among several drugs used for RT, neuroleptics and benzodiazepines are the two most commonly used.

Neuroleptics

Probably the most popular neuroleptic used in the prehospital setting today is haloperidol, a butyrophenone that can be administered by the PO, IM, or IV route.[7] This high potency neuroleptic has been shown to be effective in controlling agitation.[19] The classic regimen of administration is 5 mg IM, or IV. In extremely agitated or large patients a 10 mg initial dose can be used. The dose can be repeated every 30 to 60 minutes if needed.[20] One advantage of haloperidol is that the patient remains responsive to commands and is not sedated.[21] Onset of clinical effect is observed in 20 minutes with the IM route and in 5-10 minutes with the IV route.[22] If the patient cooperates, an oral concentrate dose (10 mg) can be used with similar effects as the IM injection.[23] Haloperidol has a low incidence of side effects. The most common is extrapyramidal symptoms (less than 10%) and it is easily reversible with diphenhydramine 50 mg IM or benztropine 2 mg IM. Extrapyramidal symptoms can occur with only one dose and up to 12-24 hours after the initial dose. Other less common side effects include akathisia, hypotension, neuroleptic malignant syndrome, and decreased seizure threshold (not proven in humans).[8,22,24,25]

Another butyrophenone that is being used for the same indications is droperidol. This medication, which is very similar structurally to haloperidol, is showing excellent results with the agitated patient as well. Droperidol can also be administered by the PO, IM, or IV route and it has a better IM absorption with a faster onset of action and a shorter half life than haloperidol. The IM absorption of droperidol is so good that its effect compares with the IV administration of haloperidol. The half-life for droperidol after IM administration is 2.2 hours compared to 19 hours for haloperidol.[26] Several studies have reported faster onset of action (3 to 10 minutes IV or IM), fewer side effects, and a decreased need for a second administration.[27-31] The usual dose for droperidol is the same as for haloperidol, 5 mg IM or IV every 30 to 60 minutes. The significant side effects with droperidol are greater sedation and orthostatic hypotension. The latter is easily treated by keeping the patient supine and giving IV fluids. Because of its faster onset of action, low incidence of side effects, and short half life, droperidol will probably become the drug of choice for RT in the prehospital environment.

Benzodiazepines

The other group of medications used for prehospital rapid tranquilization are the benzodiazepines. Diazepam has been used in the past with the limitation of an erratic IM absorption. Lorazepam and midazolam both have good IM absorption. Typical regimens would be lorazepam 0.05 mg/kg IM or midazolam 0.1-0.2 mg/kg IM every 30 to 60 minutes until symptoms are controlled (Table 16-2). The most important indication for benzodiazepines is for RT of patients in alcohol or sedative withdrawal. In these cases, benzodiazepines are the drug of choice. Significant side effects with the use of benzodiazepines are excessive sedation and respiratory depression. Patients with chronic COPD and carbon dioxide retention are especially sensitive to the respiratory depression side effect.[25,32] This represents a relative contraindication.

Benzodiazepine and butyrophenones can be used together. Several investigators have reported the use of lorazepam in combination with haloperidol with good results and an apparent synergistic effect reducing the amount required of each drug.[8,23,24] A recommended dose is 5 mg haloperidol with 2 mg of lorazepam given IM every 2-3 hours until sedated.

Pitfalls

As previously described, the scene involving a mentally disturbed patient can be chaotic. Under these circumstances, it is very easy to commit serious mistakes. One of the most common mistakes is an incomplete medical evaluation. Lack of vital sign assessment can lead to the false impression that the patient is "just nuts." This is a critical mistake with possible tragic consequences. The patient's medical condition may continue to deteriorate later on, even after EMS has left the scene. On the other hand, after medical stability has been confirmed, there is a tendency from prehospital personnel to minimize the need for intervention. There is a significant lack of empathy with psychiatric patients. This may lead

Table 16-2 Common Medications for Rapid Tranquilization[20-22]

Medication	Dose	Route	Onset of Action	Peak Effect
Droperidol	5-10 mg	PO, IM	3-10 min	30-60 min
		IV	3-10 min	30-60 min
Haloperidol	5-10 mg	PO, IM	10-20 min	30-60 min
		IV (Do not use deconate salt IV)	5-10 min	30-60 min
Diazepam	0.1-0.2 mg/kg	IV (over 1 min)	5-10 min	30-60 min
Lorazepam	0.05-0.1 mg/kg	IM, IV	15-20 min	60-90 min
Midazolam	0.05-0.1 mg/kg	IV	5-10 min	30-60 min
	0.01-0.2 mg/kg	IM	15 min	30-60 min

the crew to believe the patient is "faking" and "wasting our time." This is extremely dangerous, especially in the situation of suicidal threats. Every patient who is suspected to have suicidal ideations should be transported for psychiatric evaluation. It is better to overtreat than to undertreat.

When facing an agitated patient, it is very dangerous to rush the patient. Not spending enough time talking to the patient to establish rapport is another common mistake. Instruct the prehospital crew to give assurance and to try to gain the patient's trust. Becoming argumentative and trying to reason with a mentally disturbed patient will just cause further agitation.

If the patient is armed and agitated, order your people to leave the scene. Law enforcement agencies should be notified and assume control of the scene until it is safe for EMS personnel to proceed. Insist that they should not attempt to fight or restrain the patient without the adequate personnel and equipment. Do not subject your personnel and the patient to unnecessary injuries. After physical or chemical restraint, never leave the patient alone. Continue close monitoring of vital signs and mental status. Be careful with oversedation or side effects from pharmacotherapy.

Finally, another common and tragic pitfall is lack of interagency coordination. The approach to these patients must be very organized. Avoid arguments between rescue team members in front of the patient. Everybody should understand their role and responsibility before dealing directly with the patient.

Summary

Behavioral emergencies represent a unique challenge for the prehospital care provider. Paramedics and EMTs frequently face patients and situations that are difficult to handle given their limited training. Sometimes even their own safety is in jeopardy. Active participation from the medical director and medical control physician is important to guarantee the best quality of care for the patient and to provide assurance to the crew. Protocols and frequent training sessions with other safety agencies may yield the best results. These training sessions provide the ideal forum for practice, discussion, and improvement of communication. Only 47% of respondents to a questionnaire said they have specific protocols for handling violence in their prehospital systems. In the same study, only 9% have cross-training sessions with law enforcement authorities.[2]

As with any other medical emergency, assessment and stabilization of vital signs should be done as soon as possible. Always assume an organic etiology until proven otherwise. Under no circumstances should a person with questionable mental capacity be allowed to refuse transport and sign AMA. Familiarize yourself with local statutes for involuntary transport and be ready to use restraining techniques (physical and chemical) as needed. It is better to err on the side of transport and have the patient fully evaluated in the ED. Society expects medical professionals to be able to recognize and manage patients who are dangerous to themselves or others. This is a great responsibility that we have to be ready to assume.

S A M P L E   C A S E S

CASE # 1

"Medic command this is Medic 7. We are on the scene with a 38-year-old man with a history of HIV+. The mother says the patient has been "acting strange" since yesterday. She also says he has been vomiting and complaining of headache for 2 days. The patient is oriented in person and place but is unable to identify the date or the President of the United States. He looks lethargic, and we are having problems getting information from him due to alcohol intoxication. He has a strong odor of alcohol on his breath and his mother confirms he is drinking a lot. The patient says he doesn't want to go to the hospital and wants to sign AMA. He is not showing any aggressive behavior and denies suicidal ideas. His vital signs are: HR = 120, RR = 22, BP = 110/50, PULSE OXIMETER is 95% at room air, SKIN is warm and slightly pale, LUNGS are clear to auscultation, HEART has a regular rhythm without murmur, ABD is soft and depressible, no masses, no tender to palpation, extremities no edema or cyanosis. Doc, I believe he is just drunk. Is it OK with you if he signs AMA?"

What would you say?

Definitely you would say NO! This presentation shows multiple risk factors highly suggestive of an organic problem. First, the history of HIV+ is a warning sign for the possibility of multiple CNS complications. The behavioral changes are of acute onset and with altered vital signs (HR=120). They described the patient as being intoxicated, confused, and lethargic, so he is not mentally competent to sign AMA. You should suspect the etiology of his behavioral changes to be from an organic etiology until proven otherwise. Actually his temperature at the ED was 103.1°F and a CT scan showed a frontal lobe brain abscess.

CASE # 2

"Medic Command this is Medic 3. We were called to the scene by the sister of a 65-year-old female patient because the patient was talking about suicide. The sister says that the patient has been in a very depressed mood for the last 4 weeks. She has a history of depression in the past, including one hospitalization. At present, she is in outpatient treatment with a private psychiatrist and is taking medications (Amitriptyline). The sister says the patient told her that soon she wouldn't need to worry about her anymore. At present, the patient is alert and oriented with vital signs: HR = 90/min, BP = 120/60, RR = 16/min. She is in an obvious depressed mood but denies suicidal ideas. She is crying and upset with her sister because she called us. She says we have more important patients to see and that she doesn't need to go to the hospital. I think she is OK and she already signed the refusal for transport."

How would you proceed?

It is common for EMS systems to receive calls from a third person with concerns about a "psychiatric patient." In this example, the patient herself refused transport. The problem was that the EMS crew accepted her will without trying reasonable efforts to accomplish transport. The patient was in an "obvious depressed mood" and gave symptoms of low self-esteem when she said to the ambulance crew that they have "more important patients to see." She also had previous history of psychiatric hospitalization. These are significant risk factors that warrant further evaluation. There were no efforts to address what was the problem. They didn't try to contact the primary care physician. The patient was allowed to stay at home and 3 days later the same crew responded to the same address for a patient found in cardiac arrest secondary to amitriptyline overdose.

CASE # 3

"Doctor, this is paramedic Joe Smith. We have a problem here. We are facing a 33-year-old male patient with past history of psychiatric disorders. A neighbor called us because he heard the patient calling for help. The patient lives alone in his apartment and there is no family available. Upon arrival, we found the patient sitting at the kitchen table talking about "messages from God." He is very agitated, diaphoretic, and says we are "slaves of the devil." He is not letting us get close to him. Police are on the scene, but they say the patient is not breaking the law and they refuse to help us restrain the patient for transport."

How would you proceed?

This is indeed a relatively common scene. The acutely psychotic patient is a very challenging patient for the EMS system. Not every psychotic patient needs to be transported. Evaluate each patient individually and assess risks for violence or suicide. This particular patient is having paranoid delusions, is showing an aggressive behavior, and it is almost impossible to communicate with. This patient needs to be further evaluated in the ED and should be transported.

It is important that the rescue team show a common front to the patient; if they start arguing about what their roles are, this will only add to the pandemonium of the situation and to the patient's agitation. Coordination and communication between safety agencies are essential. Ask to talk with the law enforcement officer in charge or his or her supervisor. Explain the need for medical transport and why their intervention is important. Protocols with detailed descriptions for the role of each agency should be available and approved by the respective authorities. Frequent joint training sessions for discussion and update of protocols are recommended. This patient is a candidate for chemical restraint. If necessary, the patient may be physically restrained first. Droperidol 5 mg IM would have a sedative effect and should diminish the psychotic symptoms. If needed, a repeat dose of Droperidol 5 mg can be given in 30 minutes. Once the patient is under control, check vital signs and physical exam. He should then be transferred to the nearest medical facility with in-house psychiatric service.

References

1. Bledsoe BE: *Behavioral and psychiatric emergencies. Brady paramedic emergency care,* ed 2, 1994, Brady.

2. Tintinally JE: Violent patient and the prehospital provider, *Ann Emerg Med* 22(8):1276-1279, 1993.

3. Verdile VP: Prehospital management of the violent patient, *Prehospital Care Reports* 2(3):17-24, 1992.

4. Judd RL: Behavioral and psychological crisis in emergency medical services, *Top Emer Med* 4(4):1-7, 1983.

5. *Dorland's illustrated medical dictionary,* ed 27, Philadelphia, 1988, WB Saunders.

6. Henneman PL, Mendoza R, Lewis RJ: Prospective evaluation of emergency department medical clearance, *Ann Emerg Med* 24(4):672-677, 1994.

7. Coffman JA: Behavioral disorders: emergency assessment and stabilization. In Tintinalli JE, Krome RL, Ruiz E, editors: *Emergency medicine: a comprehensive study guide,* ed 3, Philadelphia, 1992, Lea & Febinger.

8. Goldberg RJ, Dubin WR, Fogel BS: Review: behavioral emergencies, assessment of psychopharmacologic management, *Clin Neuropharm* 12:233-248, 1989.

9. Slaby AE: Medical disease presenting as a behavioral emergency, *Top Emer Med* 4(4):24-29, 1983.

10. Greaves G, Small L: Comparison of accomplished suicides with persons contacting clinical intervention clinics, *Psychol Res* 3:390, 1972.

11. Fredrick L: Defending your life: how to manage the violent patients and scenes, *JEMS* June:64-67, 1992.

12. Lehman LS, Padilla M, Clark S, et al.: Training personnel in the prevention and management of violent behavior. In *Management of violent behavior. Washington, D.C.: Hospital and Community Psychiatry Service,* 1988, American Psychiatric Association, pp. 24-27.

13. Blumenreich P, Lippman S, Bacani-Oropilla T: Violent patients: are you prepared to deal with them? *Post Grad Med* 90(2):201-206, 1991.

14. Dagadakis CS, Maiuro RD: The assaultive patient. In Schwartz GR, Cayten CG, Mangelsen MA, et al., editors: *Principles and practice of emergency medicine,* ed 3, Philadelphia, 1992, Lea & Febinger.

15. Tardiff K: Management of the violent patient in an emergency situation, *Psychiatr Clin North Am* 11(4):539-549, 1988.

16. Sanders MJ: Behavioral emergencies and crisis intervention. In Stoy, WA, editor: *Mosby's paramedic textbook,* ed 1, St Louis, 1994, Mosby Lifeline.

17. Pilowsky LS, Ring H, Shine PJ, et al.: Rapid tranquilization: a survey of emergency prescribing in a general psychiatric hospital, *Br J Psych* 160:831-835, 1992.

18. Delbridge TR, Verdile VP, Platt TE: Variability of state-approved emergency medical services drug formularies, *Prehosp Disaster Med* 9(3), Suppl 2:55, 1994.

19. Donlon PT, Hopkin J, Tupin JP: Efficacy and safety of the rapid neuroleptization method with injectable haloperidol, *Am J Psychiatry* 136(3):273-278, 1979.

20. Benitez JG: How to control the violent patient, *UPMC Trauma Rounds* 5(3):6-7, 1994.

21. DiPiro JJ, Talbert RL, Hayes PE, et al.: *Pharmacotherapy: a pathophysiologic approach,* ed 1, New York, 1989, Elsevier Science Publishing.

22. *Physicians Desk Reference,* ed 50, Montvale, 1996, Medical Economics Co.

23. Circaulo DA: Psychotropic drug therapy in the emergency department, *Top Emer Med* 4(4):17-23, 1983.

24. Dagadakis CS: The emergent psychotic patient. In Schwartz GR, Cayten CG, Mangelsen MA, et al., editors: *Principles and practice of emergency medicine,* ed 3, Philadelphia, 1992, Lea & Febinger.

25. Dubin WR: Rapid tranquillization: antipsychotics or benzodiazepines, *J Clin Psych* 40:250-260, 1988.

26. O'Shanick GJ: Emergency psychopharmacology, *Am J Emerg Med* (2):164-170, 1984.

27. Cressman WA, Plostnieks J, Johnson PC: Absorption, metabolism and excretion of droperidol by human subjects following intramuscular and intravenous administration, *Anesthesiology* 38:363-369, 1973.

28. Neff KE, Denney D, Blachly PH: Control of severe agitation with droperidol, *Dis Nerv Syst* 33(9):594-597, 1972.

29. Resnick M, Burton BT: Droperidol vs. haloperidol in the initial management of acutely agitated patients, *J Clin Psych* 45(7):298-299, 1984.

30. Thomas H, Schartz E, Petrilli R: Droperidol vs. haloperidol for chemical restraint of agitated and combative patients, *Ann Emerg Med* 21(4):407-413, 1992.

31. Van Leeuwen AM, Molders J, Sterkmans P, et al.: Droperidol in acutely agitated patients: a double blind placebo-controlled study, *J Nerv Men Dis* 164(4):280-283, 1977.

32. Burns Stewart SM: Droperidol, *Critical Care Nurse* 7(5):86, 1987.

33. Mitchells-Heggs P, Murphy K, Minty K, et al.: Diazepam in the treatment of dyspnea in the "pink puffer" syndrome, *QJ Med* 20:178-183, 1980.

PART 3

Special Concerns

This final section describes aspects of emergency medical services systems that are taking on an ever-increasing importance in our practice as on-line medical commanders. Delivering quality medical care in the field is an expectation shared by providers and physicians alike. The process by which quality is achieved and maintained is presented succinctly. Ethical issues, such as when to honor do not resuscitate directives, when to stop resuscitation, and the limits of patient autonomy in the prehospital environment, are frequently encountered and expertly discussed in the chapter on ethics. The medicological implications of on-line medical command dovetails nicely with the ethical issues presented. The medicolegal chapter highlights many of the commonly encountered pitfalls of delivering patient care at the hands of surrogates in an uncontrolled prehospital environment. Topics, such as patients who refuse medical assistance, consent to treatment issues, and the concept of vicarious liability, are discussed.

Most on-line medical commanders seldom entertain the broader-system of emergency medical services that might affect patient care. Ambulance staffing, staging, dispatching, and levels of service provided all have ramifications on the timely delivery of out-of-hospital medical care. Air medical services, where available, must also be coordinated with the overall system to optimize use and enhance patient care. The composition of air medical teams, their capabilities, and the implications of air medical transport are all explored.

After reading this last section, the on-line medical commander should come away with a more thorough understanding of the penumbral yet critically important aspects of emergency medical services that will hopefully augment their ability to care for patients in the field.

Air-Medical Command

T he medical command physician providing direction to ALS EMT-Ps working in the air-medical environment must understand both the similarities and the dramatic differences encountered in this theater of operations. Command physicians will find the greatest similarities providing direction to EMT-Ps providing on-scene patient care for trauma and medical emergencies, which is consistent with the normal scope of practice of licensed ground providers. On the other hand, the command physician may face a dilemma when the EMT-P is involved in care and air transport of patients between hospital settings where he or she will likely meet a variety of clinical conditions not normally encountered in the prehospital arena. Here the command physician must be familiar with his air-medical crew composition (EMT-P/Nurse (RN), EMT-P/physician, or EMT-P only), level of EMT-P certification in states with more than one level, and the medications and procedures that can be administered by each flight team member in accordance with their respective scope of practice (Figures 17-1 and 17-2).

In like fashion, the command physician must be aware of the constraints placed by statute on the various members of the air-medical team. Adding to this dilemma, some medical command physicians are called on to direct medical care by an air-medical crew that flies into neighboring states that may have different statutory mandates governing the performance of EMT-Ps and nurses (RNs) with regards to patient care.

Lastly, to meet the challenges of patient care in the air-medical venue, the standard method of on-line medical direction of patient care may be unfeasible. A reliance on standing order protocols rather than contemporaneous physician input may necessarily be the norm in some flight programs because the capability of the communication equipment is likely to be insufficient in light of the helicopter's range of operation.

Crew Composition

Air-medical teams are usually made up of two medical crew members. While both may be EMT-Ps, most frequently in the United States these crews will be made up of an EMT-P and an RN. In some air-medical programs an EMT-P or an RN and a physician make up the team, and occasionally two RNs comprise the crew. In this unique setting, the physician on board may act as the command physician, as well as an integral part of the team.

MICHAEL LEICHT, MD   VINCENT P. VERDILE, MD, FACEP

DEPARTMENT OF HEALTH EMERGENCY MEDICAL SERVICES APPROVED DRUGS, MEDICATIONS AND SOLUTIONS

28 Pa. Code 1003.24(2) (v) provides a certified EMT-Paramedic may, under medical command or approved medical protocols, prepare and administer approved medications and solutions, and a list of such approved medications will be published at least annually by the Department. In addition, 28 Pa. Code 1005.11(b) (relating to licensure of advanced life support (ALS) services), provides that the Department will publish at least annually a list of drugs and medications approved for use by licensed ALS services. The following list constitutes approved drugs, medications and solutions under the above regulations.

1. Adenosine
2. Albuterol
3. Aminophylline
4. Atropine Sulfate
5. Bretylium
6. Calcium Chloride
7. Dexamethasone Sodium Phosphate
8. Diazepam
9. Diphenhydramine HCL
10. Dobutamine
11. Dopamine
12. Epinephrine HCL
13. Furosemide
14. Glucagon
15. Heparin Lock Flush
16. Hydrocortisone Sodium Succinate
17. Intravenous Electrolyte Solutions
    (a) Dextrose
    (b) Lactated Ringer's
    (c) Sodium Chloride
    (d) Normosol
18. Isoproterenol HCL
19. Lidocaine HCL
20. Meperidine
21. Metaproterenol
22. Morphine Sulfate
23. Naloxone HCL
24. Nitroglycerin Intravenous Drip (for Interfacility Transport Only)
25. Nitroglycerin Ointment
26. Nitroglycerin Spray
27. Nitroglycerin Sublingual Tablets
28. Nitrous Oxide
29. Oxytocin
30. Procainamide
31. Sodium Bicarbonate
32. Sterile Water for Injection
33. Terbutaline
34. Verapamil

Advanced life support services may carry any of the drugs above, not necessarily all of the drugs. No service, however, can exceed this list, except air advanced life support services with written approval of the Department.

Allan S. Noonan, M.D.
Secretary of Health

Source: Pennsylvania Bulletin, Vol. 22, No. 34, August 22, 1992

Figure 17-1. Sample form of approved ALS drugs.

The EMT-P/RN team provides the most common crew composition encountered. The command physician must have a working understanding of what procedures the EMT-P and the RN are each licensed to perform and what medications they are permitted to administer according to state statute. It is common in this setting for command physicians to be required to give command to the RN for drugs or procedures that are not permitted by the EMT-P and vice versa. The EMT-P often assists but cannot accept or be responsible for completing orders in areas that exceed the usual and customary scope of practice of an EMT-P. An example of this dilemma is that few states allow EMT-Ps to use neuromuscular blocking agents, but all EMT-Ps are expected to be proficient in endotracheal intubation.[1] It is good practice for the medical command physician to keep a list of drugs and procedures permitted for the EMT-P to administer near the base station for immediate reference.

In the case where the EMT-P has contacted medical command but the orders need to be carried out by the RN,

PARAMEDIC PROTOCOL MANUAL

MODULE   System Introduction

SECTION   ALS Equipment and Supplies

To receive and maintain certification as an Advanced Life Support Provider in the Susquehanna EHS Council, ALS Units are required to maintain the following minimum equipment and supplies, unless otherwise stated as OPTIONAL:

I.V. EQUIPMENT
14 G Angio-Catheters
16 G Angio-Catheters
18 G Angio-Catheters
20 G Angio-Catheters
22 G Angio-Catheters
Assorted Butterfly Catheters

Micro and Macro Administration
   Sets
Alcohol and Preps, Tourniquets
I.V. Medication Labels
Regular and Short Arm Boards
Vacutainer, Needles and Tubes

Optional
12 G and 24 G Angio-Catheters
Y-Type Blood Administration Sets

I.V. SOLUTIONS
Dextrose
Lactated Ringer's
Sodium Chloride or Equivalent

SYRINGES
1 cc, TB
3 cc
5 cc

10 cc
50 cc
Assorted Needles (for SQ and IM)

MEDICATIONS
Albuterol
Atropine Sulfate
Bretylium
Calcium Chloride
Dextrose
Diazepam Diphenhydramine HCL
Dopamine
Epinephrine HCL
Furosemide

Isoproterenol HCL
Lidocaine HCL
Morphine Sulfate
Naloxone HCL
Nitroglycerin Sublingual Tablets
Oxytocin
Sodium Bicarbonate
Sterile Water for Injection
Verapamil

Optional
Aminophylline
Dexamethasone Sodium Phosphate
Dobutamine
Glucagon
Heparin Lock Flush
Hydrocortisone Sodium
Succinate

Meperidine
Metaproterenol
Nitroglycerin Spray
Nitrous Oxide
Procainamide
Terbutaline

(continued)

Figure 17-2. Sample form of ALS equipment requirements.

PARAMEDIC PROTOCOL MANUAL

MODULE System Introduction

SECTION ALS Equipment and Supplies *(continued)*

AIRWAY MAINTENANCE

Assorted Oropharyngeal Airways
Assorted Nasopharyngeal
  Airways
Assorted Endotracheal Tubes
Esophageal Obturator Airway

Bag Valve Mask
Laryngoscope with Assorted
  Blades
Magill Forceps
Needle Cricothyrotomy Kit

COMMUNICATION AND TELEMETRY

Low-Band, Transceiver (Minimum 46.50 Mhz, 46.06 Mhz, 46.12 Mhz, 47.50 Mhz, 46.16 Mhz, 46.46 Mhz, 46.10 Mhz)
UHF Transceiver (MED Channels 1-10)
Acoustic Coupler Telephone Device

MISCELLANEOUS

Portable, Battery-Operated EKG Monitor/Defibrillator (Spare Batteries)
Portable, Battery-Operated Suction Device
Adult/Pediatric M.A.S.T.
Oxygen Supply and Adjuncts

Optional

Chem Strips
External Pacer
Mechanical CPR Devices

Nasogastric/Orogastric Tube Insertion Kits
Urinary Catheterization Kit

Figure 17-2. *(continued)*

the physician must understand what care the EMT-P can provide and where the RN must intervene, since speaking to both crew members separately is often not practical. Likewise, it is possible that in some states an RN may not be permitted to place central lines or perform endotracheal intubation; the command physician will be required to give these orders specifically to the EMT-P. More often than not, the arrangements for obtaining and carrying out physician directives will be made long before the actual patient encounter. The medical command physician must be vigilant with regard to the medical directives given and the capabilities of the individual flight crew member receiving those directives.

There is some experience with a physician as an integral part of the air-medical crew. The theoretical advantages are to have advanced clinical skills, advanced technical skills, and on-site medical direction as part of the flight crew.[2-7] The disadvantages for most flight programs are the cost and the availability of interested physicians. One study has suggested that a physician as one of two crew members offers no distinct patient care advantage in most flights although perhaps a slight advantage

for scene trauma patients.[5] Rhee found that physicians were of value in adding clinical judgment.[3] It seems as though the issue is not physician vs. nurse vs. paramedic as opposed to the training, experience, skills, and knowledge of the individual provider.

Theaters of Operation

Prehospital Transports

The most frequent prehospital setting for air-medical teams is motor vehicle related trauma. For these flights, medical command for the initial evaluation and stabilization by the RN and the EMT-P will differ very little. Trauma protocols for the care and transport of these patients are geared to allow for a rapid assessment and the adherence to fundamental resuscitative measures, with expeditious transport to a trauma center.

The two areas where protocol or medical command commonly differ between EMT-P and RN capabilities are in the administration of blood/colloid solutions and use of neuromuscular blocking agents. Many air-medical programs carry blood or colloid solutions routinely.

When the air-medical crew arrives at a scene to transport a trauma victim, it is not unusual for them to find that ALS personnel have already administered several liters of crystalloid solution. In the setting of persistent shock, the medical command physician may wish to administer packed red blood cells, a request that only the RN can execute.

Furthermore, while the EMT-P can perform endotracheal intubation, he or she is not, in most states, permitted to administer neuromuscular blocking agents.[1] Under these circumstances, to optimize patient care, in those air-medical programs that use these agents, the RN will be the flight crew member required to receive medical command and actually administer the agents. At this point, in most instances, either the nurse or EMT-P may proceed with endotracheal intubation.[1,6-11] The ability of the EMT-P to perform a surgical airway maneuver varies from state to state, and the command physician must be cognizant of the enabling statutes in his or her state.[1,12] Recently, studies have suggested that the use of neuromuscular blocking agents is safe and efficacious in the hands of non-physician flight crews.[13,14]

Unique to the use of air-medical services for the prehospital care and transport of patients is the consideration of time versus benefit. Clearly the role of air-medical services would be less useful if the time necessary to effect a ground transport of the patient would be significantly shorter than if a helicopter is used. Decisions about when and where the air-medical service will be used must, in addition to the patient's clinical condition, take into consideration the availability of ground ambulance services, the proximity to an appropriate hospital, and the time necessary to engage an air-medical service. Patients with prolonged field extrication from a motor vehicle accident or those patients requiring time dependent therapy not available at a referring hospital, such as thrombolytics for acute myocardial infarction, would usually benefit from air-medical transport. There is however, a paucity of research demonstrating the benefit of air-medical transportation for most clinical conditions. Therefore the logistics of establishing the most expeditious transport of any patient can often benefit from in-put from the on-line medical command physician. This is especially true for the trauma patient in an urban EMS enviroment.[15,16]

Interhospital Transports

The interhospital transfer of patients by air-medical services provides the greatest variety of patient types, many of whom the EMT-P is not specifically trained to treat. This is particularly true since many patients transported between hospitals in an air-medical program have already received initial resuscitative measures and are being transferred for a higher level of care. Consequently the nature and acuity of the patient's condition is often not routinely encountered by most ground prehospital care providers.[17-19]

When assisting in the care and transport of critically ill or injured patients, the ability of the EMT-P to provide airway interventions and standard ACLS care makes him or her an invaluable member of the interhospital transport team. On the other hand, certain command physician directives, such as the administration or maintenance of thrombolytic therapy, exceed the scope of practice of the EMT-P and therefore must be performed exclusively by the RN.[20]

There are potentially many such patient-care scenarios in which the EMT-P will be limited to only assisting the RN in rendering patient care. Another example might be a patient requiring vasoactive medications for maintaining a reasonable blood pressure in the setting of cardiogenic shock, which are not approved for use in the prehospital venue in the hands of EMT-Ps.

The interhospital transport of pediatric patients often presents tremendous challenges to the air-medical crew, since these patients tend to be more seriously ill or injured than those that are encountered in ground ambulance transports.[19] The command physician must be cognizant of the limitations placed upon the team members by statute with regards to the type of care that can be rendered. In many air-medical programs, the flight crew will include a specialty nurse, a physician assistant, or even a pediatrician. The composition of these specialty transport teams will usually dictate who will perform what care to the pediatric patient.[21,22]

Another challenging aspect of interhospital air-medical transports for the EMT-P is the care of those patients on predominately in-hospital equipment, such as IV infusion systems, intravascular pressure monitors, neonatal isolettes, or intraaortic balloon pumps. EMT-Ps are in most instances not permitted within their scope of practice to operate these devices. The responsibility for training on the use of these devices rests with the air-medical program. The EMT-P should develop a working understanding of these predominately in-hospital devices to be effective in the transport of these patients. Despite the additional training to EMT-Ps, medical command physicians will usually provide orders for the use of these specialized devices to the RN member of the flight crew (Figure 17-3).

MEDICAL COMMAND REPORT

DATE _____ TIME _____ HRS.

UNIT _____ PARAMEDIC _____

PHYSICIAN _____

TAPE _____ FROM-TO _____ PARAMEDIC _____

PHYSICIAN _____

INITIAL ASSESSMENT

AGE _____ SEX _____

ALLERGIES _____

C.C. & H.P.I. _____

PAST HISTORY _____

MEDICATIONS _____

PHYSICAL EXAM FINDINGS _____

VITAL SIGNS

TIME (hrs)								
BP								
PULSE								
RESP								
LOC								
EKG								

MILITARY TIME	ORDERS	TIME COMPLETED	RESULTS

NOTIFICATION OF RECEIVING HOSPITAL

DESTINATION _____ TIME NOTIFIED _____ HRS.

DATE _____

RECEIVING PHYSICIAN _____

DATE _____

COMMAND PHYSICIAN'S SIGNATURE _____

DATE _____

Figure 17-3. Sample form of an interhospital transport Medical Command Report.

Interstate Transports

The medical command physician called on to provide direction to EMT-Ps and RNs who frequently travel across state lines must be familiar with the differences that exist in state statutes regarding care allowed by prehospital care providers. While some states provide reciprocity and many states have very similar allowable lists of medications and procedures, it is important to check with adjacent state-specific EMS agencies before questions on medical command or liability issues arise. Most states also have statutes defining the scope of practice for RNs that should be clarified. Air-medical programs need to address each state's regulations to provide seamless care to the patients they transport.

Disasters

There is a great deal of literature describing the challenges and pitfalls of medical care for disasters that will not be reiterated here. A well-organized prehospital care system, including the air-medical program, can go a long way toward minimizing confusion and expediting medical care. The air-medical team should be a crucial part of any disaster management plan by providing one or more medical teams to the site, expediting transport of critically ill or injured patients, and returning to the disaster site with additional supplies or personnel. Several disaster management models have been described incorporating air-medical services.[23,24] Fortunately, disasters and mass casualty incidents are clinical venues that EMT-Ps are well-trained and certified to participate in, and medical command issues are almost nonexistent. Disaster management is one situation where the command physician responsible for triage may need to interact with an air-medical team quite apart from his or her usual practice of directing single patient encounters.

Communications

The practice of providing on-line medical direction to prehospital care providers can be difficult to accomplish routinely in an air-medical program. Often the distance from the base station, the topography, or the confines of a hospital building can prevent the contemporaneous interaction of the physician and the flight crew by either radio or cellular technology. Because of these limitations, it is essential to allow the flight crew to operate under standing order protocols that are not dependent on real-time, on-line physician communication. Standing orders, however, necessitate rigorous quality management measures after the fact to ensure safe and effective patient care.[25-28]

Aviation Physiology

It is well beyond the scope of this chapter to review all the medical ramifications of the physiological changes that occur with changes in altitude during flight. Suffice it to say that Boyle's law, temperature changes, air sickness, and other physical properties of gases in a changing altitude environment will all potentially impact the care rendered to patients in flight. It is especially important to remember that the total pressure of all gases in the air will decrease with altitude, which may, in the case of oxygen, create unexpected hypoxemia. The medical command physician must be aware of the potential implications of aviation physiology and be prepared to adjust patient care appropriately.

Along with the concerns about the impact of aviation physiology, the medical command physician must also be aware of the space and technology limitations in the helicopter. It is extremely difficult to perform a physical assessment on a patient or to perform some ALS procedures in the confines of most airborne helicopters. This requires that the air-medical crew accomplish all necessary and perhaps potentially necessary procedures before beginning transport of the patient. An example of this strategy might be the trauma patient with a small 15%-20% simple pneumothorax that might be otherwise observed, should have a tube thoracostomy performed before flight. This would be especially true if the patient was intubated and undergoing positive pressure ventilation. The inability to assess the patient's lung exam during flight, coupled with the potential for an enlargement of the pneumothorax due to altitude changes, warrants preemptive tube thoracostomy.

The same argument might be made for performing endotracheal inubation on patients with depressed level of consciousness before flight, since assessing a patient's neurological status and performing intubation during flight are nearly impossible. Indirect measurements of physiological parameters, such as pulse oximetry, are feasible, however, and can be used to guide patient management during flights.[29,30]

Summary

This chapter attempts to point out the essential principles of providing on-line medical direction to an air-medical program. The differences between ground and air ambulance services and the various health-care providers in air-medical programs are highlighted. The composition of the flight crew and the range of operation of the air-medical program often necessitate an awareness on the part of the physician providing medical direction of the specific rules and regulations governing patient care. On-line medical direction of air-medical crews is not always feasible and arrangements for standing order protocols should be made.

References

1. Lavery RF, Doran J, Tortella BJ, et al.: A survey of advanced life support practices in the United States, *Prehosp Disaster Med* 7:144-150, 1992.

2. Carraway RP, Brewer ME, Lewis BR, et al.: Why a physician? Aeromedical transport of the trauma victim, *J Trauma* (abst) 24:650, 1984.

3. Rhee KJ, Strizeski M, Burney RE, et al.: Is the flight physician needed for helicopter emergency services? *Ann Emerg Med* 15:174-177, 1986.

4. Baxt WG, Moody P: The impact of the physician as part of the aeromedical prehospital team in patients with blunt trauma, *JAMA* 257:3246-3250, 1987.

5. Hamman BL, Cue JI, Miller FB, et al.: Helicopter transport of trauma victims: does a physician make a difference?, *J Trauma* 31(4):490-494, 1991.

6. Schwartz RJ, Jacobs LM, Lee M: The role of the physician in a helicopter emergency medical service, *Prehosp Disaster Med* 5(1):31-37, 1990.

7. Meador S, Low R: Air medical transport. In Kuehl AE, editor: *Prehospital systems and medical oversight,* ed 2, St Louis, 1994, Mosby Lifeline, pp. 407-413.

8. Schwartz RJ, Jacobs LM, Lee M: The role of the physician in a helicopter emergency medical service, *Prehosp Disaster Med* 5:31-39, 1990.

9. Jacobs LM, Berrizbeitia LD, Bennett B, et al.: Endotracheal intubation in the pre-hospital phase of emergency medical care, *JAMA* 250:2175-2177, 1983.

10. DeLeo BC: Endotracheal intubation by rescue squad personnel, *Heart Lung* 6:851-854, 1977.

11. Stewart RD, Paris PM, Winter PM, et al.: Field endotracheal intubation by paramedical personnel: success rates and complications, *Chest* 85:341-345, 1984.

12. Pointer JE: Clinical characteristics of paramedics' performance of pediatric endotracheal intubation, *Am J Emerg Med* 7:364-366, 1989.

13. O'Brien DJ, Danzl DF, Hooker EA, et al.: Pre-hospital blind nasotracheal intubation by paramedics, *Ann Emerg Med* 18:612-617, 1989.

14. O'Brien DJ, Danzl DF, Sowers B, et al.: Airway management of aeromedically transported trauma patients, *J Emerg Med* 6:49-54, 1988.

15. Fox JB, Thomas F, Clemmer TP, et al.: Paramedic use of advanced life support procedures: experiences and attitude survey, *J Emerg Med* 4:109-114, 1986.

16. Murphy-Macabobby M, Marshall WJ, Schneider C, et al.: Neuromuscular blockade in aeromedical airway management, *Ann Emerg Med* 21:664-668, 1992.

17. Vilke GM, Hoyt DB, Epperson M, et al.: Intubation techniques in the helicopter, *J Emerg Med* 12:217-224, 1994.

18. Burney RE, Fischer RP: Ground versus air transport of trauma victims: medical and logistical considerations, *Ann Emerg Med* 15:1491-1495, 1986.

19. Schiller WR, Knox R, Zinnecker H, et al. : Effect of helicopter transport of trauma victims on survival in an urban trauma center, *J Trauma* 28:1127-1134, 1988.

20. Low RB, Martin D, Brown C: Emergency air transport of pregnant patients: the national experience, *J Emerg Med* 6:41-48, 1988.

21. Bellinger RL, Califf RM, Mark DB, et al.: Helicopter transport of patients during acute myocardial infarction, *Am J Cardiol* 61:718-722, 1988.

22. Goldstein B, Fugate JH, Conn AK, et al.: High risk pediatric emergency air transport, *Prehosp Disaster Med* 6:408-414, 1991.

23. Kaplan L, Walsh D, Burney R: Emergency aeromedical transport of patients with acute myocardial infarction, *Ann Emerg Med* 16:55-57, 1987.

24. Macnab AJ: Optimal escort for inter-hospital transport of pediatric emergencies, *J Trauma* 31:205-209, 1991.

25. Beyer AJ, Land G, Zaritsky A: Non-physician transport of intubated pediatric patients: a system evaluation, *Crit Care Med* 20:7:961-966, 1992.

26. Jacobs LM, Gabram SG, Stohler SA: The integration of a helicopter emergency medical services in a mass casualty response system, *Prehosp Disaster Med* 6:451-454, 1991.

27. Henninger S, Thompson J, Adams C: Guidelines for integrating helicopter assets into emergency planning, Washington, DC, 1991, Department of Transportation, Federal Aviation Association.

28. Erder MH, Davidson SJ, Cheney RA: On-line medical command in theory and practice, *Ann Emerg Med* 18:261-268, 1989.

29. Pointer JE, Osur M, Campbell C, et al.: The impact of standing orders on medication and skill selection, paramedic assessment, and hospital outcome: a follow-up report, *Prehosp Disaster Med* 6:303-308, 1991.

30. Meador S, Low R: Air medical transport. In Kuehl AE, editor: *Prehospital systems and medical oversight,* ed 2, St Louis, 1994, Mosby Lifeline, pp. 407-413.

31. Hunt RC, Buss RR, Graham RG, et al.: Standing orders vs. voice control, *J Emerg Med Serv* 7:26-30, 1982.

32. Melton JD, Heller MB, Kaplan R, et al.: Occult hypoxemia during aeromedical transport: detection by pulse oximetry, *Prehosp Disaster Med* 4:115-121, 1989.

33. Valko RC, Campbell JP, McCarty DL, et al.: Prehospital use of pulse oximetry in rotary-wing aircraft, *Prehosp Disaster Med* 6:421-428, 1991.

18

Quality Management

Quality management in EMS, especially concerning the command process, is a concept that has only recently received a good deal of attention and is a much neglected element of Quality Improvement (QI) in EMS. The EMS medical director's highest priority is to determine that proper care results in a positive outcome. It is this commitment to the examination of care given in an EMS system that ensures patients the highest quality of prehospital medicine.

The history of Quality Assurance (QA) begins with, and has traditionally been associated with, the concept of identifying deviations from a standard (usually the system protocols) and then attempting to correct these deviations in most part through punitive action. This was generally accomplished through review of trip sheets and from complaints, which could be derived from the patient up through the receiving institution.[1] This process was less than ideal, since it was rigid and failed to take into account the numerous modifying factors that frequently affect and alter prehospital care. In addition, the punitive nature of the process was often bad for morale. Thus, QA has been replaced by a system known by a number of terms, including QI, Total Quality Management (TQM), and Continuous Quality Improvement (CQI).

When the command physician participates in the QI process, there are several basic concepts that should be kept in mind. The first is that the ultimate goal is QI versus traditional QA, not to punish all of those that do not subscribe to the predetermined standard. One source has reported that in any system 85% of the problems are due to the system, with only 15% attributable to the personnel.[2,3] Problems should be viewed in this light and always with the goal of improving the overall process of delivering patient care. The second is that the process must be dynamic. No system is perfect, and not every possible situation can be predicted beforehand. Also, as prehospital care medicine evolves, the standards of care will change. A key concept in this process is involvement of the caregivers in problem solving. When an issue is identified, it is essential to solicit the views of those who are most affected, the "front line" caregivers. A good QI plan is helpful in instigating new therapies and procedures.

Thus QI, while focusing on the direction given to the prehospital care provider by a physician or nurse, should also encompass the entire medical command and control process and not just on-line contact. These areas will be discussed in detail later in the

ERIC DAVIS, MD, FACEP

chapter. Finally, the command QI program should be integrated as part of the overall EMS QI plan. This is easily accomplished and is helpful to assess the overall performance of the system.

<h2 style="background:black;color:white;display:inline-block;">Components</h2>

There are several classical models applicable to health care. Donabedian's system of structure, process, and outcome outlines the groups of components that must be addressed in a QI plan.[4] This breaks down the QI process into structure—the components of the system in place before the patient encounter; process—the actual delivery of care; and outcome—or how the structure and process affect the patient. Demming's method of continual improvement and participation of the worker in decision making also has use in the medical command QI process. However, there are three approaches that we generally use to assess the quality of care received in an EMS system: prospective, concurrent, and retrospective.

Prospective

The prospective approach is defined as the establishment of medical treatment protocols, procedures, and policies before the active patient encounter.[5,6] There are certain elements that must be in place to ensure that quality care can be achieved as early as possible. The first component of this group is communications equipment. The proper type of prehospital equipment, such as radio (UHF or VHF) or cellular telephone, should be selected depending on the area, terrain, and available equipment in your area. It must be reliable and able to make good contact with the base station in all but the most extreme circumstances. In the base station itself the prehospital contact should be easily heard and the equipment must be easily accessible and preferably isolated to aid in concentration and the ability to communicate clearly. A good writing surface and all necessary materials (such as a copy of the protocols and command sheets) must be easily accessible.

The next component that must be established before the patient encounter is the standing orders and treatment protocols. They must be thoroughly understood by both the prehospital and hospital personnel so that both sides have an equal comprehension and are able to anticipate necessary care. The manner in which the information is delivered to the command physician should be stan-dardized and follow an established format. This is beneficial in several ways since it ensures thoroughness, fosters thought processes, and allows the command physician to fill out the command sheets properly. The base station personnel must also follow the format so as not to confuse the paramedics.

The timing of base station contact should also be standardized. A useful idea is the double line concept where in each protocol there are actions that may be performed as standing orders, but any interventions beyond this point "(the double line)" require direct contact with the base station (Figure 18-1). Precisely which patients require contact with a physician and which may just be notification calls should also be decided beforehand. Generally those patients requiring any ALS care deserve command contact, and the prehospital care providers are allowed to proceed with interventions that, if delayed, could result in harm to the patient.

There are also certain specialty situations that need to be addressed. General guidelines outlining policies for receiving hospitals should be developed. There are several methods to determine general patient destination, such as patient or family request, closest hospital, etc. Specialty hospitals (such as those for trauma, burns, pediatrics) may be appropriate for direct field triage. With the proliferation of air-medical transport services, regulations as to which patients would most benefit, who is allowed to activate the transport, if and when medical command should be contacted, and what the destination should be are essential. Finally, guidelines addressing *specifically* such common events as nontransports, physician on-scene, and "Do Not Resuscitate" (DNR) situations are helpful. Medical control should be contacted in each of these instances.

Familiarity with the prehospital care providers is also a desirable, but not essential, situation. The command physician may be influenced by the competence, skill, and experience of the providers when determining the accuracy of their assessment and ability to carry out orders. This may be accomplished in various ways: by getting the command physicians involved in the training, continuing medical education, clinical time, or field time. While all of these provide the opportunity to get to know the prehospital care providers, an added advantage of field time is that the command physician gains a better appreciation of field conditions. The EMS system in San Francisco feels this is so important that they have mandated a yearly requirement for ride-alongs by all command personnel.

PROTOCOL: BRONCHOSPASM (WHEEZING)

NOTE

Bronchospasm—the reversible constriction (spasm) of the smooth muscle of the small airways (bronchioles) is a manifestation of several diseases. The most common are asthma, bronchitis and emphysema (COPD). However, congestive heart failure, pulmonary embolism and pneumonia may also present with wheezing.

INDICATIONS

1. Respiratory distress with wheezing or prolonged expiratory phase on auscultation.
2. Respiratory distress with history of asthma or COPD and no other apparent cause of dyspnea.

CONTRAINDICATIONS

Acute CHF/pulmonary edema—use Protocol #403.

PROTOCOL

1. Assist ventilation/intubate based on mental status, adequacy of air exchange, vitals, pulse oximetry.
   *NOTE: Intubation does not relieve (and may in fact worsen) bronchospasm. This should only be done when patient clearly needs ventilatory assistance or airway protection.
2. OXYGEN—as needed to maintain pulse ox reading >93%.
3. ALBUTEROL 2.5 mg in NSS 3 cc nebulized with oxygen at 6 L/min.
4. Contact Medical Command. Request EMS Physician response if patient in severe distress.
5. Monitor mental status, air exchange, vitals, pulse ox and EKG en-route to hospital.

6. Additional albuterol treatments.
7. Epinephrine 0.3 cc of 1:1000 sol. SC for patients unable to cooperate with albuterol treatment or in severe distress.
8. IV saline lock may be ordered.

Figure 18-1. Sample Protocol

A final aspect and one that is generally overlooked is to ensure the competency of the command physician. This has two components. The first is to make sure they have the requisite medical knowledge, commonly by requiring board certification/eligibility in emergency medicine. The second is to familiarize the physicians with the state, regional, local, and institutional policies and regulations. Both of these goals may be accomplished through a base-station medical command course. These courses are mandated by some states, including Pennsylvania, which requires all physicians who participate in the command process to pass a set module.[6,7]

Concurrent or Immediate Methods

This section refers to on-line communication using direct voice communication to provide direction for the pre-hospital care provider. Most systems operate with at least some direct communication, and the numerous advantages of this system will be discussed after each component.

The most identifiable component of immediate medical control and the one most pertinent to this chapter is on-line communication via radio or telephone. The benefits of this are legion. The first is to ensure the paramedics are using the proper treatment protocol. Prehospital care providers may misclassify patients, a situation enhanced by the fact that a single protocol is often selected on the basis of a single complaint. Direct real-time communication allows the command physician to mix several therapies if necessary and even to provide non-protocol treatments when appropriate (calcium in the suspected hyperkalemic patient for example). Questions may also be answered and additional information obtained to help clarify the situation. In addition, this also gives the receiving facility a more complete report on the patient. From a QI standpoint, this is a very effective way to give prompt feedback to the paramedics and serves as an educational tool.

An extension of the above concept is bedside feedback from the physician to the transporters at the receiving facility. This is the best, and possibly only, way to verify assessments and serves as a very effective educational method. Aspects of proper physical exam may also be demonstrated at this time and interesting findings pointed out.

A final aspect of concurrent QI is the use of field time. As previously stated, this is a good way to become familiar with the prehospital care providers, as well as to gain an appreciation for the conditions under which they practice. In addition this is the only method with which to determine what absolutely goes on in the field. A patient may come to the ED with an endotracheal tube in place; however, this would not be considered a successful intubation if the attempts took 5 minutes without any intermittent bag-valve-mask ventilation. The written record is not necessarily a true representation of what has transpired in the field. A field observer will get a good appreciation of how the system is functioning, if quality care is being delivered, if orders are being properly executed, and may also provide immediate, direct feedback to the prehospital care providers for purposes of education and improvement. When it is not feasible to have a physician serve in this capacity, supervisors or preceptors may fill this role. This is an especially effective tool in larger systems where a group of field supervisors may directly observe and assist in field care, using the time to teach. These supervisors should have regular contact with the medical director to ensure a current and standardized knowledge base.[8-10]

Retrospective

This method of QI, which reviews various records after the patient encounter, is the most traditional and widely used, but is fraught with problems.[6,7] It is fundamentally important that the records are accurate, complete, and available. However, even the most ideal conditions do not guarantee reliable data, which may be greatly affected by recall, transcription, and collection error. The records are all gathered together and reviewed as a whole. Those records that may be used include—

1. **Trip sheet**—This is a written record of the patient encounter and is usually reviewed as part of the overall EMS QI plan. It is of interest to medical command QI to check paramedic interventions, record of orders, and if and how the orders were accomplished. These records may be optically scanned to provide data for statistical analysis of the system concerning both overall numbers as well as trends. A new technological advancement that may have a great impact on the trip sheet is the use of a computer notebook. In this, the prehospital care provider records patient care data into the notebook, which in some configurations may have communication with patient monitoring services. This information, including a narrative if desired, can be downloaded into a computer for generation of the trip sheet. The computer can then organize this data for the aforementioned statistical analysis.

2. **Emergency department record**—This is the chart generated by the ED during the patient's stay and should include nursing notes.

3. **Command sheet**—This is a written record of what transpires during command and is filled out by the person providing command at the time of the call (Figure 18-2). It serves as both a written record of information given to the command physician to compare with the trip sheet and as a prompt for the person giving command. The use of checklist-type forms is recommended to save writing time and effort. The use of a command sheet greatly simplifies the QI process. It generates a list of calls requiring command, from which those chosen for review may be selected. By listing the orders given by a physician, it may help identify trends in patient care. Rarely a new concept in care that is proposed in the literature will first be expressed through physician orders and if consistent may warrant a change in the protocol. In addition the command sheet may serve as an earlier identifier of problem calls—the command physician may indicate his or her desire to review the case.

4. **Tapes**—Tapes of the command process may be used as part of routine QI or to help clarify the situation when a problem arises or when there is a disagreement between the prehospital and hospital personnel.

5. **Review sheet**—A review sheet combines the information gained from the above sources to evaluate the command process in the following areas:

STAT MEDICAL COMMAND SHEET

Date: _____ Flight Number: _____ Referring Facility: _____

Name: _____ ☐ Male ☐ Female Age _____ Wt. _____

Chief Complaint: _____

Brief HX: _____
_____

P: _____ R: _____ BP: _____ **Any Hypotension?** ☐

Physical Exam

Neuro: ☐ Alert ☐ Verbal ☐ Pain ☐ Unresponsive **Any LOC?** ☐ Y ☐ N

CV: _____

    Monitor: _____ Pacer ☐ EXT ☐ INT

    Settings: Rate: _____ MA: _____

Pulm: _____

    O_2 @ _____ VIA _____

    Ventilator: Rate: _____ FiO_2: _____ Vt: _____ PEEP: _____

GI/GU: _____

    NG ☐ Foley ☐

MS/DERM: _____

    2 IV's ☐ Periph _____ **(#/gauge/fluid)**

Labs: _____
_____
_____

Medications

Chronic: _____ **Allergies:** _____

Acute: _____

    Medications/Conc. on PUMPS 1 _____

    (60cc Syringes Drawn Up) 2 _____

    3 _____

Trauma Confirm:

    ☐ On Back Board ☐ C-Collar/HID ☐ MAST? ☐ Chest Tubes?

Request: ☐ Copy of Chart ☐ Face Sheets (2) ☐ Pertinent X-rays/CT (if available)

MD Orders: _____
_____
_____
_____
_____

Signature: _____ ☐ License #: on file ☐ DEA #: on file

Figure 18-2. Sample Command Sheet

A. *Answering*—Specific areas to be addressed are prompt availability of a command physician. The allowable limit should be set by the medical system, but most systems set it at 30 seconds. Situations that may require further review in case no one is available for command, no answer by the base station hospital, and those where the prehospital personnel violated appropriate standing orders/protocols. Throughout the process the personnel should maintain proper radio procedure.

B. *Basic prehospital data/patient history*—This includes full patient information including sex, age, vital signs, chief complaint, history, past medical history, medications, and allergies, documented on both the trip and command sheets. All of this data should be given in the proper format to facilitate documentation by the receiving command physician.

C. *Prehospital interventions*—This includes all actions taken by the prehospital care providers before contact with command. These interventions should be appropriate for the patient complaint and in agreement with the protocols/standing orders. When consistent errors are discovered, it usually signals a system problem and further review is usually necessary to determine the origin. Protocol revision, continuing medical education for individual or system, clinical time, etc. may be warranted based on the conclusion. Checklists are very helpful to the recording command physician to simplify and expedite the process.

D. *Physician orders*—These should be audited to determine appropriateness for the patient, that the orders follow protocol and that durations are appropriate, and that the orders documented by the command physician are in agreement with those recorded by the prehospital care provider on the trip sheet. One of the most important functions of this system is to identify changing trends in care to adjust the protocols appropriately.

The choice of how to determine which cases are to be reviewed is left to the individual systems and depends on multiple factors including run volume, case mix, and previously identified problem areas. Whatever the method,

it has been suggested that the best indicators have the following characteristics: high risk/high volume, clear case definitions, reasonable expected outcome, straightforward interventions, and that the intervention has demonstrated effect. Examples of potential audits that may fulfill these criteria are all arrests, trauma, shock, all intubation attempts, pediatric transports, etc.

Regardless of what criteria are used to select the cases for review, whenever problems are found, adequate steps must be taken to correct the deficiency, and just as important, these attempts must be documented. It is important that these efforts are not punitive but should reflect a positive intent to teach, as well as gain feedback from those being reviewed. Nevertheless, despite the best instructions and QI system, there will inevitably be those instances in which disciplinary measures must be undertaken. It is vital that before this step is undertaken all the relevant facts have been gathered, with independent confirmation of the point in question obtained whenever possible. The discipline process must be spelled out before the process, with written and readily available policies and procedures.

The person in charge of the QI plan must have an open-door policy so that people can come in with their problem—ideally before patient care is affected.

Box 18-1   QI Plan Models

Prospective

  Training

   Initial
   Continuing medical education
   Skills

  Protocols

Concurrent

  On-line direction
  Field care
  Observers
  Assessment

Retrospective

  Trip sheets
  Command sheets
  Audio tapes

Summary

Quality improvement should be a positive experience, with the ultimate goal of continually improving medical command. All personnel involved in the process, including both prehospital care providers and the command physician, should be involved in the process. When problems are discovered, the response should not be punitive but looked upon as a method to teach and to gain input about the system. Most continual problem areas are due to system flaws rather than with personnel. Efforts at correcting the problems must also be documented.

Remember: "The successful quality improvement program greatly increases the likelihood for the ongoing safe, ethical, clinically sound, and cost effective practice of medicine in the field."[5] More information on this important topic can be found in texts published by both the National Association of EMS Physicians[5] and the American College of Emergency Physicians.[11]

References

1. Libby M, Vahradian S: Investing in your people: improvement from within, *JEMS* 6:24-33, 1994.

2. Warton M: *The Deming management method,* New York, 1986, Putnam Publishing.

3. Deming WE: *Out of the crisis,* Cambridge, MA, 1982, MIT Publishing.

4. Donabedian A: *The definition of quality and approaches to its assessment,* 1980, Health Administration Press.

5. Holyrody B, Knopp R, Kallsen G: Medical control: quality assurance in prehospital care, *JAMA* 256:1027-1031, 1986.

6. Swor R, editor: *Quality management in prehospital care,* St Louis, 1993, Mosby Lifeline.

7. Kuehl A, editor: *Prehospital systems and medical/oversight,* ed 2, St Louis, 1994, Mosby Lifeline.

8. Berwick DM, Godfrey AB, Roessnor J: *Curing health care: new strategies for quality improvement,* San Francisco, 1990, Jossey-Bass.

9. Pepe PE, Stewart RD: Role of the physician in a prehospital setting, *Ann Emerg Med* 15:1480-1483, 1986.

10. Pepe PE: The impact of intense physician supervision on the effectiveness of an emergency medical services system, *Ann Emerg Med* 17:752, 1988.

11. Polsky SS, editor: *Continuous quality improvement in EMS,* Dallas, 1992, ACEP.

19

Ethical Issues

The topic of ethics usually brings to mind philosophical, abstract notions. Emergency physicians in particular might believe that ethical issues are far removed from the daily reality of swift patient assessment, diagnosis, and intervention. Experienced physicians know, however, that ethical issues are common in the prehospital setting. These dilemmas are not theoretical but are concrete and sometimes dramatic. It will be these dilemmas that present tough questions and memorable cases. Both the physicians and prehospital care providers must develop skills to make reasoned analyses of these difficult situations to navigate smooth resolution of the conflicts. Prehospital care providers also must understand basic legal concepts, many of which are addressed in Chapter 20. In this chapter, ethical dilemmas common to the prehospital environment are discussed so that the provider can recognize the conflict and understand some of the basic ethical issues involved. Nothing said here should be interpreted as legal advice. State laws vary, legislation changes, but a well-grounded ethical approach to problem solving will assist in negotiating a solution. Adequate resolution of these problems depends on recognition, clear understanding of the issues at hand, and a solid, acceptable analysis.

All situations presented in this chapter are based on true cases and point out dilemmas that occur relatively commonly in a busy EMS.[1] While familiarity with state statutes or case law can help guide some difficult decisions, legislative direction may be inadequate. Personal judgment, effective policy, and well-trained EMTs will be important for appropriate resolution of these conflicts. Also important is a legal consultant experienced in EMS law. Knowing when to involve this consultant is also a critical judgment for the EMT and physician and will be discussed.

Refusal of Treatment and Transport
CASE # 1

A 30-year-old male was shot in the left lower abdomen. The paramedics noted a tense, rigid abdomen. He refused placement of an IV line and said he did not want to go to the hospital, while intermittently yelling, "The Iceman got me" and thrashing and rolling in obvious discomfort.

JAMES G. ADAMS, MD, FACEP

The patient may have identifiable fears that make him reluctant to accept care. Fear of further pain, fear of being arrested, or irrational denial of the severity of the injury may have played a role in his impulsive refusal. We can argue that this refusal is not made with clear understanding of the risks of refusing care and further say that refusal is not informed. An uninformed refusal, when a person's life is at stake, cannot ethically be accepted. We must recognize also that the EMTs, along with society and the legal system, have an overriding interest in the preservation of life and health. There are many good arguments for treating the patient, but we must make the right decision via the right reasoning.

For a person to either consent to or refuse medical care, the patient must understand several facts: 1. the nature of the illness or injury, 2. the risks and benefits of treatment, 3. alternative methods of treatment and their risks and benefits, and 4. the risks, benefits, and prognosis of no treatment at all.[2,3]

Can this patient meet these criteria? Should the EMTs even become involved in such discussions? The patient in this case was alert but refusing care and not at all inclined to discuss the reasoning behind his refusal. The EMTs confronted an ethical choice between the patient's right to self-determination (autonomy) and the paramedic's obligation to provide patient care (beneficence). In this scenario, the obligation to attempt to care for the patient must take precedence over the patient's possibly irrational attempt at self-determination. The EMT must make every reasonable attempt to provide for the best interest of the patient, within the limits of a competent patient's acceptance. This is the key to ethical resolution: every reasonable attempt at care must be made. Issues of decision-making capacity confound the issue, as we see in the following scenario.

"Incompetent" Patient
CASE #2

EMTs responded to the scene of a female who fell, hit her head, and sustained a short period of unconsciousness. The patient was found to be staggering down the street, refusing any intervention. She appeared intoxicated. In a nearby locked car, presumably the patient's, needles were evident. The patient adamantly and violently refused care and continued to stagger away.

Medical professionals in the prehospital setting must make determinations of decision-making capacity when a patient refuses important medical care. A high degree of understanding and reasoning must be exhibited if the patient is to refuse care. This patient appeared to the EMTs to lack the capacity to make any form of rational decision. This patient, violently and clearly, refused treatment and transport, but she fulfilled none of the requirements to indicate that it was informed. Based upon the obligation to promote the health and well-being of the patient, the EMTs should use whatever means they have available to safely evaluate this patient. In this instance, the police might become involved to assist in restraint and transport of the patient. Commonly, the police will not become involved unless a crime may have been committed. The EMTs themselves, though, have no ethical obligation to place themselves at risk to accomplish the evaluation. They do, however, have an obligation to do their best to attempt to provide for the safety of this individual. Impatience, frustration, or prejudice should not interfere with responsible care for the individual.

In general, the on-line physician should be contacted when a patient's refusal of care could result in harm. Such contact may help ensure that all that can be done to care for the patient is done. Frequently, a satisfactory conclusion can be reached when an on-line physician discusses risks of refusal with a lucid but reluctant patient. When the patient does not appear lucid or is uncooperative, the on-line physician can help ensure that maximal safe attempts are made to evaluate and care for the patient, including requesting peace officer assistance.

Informed Refusal
CASE #3

A 68-year-old man called the paramedics because of crushing substernal chest pain. The medics found him diaphoretic and in acute distress. A single sublingual nitroglycerin provided some relief. He refused to go to the hospital, however, until his wife returned from shopping. He understood that the delay could risk his life.

This patient appeared clearly lucid but also appeared to be making a dangerous decision. As the case unfolded, it was discovered that the patient had a large sum of money in a dresser drawer that he wanted to give to his wife. He was afraid that his son would take the money otherwise. Once this issue was identified, a resolution was easily achieved as the money was secured for the wife and the patient transported.

Appropriate care of this patient would be facilitated by taking time to discuss the patient's reasons for refusing care. If he is unable or unwilling to clarify his desires, then every effort must be made to convince the patient to accept transport to the ED. Maximal effort must be made to provide for the care of this individual, within the limits of acceptance of the patient, who apparently possesses full decision-making capacity. The EMTs might contact the family physician or a relative to discuss the issue with him. If the patient is lucid and meets the criteria necessary for an informed refusal, the EMTs cannot force transport. On the other hand, some ethicists would argue that the infringement on the patient's autonomy would be relatively small when compared with the potential harm. This is, at best, a precarious legal argument. Legal consultation might be sought when such high-risk scenarios occur.

Most states have no statutory support for the involuntary transport of patients except those with psychiatric disease and those with legal declarations of incompetence. Few states allow transport so that further ED evaluation can occur when there is a question regarding decision-making capacity. Careful documentation of the scenario, including identification of the difficulties and explanation of the reasoning behind the decision, is always necessary.

Informed Refusal and Family Conflict
CASE #4

A 70-year-old debilitated female with a history of COPD called the paramedics because of SOB. Upon arrival, the paramedics found her in significant respiratory distress. Her pulse was 120 and her blood pressure was 95 systolic. Low-flow oxygen was applied, and an aerosolized albuterol treatment was administered in the patient's home. The treatment provided significant relief. The patient subsequently refused transport to the hospital. The family demanded that she be taken to the ED.

Should the paramedics allow the patient to refuse further therapy and risk a bad outcome? Although the patient seemed "competent", the paramedics worried that the patient could suffer a respiratory arrest without further

care. They also wondered about their duty to the family, the caretakers.

It would seem prudent to first explore the patient's reasons for refusing care. As a general rule, if a person possesses full decision-making capacity, the person cannot be transported against his or her will. The outcome of this case was dictated by the patient, who, in her home hospital bed, with her home oxygen and nebulizer machine, emphatically refused to be transported. Of the past 160 days, she had spent 117 in the hospital, according to her careful count. She knew she did not have long to live and preferred to die at home. She accepted the warning that this episode could worsen and she might die. The patient noted that it was the family, not her, who called the EMTs and it was they who were having difficulty dealing with the situation. Does this argument clarify the obligation to the patient? In the end, the patient was judged to possess full capacity to make this decision, the family was advised to call the patient's physician and discuss the situation, and the patient was not transported. The discussion with the patient was documented in detail and the legal consultant was notified.

Conflict of Hospital Destination
CASE #5

Mrs. R. complained of crushing substernal chest pain and SOB. Her blood pressure was 85/40 and pulse was 80. She requested to be taken to a local community hospital with no cardiac care unit. The paramedics felt she would be better cared for at the tertiary center approximately 1½ miles further.

One of the fundamental premises of prehospital care includes rapid transport of patients to an appropriate medical facility of the patient's choice. This policy generally presumes that the facility has the technical capability to appropriately treat the illness. Ethical conflict can arise for prehospital care providers when the patient or the family insists on transport to facilities that the health care professionals feel is suboptimal. Should the EMTs influence this patient? The paramedics felt that this patient was making an uninformed decision. Do paramedics have a right, or an ethical obligation, to recommend facilities that they feel would provide the best care? In fact, the obligation of the EMTs is to provide for the best interests of the patient. This may include an offer of factual information in an unbiased, non-judgmental manner, conforming to existing policies that govern such decisions. Standard policies may exist regarding trauma center referral or transport of critically ill patients to the nearest facility. Intuitive opinions as to the best destination, however well intended, may not be correct. For example, an EMT might say that one hospital has a special chest pain center. This may not indicate that a higher level of care is offered and it certainly does not promise a better outcome. In the scenario described, however, it was well known to the EMTs that the hospital transferred critically ill cardiac patients. This information was shared with the patient and the family, who opted for transport to the facility with greater capabilities. The family called the private physician who retrospectively concurred with the decision. If the patient and family had insisted on transport to the other facility, the EMTs should have offered the factual information that they knew, notified the facility of the pending arrival (perhaps discussing the issue), and if the facility was willing, the patient should have been taken to the preferred hospital. The willingness of the facility to receive the patient implies that they feel that they have the capability. Additionally, the back-up physician would be valuable in resolving conflict or answering questions, but ideally, EMS policy should help by addressing these issues.

Treatment of Minors
CASE #6

A 14-year-old patient called the paramedics because she had severe lower abdominal pain and vaginal bleeding. Her blood pressure was 95/70 and her pulse was 90. The paramedics wished to initiate an IV line and transport the patient to the ED, but wanted to know if parental consent was required.

The emergency exception to informed consent allows treatment necessary to prevent mortality or serious morbidity.[3] Usually when the "emergency rule" is invoked, the illness is obvious and the situation grave. Even in the care of minors, the prehospital care provider must err on the side of providing necessary care and transporting the patient for definitive evaluation at the ED, although effort to contact a parent or guardian must proceed as well if the minor is not "emancipated" under state law. The rules governing emancipation vary but often encompass minors who are married, pregnant, or seeking care for sexually trans-

mitted diseases. Acting in the best interest of the patient, according to the needs of the patient, especially with a minimal chance of harming the patient, will minimize conflict. It is important to request parent or guardian permission before treating non-emancipated minors, but emergency care should never be withheld when the delay could present harm to the patient. Important needs must be met, while attempts are undertaken to contact the responsible adult, especially if a minor's life is at risk. Less urgent issues must wait for the parent's permission.

Coercion of Uncooperative Patients
CASE #7

Paramedics arrived at the scene of a single motor vehicle accident and encountered an obviously intoxicated, unrestrained driver who had been ejected from the vehicle. The patient was thrashing and cursing. The paramedics attempted unsuccessfully to calm the patient. The patient attempted to punch one of the paramedics, at which point the team of paramedics held down the patient's arms and legs and forcefully told him that if he didn't calm down they would give him medicine to paralyze him and would put a plastic tube down his throat to breathe for him. The patient became cooperative enough for the paramedics to proceed with the evaluation, immobilization, and rapid transport.

The EMT committed assault by threatening the patient. Holding the patient down may have been battery. Are these actions ever justified to ensure compliance? Does the severity of the patient's illness affect the justification? What limitation should be placed on paramedics' ability to "convince" patients to submit to care? Usually there are less aggressive means to encourage care and, very often, agitation is a sign of a medical rather than personal pathology. This patient was clearly in need of medical evaluation. The emergency rule supports the treatment necessary to remedy the emergency condition. This begins with thorough evaluation. Some might argue that whatever provides for the necessary evaluation is in the patient's best interest if it promotes efficient care and lessens the risk to the patient and EMTs. Above all, such action can never be punitive, can never be excessive, and must provide for the best interest of the patient. Hostility, impatience, or impulsive reaction on the part of the EMT is not beneficial to the patient and must be avoided, although a reasoned, decisive, authoritative instruction might be important in some scenarios. It is important for the EMT to avoid uncontrolled emotional reactions.

Advance Directives
CASE #8

An 83-year-old woman was found by paramedics to be asystolic after she suffered a cardiac arrest that was witnessed by the family. The family presented a paper to the paramedics, signed by a physician, noting that the patient was not to be resuscitated in the event of cardiac arrest. No resuscitation was undertaken. The police were notified that the patient was "dead on arrival".

Under what circumstances can paramedics honor advance directives to limit resuscitation attempts? Some EMS have developed explicit protocols for advance directives.[4] How should the prehospital care provider respond if the advance directive varies from the policy? The first rule is that the decision to withhold resuscitation cannot be a spontaneous decision by the family. Any decision to limit resuscitation must be thought about in advance of the time of crisis, ideally by the patient herself. The directive should also be in writing. If no written document can be produced that specifies limits of resuscitation, then full resuscitation must be attempted in the prehospital setting.

Some people go to great lengths to devise a written document to limit resuscitation. Some EMS systems accept different types of written documents as long as the patient's (or designee's) signature and personal physician's signature are present. Each EMS system must decide what type of documents to accept: a standard form devised and distributed by the system is best because it is recognizable. The role of the EMT is not to make judgments about the validity of documents, the prognosis of the patient, or the appropriateness of resuscitation. Decisions must be immediate. Only if the EMS system has clear and well-recognized guidelines for limitation of resuscitation should EMTs withhold resuscitation attempts.

Decisions to Limit Resuscitation
CASE #9

A 67-year-old woman "passed out" in a restaurant. Paramedics found her in ventricular tachycardia. Her husband reported that she had metastatic lung cancer.

He produced a "Living Will", which was officially notarized and signed by a physician and attorney but not currently protected by state law. Resuscitation had already been initiated and after two defibrillation attempts the patient was in a pulseless rhythm with electrical activity. The paramedics asked the medical command physician if they should cease resuscitation attempts. The physician advised the paramedics to continue.

Current medical, legal, and ethical thought widely recognizes that patients have the right to limit resuscitation attempts in the event of cardiopulmonary arrest.[5-7] This case illustrates the difficulties "Living Wills" may present in an emergency setting. It is difficult to attempt to interpret the validity of any advance directives in this setting, and documents such as living wills are particularly troubling. We must keep in mind, though, that most living wills were not meant for prehospital use, so this patient should undergo resuscitation attempts. Even with the document in hand, her wishes in this specific, unpredictable circumstance would not be known. The living will provides limits for hospital and long-term care, and unless a recognizable "do not attempt resuscitation" provision is clearly evident, resuscitation attempts should proceed. When a Do Not Resuscitate (DNR) order is established according to authorized guidelines, then resuscitation should be withheld. A living will is not necessarily a DNR order, however, unless it contains an explicit provision within the document to make it so.

Terminating Resuscitation in the Prehospital Setting

This case also raises difficult questions about deciding to terminate resuscitation in the prehospital setting. This decision is more medical than ethical. If further resuscitation attempts will be futile, there is no good argument for continuing.[8-10] Each system must determine the medical, ethical, and operational approach that will be most appropriate in the setting. Families seem to be satisfied with field termination of resuscitation.[11] No single answer will suffice. Termination of resuscitation attempts without transport to the hospital may be appropriate with sound medical decision making, adequate physician participation, cooperation of the coroner and police, and sound legal guidance. In the case, as presented, however, a full and adequate trial of ALS was not offered, and so, resuscitation attempts and transport should continue.

Triage Decisions
CASE #10

While responding to a call for "a lady who sat on broken glass and is bleeding," EMTs encountered a motor vehicle accident. There were people with obvious injuries. The EMTs had no more information about the patient who sat on the glass.

Should the paramedics stop at the new scene, where they are sure their assistance is needed? Under what circumstances does the obligation to a second patient supersede the obligation to the original patient who requested aid? Most EMS systems have worked out procedures for circumstances such as this so that prompt care can be rendered to all those in need. Efficient dispatch is necessary to contact another medic unit while the original unit proceeds to the initial call. For the individual EMT, however, a sense of conflict might persist. If an immediate and life-threatening need is apparent, such as severe active bleeding or acute airway obstruction, it would be reasonable to stop and render aid. The EMTs must keep in mind that the original patient may have a similar life-threatening injury or may have a trivial problem, so sophisticated crew coordination is called for. The responding unit has an obligation to the original call until significant evidence of disproportionate severity dictates that a second need be answered first.

Confidentiality
CASE #11

A 32-year-old male in a motor vehicle accident was transported to the regional trauma center. His vital signs were stable and his sensorium was clear. The EMTs did not smell alcohol but asked if he had been drinking or taking drugs. The patient admitted to "a beer or two" and "a little cocaine" about 30 minutes before the accident. The patient asked that this be kept confidential. At the trauma center the police asked the EMTs if the patient had been drinking. The response would likely have determined whether the police would have requested a serum alcohol level and would have pursued a "driving under the influence" investigation.

Physicians have the ethical and legal obligation to maintain the confidentiality of patient information. EMTs also share this duty. Sometimes, however, the EMT's medical or societal obligations conflict with their oblig-

ation to maintain patient confidentiality. Do the EMTs have a duty of confidentiality to this patient? Do they have a larger duty to society? The EMTs must be trustworthy and have the confidence of their patients, yet must also work closely with police and public agencies. Peace officers should consider their legal authority to request a blood alcohol determination and proceed according to their established guidelines. The EMTs should professionally defer from involvement in issues outside their scope of practice, including the notoriously unreliable prediction of legal intoxication and suggest that the police gather such important information by exercising their usual and customary authority.

CASE #12

A city public official suffered a cardiac arrest while at work. EMTs arrived, initiated resuscitation, and transported the patient to the nearest hospital. The media arrived and asked the EMTs for information.

Should the EMTs speak to the media? How much should they say? Is the duty to keep confidence different when caring for a public official? The best policy is to designate a spokesperson for the EMS who is experienced in media relations. Care must be taken not to volunteer information beyond the realm of EMS involvement or expertise. Guidance should be offered to EMTs regarding media relations, especially regarding patient confidentiality and the significance of assuming responsibility as spokesperson for the system.

Truth-Telling
CASE #13

EMTs responded to a 78-year-old patient with severe abdominal pain. The family stated that he had recently been diagnosed with stomach cancer but did not know it.

EMTs have a duty to be honest with patients and must honor the trust placed in them. What is the duty of the EMT in this case? Should such secrets be kept? What if the patient asked about his illness? In this case, the EMTs have little knowledge of the medical history, know few details about the illness, the family, the patient's values, or the psychosocial implications of such information. Medical and ethical judgment suggest that conversations relating to a chronic medical condition be deferred to the primary care physician. The EMTs can professionally and appropriately defer comment and focus on the issue, the abdominal pain.

Personal Risk
CASE #14

EMTs arrived at a scene where a man reportedly was "beat up and bleeding". He was inside a tavern, where bystanders were shouting and screaming at each other. A person spotted the ambulance pull up and ran to the unit yelling, "my man's hurt in here, come on in and help him". Police were not on the scene.

EMTs' duties to patients are sometimes constrained by other concerns. For example, their ability to help a patient may be limited by a concern for their own health or safety. The extent of responsibility of the paramedics to other parties is sometimes unclear and presents ethical conflict.

How much risk should the EMT assume? Should the EMT enter the tavern without police assistance? The EMT must evaluate the safety of the scene and make a judgment. The EMT must not be encouraged to take risks in the name of bravado or heroism. Assistance of peace officers should be available. The immediacy of the friend's request pressures the EMTs but does not change the ethical obligation. There is no requirement to be a battlefield medic and put oneself in harm's way to rescue people from in the midst of conflict. A safe scene, preventing additional casualties, is a fundamental premise of civil EMS. This does not mean that EMTs can avoid all danger and prevent all risk. One must only minimize risk and calculate reasonable actions, avoiding conflict for which one is not trained.

CASE #15

The paramedics encountered a 28-year-old man with a "high fever". The patient was disoriented. A friend told the paramedics that the patients has AIDS. Medical command advised oxygen and an IV line of lactated Ringer's solution. The paramedics responded that "This patient seems pretty stable and we are on our way to the hospital and I am not sure he has very good veins".

Is it reasonable to alter recommended interventions in the patient with an infectious disease? While unwar-

ranted fear or prejudice must never bias appropriate prehospital care, there are reasonable medical considerations that might affect prehospital practices. Starting an IV on an AIDS patient in the back of a moving ambulance entails some degree of personal risk. Barrier precautions should be used in the care of every patient. IV lines might be started with the ambulance stopped. The EMTs should not assume unreasonable risks, nor should they let predictable risk and irrational fear negatively impact patient care. Patients with AIDS can and should be safely cared for. Patients with any communicable disease (tuberculosis, hepatitis, etc.) should be cared for so that transmission does not occur, including the scrupulous use of precautions (masks, gloves, and other barriers as indicated).

Societal Obligations
CASE #16

EMTs responded to a call for a child who "fell down". Upon arrival, a 5-year-old with multiple bruises and contusions on three extremities was encountered. The EMTs felt these injuries were inconsistent with the stated history. The EMTs did not mention this to the parents. The parents refused transport or further evaluation of the child.

Conflict arose because the EMTs wanted to protect the child by transporting him to the hospital, where social service agencies would become immediately involved. The EMTs felt that there was an imminent threat to the child's health. Should they insist on transporting this child? Every state has legal requirements to report suspected child abuse. Knowledge of legal requirements would limit the ethical conflict in most situations. In this circumstance, the EMT could provide for the child's safety by calling the social service agencies and requesting immediate family evaluation. Physician back-up can assist in providing guidance in this scenario.

Training
CASE #17

Paramedics attempted resuscitation of an 88-year-old cardiac arrest victim. Efforts were discontinued after 35 minutes. One of the paramedics asked if anyone would mind if he extubated and re-intubated the patient to practice. The other paramedics said that was not appropriate.

It is imperative that paramedics develop and maintain procedural skills, such as intubation and IV line placement, to effectively care for patients. During the prehospital care of patients, however, it is not appropriate to deviate from the accepted procedures. Standards of training must be in place, continuing education should be available, as needed, and if this was to be done, a system-wide policy should be developed. There is significant debate in the emergency medicine literature regarding using the recently deceased for training. It is generally agreed that if the practice occurs, there should be open and honest admission that it occurs. Many authors advocate asking for family permission, an issue not widely addressed in the prehospital setting. In general, most EMS systems might be uncomfortable with the practice, even though there is no medical or ethical consensus on the matter.

Summary

Medical ethics has traditionally focused on the role of the physician as the direct health-care provider. In the prehospital environment, however, EMTs, under the auspices of a remote physician, provide the medical care. Medical protocols guide the EMTs' actions and on-line medical command physicians may further direct therapy.[12] This chapter discusses many of the ethical conflicts that are likely to occur.

Issues of informed consent and limitation of resuscitation highlight the important role that ethical decision making plays in prehospital care.[13] It is imperative that EMTs be trained to skillfully handle the patient who refuses care or the family that requests no CPR for their loved one in cardiac arrest. One cannot assume that all have the ability to identify conflicts, assess competing values, and make reasoned judgments. Training in ethics might better equip prehospital care providers to deal with these issues. Such training could promote appropriate, efficient, and optimal care of the prehospital patient. Medical command physicians must have equally comprehensive training regarding the conflicts they may be asked to help resolve. Policy must also be developed to promote adequate resolution for difficult situations, such as refusal of care, DNR orders, and informed consent. Appropriate resolution of ethical conflicts in the prehospital setting will be promoted when the EMT and medical command physician can identify the conflicts and when effective policy is developed to provide a guiding framework.

References

1. Adams JG, Arnold R, Siminoff L, et al.: Ethical conflicts in the prehospital setting, *Ann Emerg Med* 21:1259-1265, 1992.

2. Applebaum PS, Grisso T: Assessing patients' capacities to consent to treatment, *N Engl J Med* 319:1635-1638, 1988.

3. Beauchamp TL, Childress JF: *Principles of biomedical ethics,* ed 2, New York, 1983, Oxford University Press.

4. Sprung CL, Winick BJ: Informed consent in theory and practice: legal and medical perspectives on the informed consent doctrine and a proposed reconceptualization, *Crit Care Med* 17:1346-1354, 1989.

5. Miles SH, Crimmins TJ: Orders to limit emergency treatment for an ambulance service in a large metropolitan area, *JAMA* 254:525-527, 1985.

6. *President's Commission for the Study of Ethical Problems in Medicine and Biomedical and Behavioral Research: Deciding to forego life-sustaining treatment: a report on the ethical, medial and legal issues in treatment decisions,* Washington, D.C., 1983, U.S. Government Printing Office.

7. Mehling A: *Prehospital provider and the right to die: National EMT Conference,* Reno, Nevada, December 1988.

8. Miles SH: Advanced directives to limit treatment: the need for portability, *J Amer Ger Soc* 35:74-76, 1987.

9. Weir RF, Gostin L: Decisions to abate life-sustaining treatment for non-autonomous patients, *JAMA* 264:1846-1853, 1990.

10. *Standards for cardiopulmonary resuscitation and emergency cardiac care. Part VIII. Medicolegal considerations and recommendations, JAMA* 255:2979-2984, 1986.

11. Delbridge TR, Fosnocht DE, Garrison HG, et al.: Field termination of unsuccessful out-of-hospital cardiac arrest resuscitation: acceptance by family members, *Ann Emerg Med* 27(5):649-654, 1996.

12. Sprung CL: Changing attitudes and practices in foregoing life-sustaining treatments, *JAMA* 263:2211-2215, 1990.

13. Adams JG: Ethical issues. In Kuehl AE, editor: *Prehospital systems and medical oversight,* ed 2, St Louis, 1994, Mosby Lifeline.

Medicolegal Principles

$\mathbf{T}$he physician responsible for providing EMS medical direction must be acquainted with various legal principles pertaining to scope of responsibility and risk management. Medical command entails the formal acceptance of legal obligation by medical control[1] and is promulgated by local regulations or laws. Since a formal physician-patient relationship is established, the medical command physician should apply sound patient care principles to each encounter. The medical command physician is compelled to become familiar with local policies and procedures governing the situations discussed in this chapter. The following discussion serves as a general review of some potential medicolegal pitfalls with suggested means of remediation. The information contained in this chapter is intended as a general discussion and should augment, but not replace, requirements within your EMS system. Please refer to Chapter 19, Ethical Issues, for a parallel discussion on refusal of service, nontransports, consent, competence, treatment of minors, termination of prehospital CPR, DNR orders, and hospital destination. The medical command physician will minimize the risk of medicolegal error if decisions based on the ideals of optimal patient care guide the interpretation of applicable legal principles.

Medical Direction

The nomenclature of medical direction has not been resolved. The terms on-line, direct, and concurrent medical control have all been used to describe the process whereby physicians direct patient care remotely via telecommunications. Despite the use of varying terms to describe directed patient care, the fundamental concept of EMS as a form of delegated practice has endured this changing terminology and "requires the exercise of medical direction and physician control over the EMS system and prehospital providers."[2] In providing medical control to prehospital care providers, the base station physician is essentially guiding patient care based on information received from the field. Medical direction is unique in that the physician becomes responsible not only for his or her actions, but also for the actions of EMS providers carrying out physician orders. For this reason, the term 'direct medical control' may be preferable since

ROBERT E. O'CONNOR, MD, FACEP

it connotes an orchestration of patient care in immediate response to information conveyed from the scene.

Studies in Prehospital Litigation

When assuming medical direction, the physician assumes the legal obligation to obtain necessary information, to make appropriate medical decisions, and to oversee the general care provided to the patient. Failure to elicit certain history or to provide specific orders may theoretically breach the standard of care and expose the physician to individual liability. The medical control physician must therefore be aware of standards of patient care and recognize the capabilities and shortcomings of their system.

In delegating patient care to EMS providers, the medical command physician may also assume vicarious liability for treatment rendered in the field. The concept of vicarious liability holds the medical control physician responsible for the actions of others carried out by physician order. Negligence on the part of EMS may become the responsibility of medical control, even in the absence of direct involvement. [2]

The frequency of litigation by patients against EMS appears to have been less than for ED treatment.[3-5] Prehospital claims generally involve allegations of improper treatment and frequently do not involve the physician. Failure to transport is the most common cause of actions, while improper treatment, such as failure to provide cervical immobilization, is a less common cause.[5] According to the three published studies of patient care claims, most suits are filed against the EMS agency and the providers themselves. A physician is named as co-defendant less than 10% of the time.[3,4,6]

The frequency of litigation in EMS has been reported to be approximately one suit per 27,000 patient contacts.[4] The medical director of the EMS service was a defendant in one case per 900,000 contacts, while the medical command physician was named in one case per 1.8 million contacts.[4] Despite the much lower risk of litigation compared with the ED, EMS physicians have a medicolegal obligation to the EMS service and owe an ethical duty to the patient in providing care. Physicians staffing a medical control facility should not become so overly concerned with litigation that they refuse to direct prehospital care. Failure to provide medical direction may constitute a greater act of negligence than could ever be incurred through medical direction given in good faith.

Details of liability coverage should be defined in the medical director's contract.[7] There should also be a policy pertaining to the shared responsibility of the medical command physician and the EMS agency's medical director. While medical command physicians are usually covered under their individual malpractice policy, it may be wise to verify this coverage with the carrier before assuming EMS responsibility. Many EMS jurisdictions have placed limits on liability for their personnel, including the medical control physician, however, there is little uniformity in these limitations between jurisdictions. If a suit is filed, it is the medical control physician's responsibility to establish the existence of immunity from liability. It is of paramount importance for the medical control physician to become familiar with local laws and regulations governing liability.

Duty

When EMS coverage is provided to a jurisdiction, certain obligations are accepted regarding coverage and the response to calls for assistance. Whenever a request for EMS response is received, personnel should be dispatched. Denial of an EMS response based on location within the coverage area, financial factors, or perceived non-emergency is unacceptable. Coverage should be maintained at previously agreed upon levels of staffing and training. Part-time coverage or the use of variably trained personnel may be a violation of the duty to serve the public, if the net result breaches previously established levels of service.[8]

Consent

Consent to treatment is usually presumed when EMS is accessed by a competent adult. Even if EMS is accessed by someone other than the patient, acceptance of treatment by a competent patient on EMS arrival constitutes consent. A problem exists whenever a competent patient who initially requests treatment subsequently withdraws consent. A case-by-case determination should be made in these circumstances using principles discussed in the Refusal of Service and Competence and Impairment sections of this chapter. The medical command physician should keep in mind that consent can also be obtained in certain situations that do not require a competent adult or guardian, as in the case of minors (Box 20-1).

Implied consent permits emergency personnel to treat patients who are unconscious or incompetent.

Minors who are pregnant, emancipated, married, or seek treatment for a suspected venereal disease are capable of consenting to treatment.[2] Consent to treatment by a parent or guardian is required for the treatment of minors. If parental consent is unavailable, EMS personnel should be governed by the principle that the potential liability for nontreatment greatly exceeds the potential liability for treatment of a minor without parental consent.[2] Parents are not permitted to withdraw or refuse consent to treatment in emergency situations involving a minor, hence such requests should not be honored. Health-care professionals are therefore compelled to administer essential treatment to minors.[9] Minors should always be treated for an injury or illness, which if left untreated, could possibly constitute a threat to life, limb, or function.

Competence and Impairment

A competent and conscious adult has the right to withdraw consent or refuse treatment by EMS personnel. Minors, or adults impaired by trauma, medical illness, drugs, alcohol, or psychiatric disturbances[2], cannot refuse treatment. The risk of violence or incurring a charge of false imprisonment or assault and battery must be weighed against the risk of allowing an incompetent person to refuse treatment. As in the case of minors, the potential liability for nontreatment greatly exceeds the potential liability for treatment against an incompetent patient's will. The medical command physician should try to act in the patient's best interest. The safety of prehospital care providers, being the utmost priority, may preclude patient transport in certain instances.

The issue of competence is defined by the context in which it is determined. Competence is not an issue of stark polarity but instead is a continuum. Certain patients may refuse all care, others may be competent to refuse certain specific elements of their care, while others are not competent at all.[10,11] The continuum may range from incompetent to impaired to competent. In addition, determination of competence is a dynamic process that may change abruptly. For example, a patient who is unconscious due to hypoglycemia may not be competent to refuse dextrose yet may become competent after treatment and refuse transport.

Box 20-1 Informed Consent or Refusal Terminology

- **Informed consent.** Information that the average patient, possessing reasonable intelligence, would need to know to make an informed decision regarding medical treatment, thereby preserving the patient's right to self-determination.
- **General consent.** Consent to overall evaluation and treatment excluding invasive procedures and unusual treatments.
- **Special consent.** Consent to specific invasive procedures and unusual treatments.
- **Exemptions to the requirement for informed consent:**
  1. Incompetent adults and minors, unless emancipated, are deemed legally unable to give consent. Consent must be given by a legal guardian or surrogate, unless the requirements for an emergency exemption to informed consent are present.
  2. Emancipated minors may legally provide or withdraw consent. Minors are usually considered emancipated if they have graduated from high school, have been pregnant, have a child, have been married, or have lived on their own.
  3. Minors may also consent to treatment for mental illness, substance abuse, pregnancy, and veneral disease.
  4. Neither parents, legal guardians, nor surrogates may refuse necessary medical treatments, especially if lifesaving.
  5. The principle of emergency exemption to informed consent is invoked when an immediately life- or limb-treatening problem exists and the patient is unable to give consent. Consent under these circumstances is implied. The emergency exemption is predicated on the assumption that the average, reasonable patient would consent to emergency treatment if they were able.
- **It is the responsibility of the provider to determine if an emergency exists.** If unable to obtain informed consent, the decision whether to treat should be made with the protection and health of the patient uppermost in the mind of the provider.

If the patient is incompetent, every effort should be made to transport the patient to the ED for evaluation. For the prehospital patient who refuses care to be deemed competent, he or she must understand the situation, be informed of the potential diagnosis, be informed of possible consequences resulting from refusing service, be provided with reasonable alternatives to care, and then be asked to sign a Refusal of Service form. Since determination of patient competence requires a judgment call by the emergency physician, the decision should be made to transport if there is any doubt.[12]

Patient's Refusal of Service

The competent patient's right to refuse treatment creates one of the most difficult liability quandaries the medical command physician faces. In general, refusal of service embodies many of the principles of leaving the hospital Against Medical Advice (AMA) including testing for patient competence before granting refusal. One might assume that requests for EMS assistance nearly always result in patient transport, but this is not the case. Depending on the structure of the EMS system, anywhere from 25%-75% of all EMS activations do not result in transport to the hospital.[13-17] These figures include cases where patients refuse service against the advice of EMS personnel, as well as cases where EMS providers do not transport the patient after judging that no emergent condition exists (Table 20-1).

The situation where an incompetent patient's family insists on withholding care is difficult and deserves mention. In general, the law does not permit the family to refuse treatment on behalf of a patient who is incompetent, unless a court order to that effect has been obtained. EMS physicians will seldom encounter this type of court order and should recognize that EMS may serve the best interests of the patient to treat and transport until further determinations can be made at the hospital. The medical control physician may elect to speak directly with the family and explain the medicolegal requirements governing the decision to treat.[2]

In situations of refusal of service, the medical control physician is an indispensable resource who should be consulted liberally by EMS personnel. Mitigating circumstances, such as hostile crowds and the need for police back-up or physical restraint, can be identified. Direct conversation between the physician and patient has been successfully used to reconcile tense situations, further establish competence, and encourage patient cooperation.[12] The medical control physician should at all times work with EMS providers to guarantee their safety and to act in the best interests of the patient. Ideally, all refusal of service calls should be documented by the providers and base physician. If audio recordings are made, these should be available to the medical director for review.

Medical control should be contacted for refusals of service because of the potential liability incurred. Anywhere from 50%-90% of litigation against EMS personnel involves cases of nontransport or refusal of service.[3,18] Taking into account that approximately two thirds of these cases are inadequately documented[16], involvement of medical control should serve to improve documentation, decision-making, and quality of care.

The risk of litigation for refusal of service is high because of a number of factors. Although a direct cause and effect with refusal of service has not been demonstrated, serious and even fatal outcomes have followed.[18] While follow-up of these patients studied was not optimal, one third required physician care and between 6%-9% required subsequent hospital admission.[18,20] Without a stipulated protocol, medical control is contacted at a rate that may be as low as 5%.[20] Patients and their families do not recall the explanation of the risks of their decision to refuse service in 30% of cases.[19]

The adage "if it isn't documented, it wasn't done" is underscored by the patient's low rate of recall of explained risk. Use of a standard refusal of service form (Figure 20-1) may greatly facilitate documentation and will be an asset to the defense of a case should litigation ensue. EMS personnel, family members, and patients simply may not remember the details of contact with EMS, thus making it difficult to reconstruct events surrounding the call. Refusals of service therefore require attention to thor-

Table 20-1 Transport Outcomes[11]

		Patient Consents to Transport	
		Yes	**No**
EMS Determines Transport is Necessary	**Yes**	Patient transported	Refusal of service
	No	EMS nontransport	Refusal of service nontransport

ough documentation because of the inherent risk of litigation and bad outcome

Nontransports and Releases

In most EMS systems, all calls for assistance result in dispatch of a provider, who when dispatched, is effectively taken out of service for the remainder of the coverage area. While call-takers attempt to ascertain the level of response required by the caller, EMS crews may sometimes be dispatched to scenes where they are not absolutely required. In certain systems, prehospital care providers are permitted to refuse to transport the patient to the hospital after determining that no emergent illness or injury is present.

Refusal of Prehospital Treatment and Transport Patient Information Sheet

Please read this form and retain a copy.

This form has been given to you because you wish to refuse treatment and/or transport to the hospital by Emergency Medical Services (EMS). Please understand that your health and safety are our primary concern. Since you are declining further treatment, consider the following:

1. The EMS personnel have determined that medical evaluation and treatment is necessary in order to diagnose and treat your condition.

2. The evaluation and/or treatment provided to you by the EMS squad is not a substitute for evaluation and treatment by a medical doctor. We wish to transport you to the hospital so that you may be evaluated and treated by a doctor.

3. Your illness or injury may not seem as bad to you as it actually is. Without treatment you could become worse. Refusing treatment and transportation by EMS will delay your treatment. This delay may worsen your illness or injury.

4. If you change your mind and wish EMS treatment and/or transport to the hospital, call us back by dialing 911. We will return to help you.

I have read and understand the above information.

Patient (or guardian) signature: _____

Translator signature (if applicable): _____

Name(s) Printed: _____

Date: _____   Patient Telephone #: _____

Time: _____   *(for QI purposes only)*

Identification (county & case) #: _____

EMS Personnel signature: _____

Case #:_____

Names of family members or witnesses present *(include relationship)*: _____

_____

_____

Figure 20-1. Sample Refusal of Service-EMS Patient Form (continued on p. 258.)

Refusal of Service — EMS Patient Checklist

Patient Name:_____ Age:_____ Date: _____

Location: _____ Report #: _____ Unit #: _____

Patient Assessment: (circle all that apply)
1. Orientation?   person   place   time   situation
2. Altered level of consciousness?   yes   no
3. Head injury?   yes   no
4. Alcohol or drug ingestion?   yes   no

Medical Control: (circle all that apply)
1. Mode of contact?   phone   radio
2. Time of contact? _____
3. Orders given   _____   Treatment and transport may be refused by the patient.
                  _____   Transport may not be refused by the patient.
(initiate 24 hour psychiatric commitment form if patient to be transported against their will)
4. Base Station Physician #: _____

Patient Advised: (circle yes or no)
Yes   No   Medical evaluation and treatment needed
Yes   No   Ambulance transport recommended
Yes   No   Further harm could result without medical evaluation and treatment
Yes   No   Patient understands refusal of service instructions
Yes   No   Patient given refusal of service instructions

Disposition: (check all that apply)
_____   Refused all EMS services
_____   Refused transport after field treatment initiated
_____   Refused field treatment but accepted transport
_____   Released to own custody
_____   Released to custody of law enforcement

Agency: _____ Officer:_____

Name(s) of relatives, family, or friends present:_____

_____

_____

EMS Personnel signature:_____

EMS I.D.#:_____

*Comments*_____

_____

_____

_____

Figure 20-1. (continued)

The previous example of a diabetic patient presenting with hypoglycemia comprises one such group in which it may be appropriate for paramedics not to transport the patient after treatment with dextrose and return of normal mentation.[21]

As mentioned earlier, refusal of service and non-transport are inherently risky since they account for 50%-90% of all lawsuits against EMS.[3,18] While EMS litigation data do not distinguish between these two areas, non-transport cases may be a greater risk due to concomitant issues of incomplete assessment, improper treatment, and abandonment. If the EMS system in which you serve as base station physician requires medical control notification or approval, the medical control physician should take a number of points into consideration before releasing the EMS crew.

Based on the results of one study, as many as 22% of patients not transported are subsequently admitted to the hospital, including those who are ultimately admitted to the intensive care unit and even die.[19] These data do not indicate an error on the part of EMS, since subsequence cannot be distinguished from consequence. Even in the absence of proximate cause, the frequency of hospital admissions in the nontransport group is of concern because these patients may be inclined to sue if they feel care had been inadequate.

Zachariah et al. reported another factor which, on further examination, may increase liability exposure for EMS. Nine of 50 nontransport patients expressed dissatisfaction with the paramedic's assessment and the care rendered and included 6 patients who were subsequently admitted.[19] It seems reasonable to expect that dissatisfied patients may be inclined to litigate, especially if there is an adverse outcome.

One should be wary of nontransports motivated by the patient's request for transport to a hospital outside of their jurisdiction, especially if such a transport would remove the unit from service for an unacceptably long time. Transport to a hospital within the area of jurisdiction with subsequent interhospital transfer might be offered, and if refused, may be handled as a refusal of service. It makes the most sense to transport patients requiring treatment to a mutually acceptable facility rather than forcing them to refuse service since any hospital is probably better than no hospital. If the patient is deemed unable to refuse transport, the benefit of forcibly transporting a patient to a hospital they do not want to go to must be weighed against the risk of false imprisonment.

Medical control should carefully gauge the potential for serious illness based on the chief complaint, age, vital signs, and other factors. If any doubt exists, the patient should be transported.

Abandonment

Abandonment occurs when the provider unilaterally terminates care without affording the patient sufficient time to secure alternate treatment.[2] In light of the preceding discussion of nontransports, EMS systems should be wary of abandonment, especially if the patient who is deemed to have a condition not requiring ALS subsequently deteriorates and suffers harm due to the same condition.

Abandonment may also apply to cases where ALS is called to assist a patient and, following their evaluation, care is turned over to lesser trained personnel. This transfer of care releases responsibility to BLS and should ideally occur with agreement from medical control that the patient does not indeed require an ALS level of care. If the patient who is released to BLS subsequently deteriorates and suffers harm that may have been prevented by having ALS personnel in attendance, abandonment may be alleged.[19] On the other hand, the EMS system will function best if ALS remains free to respond to ALS-level calls. A mechanism must therefore be in place to permit ALS to turn care over to other providers when appropriate. The base station physician must remain extremely wary of the potential for abandonment with both nontransports and BLS releases, permitting them when appropriate and prohibiting them if the patient has the potential for requiring ALS.

Choice of Destination

Most EMS systems attempt to accommodate patient requests for a specific hospital unless the hospital is outside of the EMS coverage area or is an inappropriate destination given the patient's condition. EMS systems cannot afford to have units out of service for extended periods of time transporting to distant hospitals merely for the patient's or private physician's convenience. The EMS system should have rules governing or restricting these transports. If medical control is contacted regarding a patient's request for transport to a distant hospital, the impact of having a unit out of service, as well as the risk of prolonged transport time to the patient, should be evaluated. In most instances, it is more appropriate to transport the patient to a hospital within the EMS coverage area for stabilization, followed by interhospital transport to the initially requested hospital, should the patient still desire treatment there.

Another reason not to transport a patient to the hospital of their choice occurs when the hospital is not appropriate to care for their condition. Many EMS services have policy, protocol, or legislation permitting bypass of the nearest facility in favor of a specialty care facility if the patient's condition warrants. In these circumstances, the patient's medical needs should supersede any request for a specific hospital if those needs cannot be met at the requested facility. For instance, regional trauma protocols may require patients meeting field triage criteria to be taken to a specific trauma center. In other cases, burn centers or pediatric hospitals may be more suitable destinations than the hospital requested by the patient or their family. In cases where EMS personnel encounter resistance from the patient or their family, medical control should be consulted. Medical control must carefully assess the medical or EMS system need for transport to a hospital that the patient does not want to go to.

Diversion and Bypass

Diversion and bypass serve distinct roles in EMS and have drastically different medicolegal implications for the base station physician. EMS diversion is defined as the temporary rerouting of patients from one hospital to another when conditions at the hospital 'on diversion' reduce the ability to provide patient care. Reasons for EMS diversion include overcrowding, equipment failure, fire, and other transient events. Diversions are temporary, dynamic, and flexible, thus requiring base station physician interaction. On the other hand, bypasses are fixed policies that redirect patients to specialty care facilities using field triage criteria, and require little or no input from base station physicians. Bypass policies require the base physician to refer to local protocols since they are not used by all EMS systems and, when used, are extremely variable.

Of special interest to this discussion are the federal patient transfer law, sometimes known as EMTALA. Violations of EMTALA statutes may result in fines of up to $50,000 per incident and do not indemnify the alleged violator from concomitant civil action. In addition, EMTALA violations involve strict liability only, that is, proof of negligence is not required; statutory violation is all that is needed to prove liability.

Patients arriving on hospital property who request treatment cannot be turned away or diverted. The definition of hospital property has been expanded to include such property as ambulances owned and operated by the hospital, even if the ambulance is nowhere near the hospital. Patients who are placed in a hospital owned ambulance cannot be diverted. If a patient is transported by an ambulance not owned by the hospital, they are not considered to be on hospital property, even if communications have been established between hospital and ambulance personnel. The patient may be subsequently denied access to the ED when on diversionary status. If EMS personnel ignore the diversionary status of the hospital and transport the individual onto hospital property, the individual is then considered to have arrived on hospital property and must be treated.

Patients who arrive on hospital property, regardless of the means, cannot be turned away or diverted without first having an initial screening examination performed as specified by federal regulations.[22] Federal regulations do not prohibit transfer per se, providing the requirements for medical screening and stabilization have been satisfied before transfer. Once a screening exam has been performed and the patient has been stabilized, he or she may be transferred if appropriate. Since the application of EMTALA to diversion is currently undergoing scrutiny in the courts, new developments should be carefully monitored.

The basic tenet of diversion is to ensure adequate care of patients already within the hospital, those who arrive during the period of diversion, and those who are diverted elsewhere. The base station physician can use the principles of patient advocacy to govern all actions pertaining to diversion.

Triggering mechanisms must be developed to "identify situations in which necessary resources are not available and temporary ambulance diversion is acceptable."[23] Patients should not be diverted unless the ED is unable to maintain an acceptable level of care, providing medically appropriate alternatives are available within a reasonable proximity. The goal of diversion is to "provide for the safe, appropriate and timely care of patients who continue to enter the EMS system during these times of diversion."[23]

There are a number of situations where diversion cannot apply. Critical or unstable patients, whose condition might be jeopardized by diversion, should be taken to the nearest facility. A specialty care facility, such as a pediatric, burn, or trauma center, should not divert patients requiring specialty care to less capable facilities.

The On-Scene (Bystander) Physician

One of the more stressful situations in EMS arises when a physician stops to render assistance at the scene of an accident or medical emergency and attempts to wrest control of patient treatment. Having a physician stop to render assistance is deemed helpful to the paramedics in less than 10% of cases.[24] If the physician attempts to direct the paramedics' actions in a manner contrary to training, protocol, or general principles of prehospital care, the patient may be compromised. Paramedics should recognize that physician orders for gross deviation from protocols are usually the result of ignorance, arrogance, or both. The paramedic should attempt conflict resolution by contacting the medical control physician so that the two physicians might see the disagreement to resolution.[25] Many systems provide cards for paramedics to issue to bystander physicians officially prohibiting interference with paramedics performing their duties. Authority to issue these cards varies between systems but requires regulatory or legislative backing.

Physicians and allied health professionals are encouraged to stop and help, since all 50 states have enacted "Good Samaritan" laws (Box 20-2). These laws limit professional liability for the on-scene physician to gross, willful, or wanton negligence. A physician acting in good faith, without intent of doing harm, and in accordance with his or her training, may seek indemnity from subsequent legal tort if the local statute limits liability to gross, willful, or wanton negligence. The premise of these laws hinges on the requirement that the physician volunteer emergency assistance. Protection afforded by the Good Samaritan laws is negated if the on-scene physician bills for services, or if the physician renders assistance as part of his or her professional duties.[12, 26]

When the paramedic contacts medical control for assistance, the medical control physician must safeguard the well-being of the patient (Box 20-3). EMS personnel should not deviate from preexisting orders. If orders are given by the bystander physician that deviate from standard protocol, the medical control should attempt to resolve control issues by explaining any laws or policies governing medical control. Some jurisdictions have laws stipulating that EMS providers receive medical direction from base sta-

---

Box 20-2 General Components of the Good Samaritan Law

- Purpose: to encourage emergency assistance by health-care providers
- Variable definitions by state regarding who is protected (i.e., laypersons, physicians, nurses, EMTs)
- Variable definitions by state regarding standard of negligence (i.e., gross, willful, standard of care)
- Does not apply to practice of emergency medicine in a ED
- May not apply to regular job duties
- Physician must not have a pre-existing duty to treat
- Requirement to render emergency assistance is void if care is already being provided by others
- Requirement to render emergency assistance is void if care endangers the health-care provider
- Generally applies only to sudden, unexpected, prehostpital emergencies
- Rescuer does not request a fee

Box 20-3 Basic Ways for Prehospital Personnel to Limit Liability

- Freely consult supervisors and medical command physicians.
- Document extensively.
- Always be guided by the patient's best interest.
- Never use excessive force.
- Never be punitive
- The health-care provider's health and safety takes precedence.

---

tion physicans only. Most tense situations can be defused with physician-to-physician discussion. Relinquishing medical direction to an on-scene physician is illegal in some states and is otherwise not recommended, even if permitted by local statute. If the base station physician relinquishes control and an untoward event occurs, the bystander physician may be covered by the Good Samaritan statute, whereas the base station physician would not be protected since medical direction is part of the regular job duties.

Do Not Resuscitate Orders

EMS systems emphasize rapid response and immediate initiation of treatment, especially in cases of cardiac arrest.[27] This fundamental tenet of EMS must be tempered by the widely accepted belief that patients who are terminally ill have the right to "forego futile or useless treatment."[28] EMS providers are usually required by local protocol to initiate resuscitative efforts, since they are rarely able to verify the validity of a DNR order rapidly enough. Most jurisdictions do not address the prehospital DNR problem. In a 1991 survey, 8 states permitted prehospital DNR orders and 23 more were working on their development.[28]

In the absence of a written DNR order or a local protocol enabling prehospital DNR orders, the base station physician must recognize the need to initiate resuscitative efforts unless death can be determined at the scene. Living wills specifying that medical treatment should not be initiated unless there is a reasonable hope of recovery generally do not apply to EMS patients since no prior physician-patient relationship existed. It would be difficult for a base station physician to determine prognosis if unfamiliar with the patient. Hence the living will should not be construed as a valid DNR order.

Prehospital Termination of CPR

Many EMS agencies are reluctant to implement policies permitting paramedics to terminate CPR before hospital arrival.[30, 31] As discussed in the context of prehospital DNR orders, there is a reticence on the part of those involved in EMS to 'do nothing'. EMS treatment emphasizes rapid stabilization and transport with aggressive treatment of life- or limb-threatening illness, such as cardiac arrest.

The preponderance of scientific data indicates that the outcome for patients who were unable to be resuscitated in the field, but on whom resuscitative efforts were continued on arrival to the hospital, is dismal.[27] The reported rate of discharge from the hospital with intact neurological status has been reported to be in the range of 0.2% to 0.5%[29-38], with a cumulative discharge rate of 0.47%.[28] Despite these data, termination of CPR in the field is approached with reluctance and trepidation owing to fears of not meeting the expectations of the public and facing presumed legal repercussions.

Prolonged unnecessary CPR may endanger the public, since the paramedics are prevented from responding to other calls while CPR is in progress. Rapid transport may also place the public at risk for collisions. EMS systems should consider adopting protocols that permit termina-

tion of CPR in the field if ordered by medical control based on refractory cardiac arrest despite comprehensive and prolonged ALS therapy.[38] The base station physician is cautioned to adhere to local EMS regulations however.

Summary

EMS litigation involving physicians providing medical direction is extremely rare relative to emergency medicine as a whole. Malpractice litigation against EMS providers alleging improper care is less common than litigation alleging improper vehicle operation resulting in motor vehicle accidents and personal injury. Nonetheless, the physician who provides medical direction for prehospital care providers should be aware of their duties, responsibilities, and potential medicolegal pitfalls. By anticipating these potential pitfalls, the base station physician may not always prevent litigation but will provide medical direction in a manner promoting optimal patient care to benefit the public.

References

1. Braun O, Callahan ML: Direct medical control. In Kuehl AE, editor: *EMS medical directors' Handbook*, St Louis, 1989, Mosby, pp. 175-212.

2. Frew SA: Emergency medical services legal issues for the emergency physician, *Emerg Med Clin N Am* 8:41-55, 1990.

3. Soler JM, Montes MF, Egol EB, et al.: The ten year malpractice experience of a large urban EMS system, *Ann Emerg Med* 14:982-985, 1985.

4. Goldberg RJ, Zautcke JL, Koenigsberg MD, et al.: A review of prehospital care litigation in a large metropolitan EMS system, *Ann Emerg Med* 19:557-561, 1990.

5. Ayres RJ: Legal considerations in prehospital care, *Emerg Med Clin N Am* 11:853-867, 1993.

6. Morgan DL, Wainscott MP, Knowles HC: Emergency medical services liability litigation in the United States: 1987 to 1992, *Prehosp Disaster Med* 9:214-221, 1994.

7. The American College of Emergency Physicians: Medicolegal issues. In *Medical direction of emergency medical services*. Dallas, 1993, The American College of Emergency Physicians.

8. Aranosian RD: Medical-legal concerns in EMS. In Roush WR, editor: *Principles of EMS systems*, Dallas, 1989, American College of Emergency Physicians, pp. 165-174.

9. Selbst SM: Leaving against medical advice, *Pediatr Emerg Care* 2:266-268, 1986.

10. Drane JF: Competency to give informed consent: a model for making clinical assessments, *JAMA* 252:925-927, 1984.

11. Buchanan AE: The question of competence. In Iserson KV, Sanders AB, Mathieu DR, et al., editors: *Ethics in emergency medicine*, Baltimore, 1986, Williams & Wilkins, pp. 52-56.

12. Megargel RE, Dickinson ET: Prehospital care. *foresight: Risk Management for Emergency Physicians*, July 1992 Issue 23. Dallas, The American College of Emergency Physicians.

13. Stark G, Hedges J, Neeley K, et al.: Patients who initially refuse prehospital transport and/or therapy, *Am J Emerg Med* 8:509-511, 1990.

14. Carmichael D, Mohler J: Refusal of care, *JEMS* April: 36-38, 1985.

15. Holroyd B, Shalit M, Kallsen G, et al.: Prehospital patients refusing care, *Ann Emerg Med* 17:957-963, 1988.

16. Seldan BS, Schnitzer PG, Nolan FX: Medicolegal documentation of prehospital triage, *Ann Emerg Med* 19:547-551, 1990.

17. Mottley LL: Refusal of medical assistance in the field, In Kuehl AE, editor: *EMS medical Directors' Handbook*, St Louis, 1989, Mosby, pp. 261-265.

18. Ayers JR Jr: *The law and you: causes of lawsuits: emergency medical update*, vol 1, Winslow, Washington, 1988, Ellen Lockert, p 4.

19. Zachariah BS, Bryan D, Pepe PE, et al.: Follow-up and outcome of patients who decline or are denied transport by EMS, *Prehosp Disaster Med* 7:359-364, 1992.

20. Sucov A, Verdile VP, Garettson D, et al.: The outcome of patients refusing prehospital transportation, *Prehosp Disaster Med* 7:365-371, 1992.

21. Thompson RH, Wolford RW: Development and evaluation of criteria allowing paramedics to treat and release patients presenting with hypoglycemia: a retrospective study, *Prehosp Disaster Med* 6:309-313, 1991.

22. 42 USCA Section 13955 dd (Supp 1991)

23. American College of Emergency Physicians Position Statement: *Guidelines for ambulance diversion/destination policies*, November 1991.

24. Mellick LB, Yurong H, Haley K, et al.: Paramedic perceptions of the on-scene physician, *Prehosp Disaster Med* 6:331-334, 1991.

25. Frew SA: *Street law: rights and responsibilities of the EMT*, Reston, VA, 1983 Reston Publishing, pp. 57-59.

26. American College of Emergency Physicians: Control of advanced life support at the scene of medical emergencies, *Ann Emerg Med* 13:547-548, 1984.

27. National Association of Emergency Medical Services Physicians (NAEMSP): Consensus document on resuscitation decisions in the prehospital setting: special bulletin, *NAEMSP*, 1989.

28. Kellermann AL: Criteria for dead-on arrivals, prehospital termination of CPR, and do-not resuscitate orders, *Ann Emerg Med* 22:47-51, 1993.

29. Sachs GA, Miles SH, Levin R: Limiting resuscitation: emerging policy in the emergency medical system, *Ann Intern Med* 114:151-154, 1991.

30. Eisenberg MS, Cummins RO: Termination of CPR in the prehospital arena (editorial), *Ann Emerg Med* 14:1106-1107, 1985.

31. Kellermann AL, Hackman BB: Terminating unsuccessful advanced cardiac life support in the field. (editorial), *Am J Emerg Med* 5:548-549, 1987.

32. Bonnin MJ, Pepe PE, Clark PS: Key role of prehospital resuscitation in survival from out-of-hospital cardiac arrest (abstract), *Ann Emerg Med* 19:466, 1990.

33. Lewis LM, Ruoff B, Rush C, et al.: Is emergency department resuscitation of cardiac arrest victims who arrive pulseless worthwhile? *Am J Emerg Med* 8:118-120, 1990.

34. Bonnin MJ, Swor RA: Outcomes in unsuccessful field resuscitation attempts, *Ann Emerg Med* 18:507-512, 1989.

35. Gray WA, Capone RJ, Most AS: Unsuccessful medical resuscitation: are continued efforts in the emergency department justified? *N Eng J Med* 325:1393-1398, 1991.

36. Kellermann AL, Staves DR, Hackman BB: In-hospital resuscitation following unsuccessful prehospital advanced cardiac life support: heroic efforts or an exercise in futility, *Ann Emerg Med* 17:589-594, 1988.

37. Markovchick VJ, Cantrill SV, Pons PT, et al.: Identification of those nontraumatic cardiac arrest patients for whom ED resuscitation is futile (abstract), *Ann Emerg Med* 19:460, 1990.

38. Bonin MJ, Pepe PE, Kimball KT, et al.: Distinct criteria for termination of resuscitation in the out of hospital setting, *JAMA* 270:1457-1462, 1993.

Index

B

Bag-valve-mask, ventilation and, 30-31
Base station remote, communication and, 15
Basic life support (BSL), 1, 5
Bedside feedback, quality improvement and, 240
Bedside report, 23-24
Behavioral emergencies, 213-223
    anxiety disorders, 214
    bipolar disorder, 214
    chemical restraint in, 219-220
    depression, 214
    initial assessment and intervention in, 214-220
    organic disorders with behavioral manifestations, 215
    physical restraint in, 218-219
    psychiatric conditions, 214-220
    sample cases of, 222-223
    schizophrenia, 214
    suicidal patient, 216-217
    violent patient, 217-218
Benzodiazepine antagonists, 74-75
Benzodiazepines, 46, 220
Beta-adrenergic agents, 71
Beta-agonist aerosols, 45
Bipolar disorder, 214
Bleeding; *see* Hemorrhage
Blunt trauma, 161
Board splints, 50
Bradycardia, 48
Breath, shortness of; *see* Shortness of breath
Breathing in pediatric emergencies, 191
Breech presentation, 176, 186
    protocol for, 186
Bretylium, 70
Bronchodilators, 45
Bronchodilators
    inhaled, 71
Bronchospasm
    chest pain and, 115
    protocol for, 110, 239
    shortness of breath and, 102-103
BSL; *see* Basic life support
Butorphanol (Stadol), prehospital analgesia and, 86
Butyrophenones, chemical restraint and, 220
Bypass, medicolegal principles and, 260-261
Bystander physician, medicolegal principles and, 261-262
Bystanders in prehospital environment, 20

C

Calcium, 77
Calcium channel blocking agents, 77
overdose of, 207
Calcium chloride, 77
Calcium gluconate 10%, 77
Capillary refill, hypovolemia and, 150-151
Cardiac arrest, 135-147
    care after resuscitation, 139
    cessation of resuscitation efforts vs. hospital transport in, 139-140
    chain of survival, 136
    hypothermic, protocol for, 145-146
    off-line command and, 135-137
    on-line command and, 137-138
    poisoning and drug overdose in, 205-206
    protocols for, 137, 142-147
    quality improvement and, 137
    rapid response to, 136
    sample cases of, 140-142
    standing orders for, 137, 142-147
    training in interventions for, 136-137
    traumatic, protocol for, 145
Cardiac pacing, external, 48
Cardiac procedures in advanced life support, 47-49
Cardiogenic shock, 151
Catapress (Clonidine), overdose of, 201
Cellular telephones, 13-14
Central venous access, 43
Cephaeline, poisoning and drug overdose and, 204
Cervical collars, 49
Cervical immobilizers, 50
Cervical spine movement, endotracheal intubation and, 33, 34
Charcoal, activated, 76, 204-205
Chemical restraint, 219-220
    benzodiazepines in, 220
    neuroleptics in, 219-220
    rapid tranquilization, 219, 220
Chest, flail, protocol for, 165-166
Chest decompression, 41-42
Chest pain, 113-123
    dysrhythmia suppressants, 117
    atypical, 118
    causes of, 114-116
    differential diagnosis of, 114-116
    dysrhythmias and, 126
    in elderly patients, 118
    historical aspects of, 114
    hyperventilation and, 119
    hypotension and, 119
    pleuritic, 115-116
    protocols for, 122
    relief of, 116-117
    "safe" transport of patient with, 116
    sample cases of, 120-121
    silent myocardial infarction, 118
    suspected ischemia and, 114-115
    thrombolysis, 118
Chest trauma, protocol for, 165-166
Chest wound, sucking, protocol for, 166
CHF; *see* Congestive heart failure
Children; *see* Pediatric patients
Choice of destination; *see* Destination, choice of
Chronic obstructive pulmonary disease (COPD), shortness of breath and, 105
Circulation in pediatric emergencies, 191
Clonidine; *see* Catapress
COBRA/OBRA, 260-261
Cocaine
    chest pain and, 115
    overdose of, 208
Coercion of uncooperative patients, ethical issues and, 248-249
Colloid infusions, 47
Coma cocktail, 73, 74, 75
Command sheet, quality improvement and, 240, 241
Communication, 13-25
    air-medical command and, 235
    bedside report and, 23-24
    in crime scenes, 21
    Duplex, 13, 17
    emergency medical services, for base station physician, 13-18
    emotions and, 23
    equipment for, 13-17
    indirect means of, 22
    medical command, interpersonal aspects of, 19-25
    "Oh—By the Way," 21
    with other physicians on-scene, 21
    prehospital analgesia and, 88
    prehospital environment and, 19-20
    presentation of living will and, 21
    radio etiquette, 17
    sample cases of, 16-17, 25
    Simplex, 17
    tape recorder and, 22
    types of, 17
    weapons and, 21
Competence, medicolegal principles and, 255-256
Concurrent approach to quality management, 239-240, 242
Confidentiality, ethical issues and, 250
Congestive heart failure (CHF)
    protocol for, 111
    shortness of breath and, 103-104, 106
Consciousness, altered level of; *see* Altered level of consciousness
Consent, informed, medicolegal principles and, 254-255
Contamination reduction zone, hazardous materials and, 208
Contemporary medical direction; *see* Medical direction, contemporary
Continuous quality improvement (CQI), 237-243

non-trauma, 109
for spinal cord injury, 164
for sucking chest wound, 166
for tension pneumothorax, 166
for trauma patient, 162-168
for traumatic cardiac arrest, 145
for upper airway obstruction, 109-110
for ventricular fibrillation, 143-144
for wheezing, 110, 239
Psychiatric conditions, 214-220
anxiety disorders, 214
bipolar disorder, 214
chemical restraint in, 219-220
depression, 214
panic attack, 214
phobia, 214
physical restraint in, 218-219
schizophrenia, 214
suicidal patient, 216-217
violent patient, 217-218
PTL; *see* Pharyngo-Tracheal Lumen Airway
Pulmonary edema, acute, protocol for, 111
Pulmonary embolism (PE)
chest pain and, 115
shortness of breath and, 105
Pulse oximetry, 40
Pulseless electrical activity (PEA), 48
protocol for, 144-145
Pulseless ventricular tachycardia
protocol for, 143-144
PVCs; *see* Premature ventricular complexes

Q

QA; *see* Quality Assurance
QI; *see* Quality improvement
Quality Assurance (QA), 237-243
Quality improvement (QI), 137, 237-243
Quality management, 237-243
components of, 238-242
concurrent method of, 239-240, 242
immediate method of, 239-240
prospective approach to, 238-239, 242
retrospective approach to, 240-242

R

Radio communication, 7, 14-15
cardiac arrest and, 138
etiquette of, 17
quality improvement and, 239-240
Rapid fluid infusion in treatment of
hypotension and shock, 152, 153
Rapid tranquilization (RT), chemical
restraint and, 219, 220
Rectal administration of medications, 44,
45, 65-66
Refusal

of transport; *see* Transport, refusal of
of treatment; *see* Treatment, refusal of
Releases, medicolegal principles and, 257-259
Repeaters, communication and, 15
Residency program for EMS physicians, 4
Respiratory arrest in children, 191-193
Respiratory distress
in children, 191-193
non-trauma, protocol for, 109
protocol for, 105
Restraint
chemical, 219-220
physical, 218-219
Resuscitation
care after, 139
fluid, trauma and, 161
prehospital termination of
ethical issues and, 249
versus hospital transport, 139-140
medicolegal principles and, 262
protocol for, 146-147
Retrospective approach to quality management, 240-242
Review sheet, quality improvement and, 240-242
Rhythm strips, dysrhythmias and, 130
Risk, personal, ethical issues and, 251
Routes of administration of medications, 64-66
RT; *see* Rapid tranquilization

S

SAEM; *see* Society of Academic Emergency Medicine
Sandbags, immobilization and, 50
Satellite technology, communication and, 15
Schizophrenia, 214
Sedation during countershock, dysrhythmias and, 130-131
Sedative-hypnotics, overdose of, 207
Seizures
altered level of consciousness and, 95
in children, 196-197
Seldinger technique, 39
Self-Inflating Bulf (SIB), 37
Sellick maneuver, 30
Semi-automatic defibrillators, 47
Serum glucose measurements in altered
level of consciousness, 93
Shock
anaphylactic, protocol for, 111-112
cardiogenic, 151
in children, 193-194
definition of, 149
distributive, 151
etiologies of, 151
and hypotension; *see* Hypotension and
shock

obstructive, 151
signs and symptoms of, 150
treatment of, 151-152
Shortness of breath (SOB), 101-112
asthma and, 102-103
bronchospasm and, 102-103
congestive heart failure and, 103-104, 106
COPD and, 102-103, 106
differential diagnosis of, 101-102
non-traumatic etiologies of, 102
objective measures of, 102
peak expiratory flow rate and, 102
pneumonia and, 104
pneumothorax and, 107
protocols for, 105, 109-112
pulmonary embolus and, 105
sample cases of, 106-107
upper airway obstruction and, 104
Shoulder dystocia, 176-177
SIB; *see* Self-Inflating Bulf
Silent myocardial infarction, chest pain
and, 118
Simplex communication, 17
SOB; *see* Shortness of breath
Societal obligations, ethical issues and, 251
Society
for Academic Emergency Medicine, 5
of Academic Emergency Medicine
(SAEM), 4
Sodium bicarbonate, 70-71
overdose of, 207
Spinal cord injury, protocol for, 165
Spinal immobilization, 49-50
Spine boards, 49-50
Splints, extremity, 50-51
SQ; *see* Subcutaneous administration of
medications
Squelch, communication and, 15-17
Stadol; *see* Butorphanol
Standing orders
for cardiac arrest, 137
direct medical control and, 5-6
Stat medical command sheet, 240, 241
Stifneck collar, 49
Subcutaneous (SQ) administration of medications, 44, 45, 64
Sublimaze; *see* Fentanyl
Sublingual administration of medications, 44, 45, 64
Sublingual injections, 44, 45-46
Succinylcholine, 46, 72
Sucking chest wound, protocol for, 166
Suicidal patient, 210, 216-217
Synchronization during countershock,
dysrhythmias and, 130-131
Syringe pumps, 46-47
Syrup of ipecac, 75-76, 204